Arthropod-borne Infectious Diseases of the Dog and Cat

Second Edition

MICHAEL J. DAY, BSc, BVMS(Hons), PhD, DSc, DiplECVP, FASM, FRCPath, FRCVS

Professor of Veterinary Pathology
School of Veterinary Sciences
University of Bristol
Langford, Bristol, UK

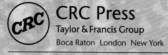

CRC Press
Taylor & Francis Group
Boca Raton London New York

CRC Press is an imprint of the
Taylor & Francis Group, an **informa** business

CRC Press
Taylor & Francis Group
6000 Broken Sound Parkway NW, Suite 300
Boca Raton, FL 33487-2742

First issued in paperback 2020

© 2016 by Taylor & Francis Group, LLC
CRC Press is an imprint of Taylor & Francis Group, an Informa business

No claim to original U.S. Government works

ISBN 13: 978-0-367-57493-2 (pbk)
ISBN 13: 978-1-4987-0824-1 (hbk)

Visit the Taylor & Francis Web site at
http://www.taylorandfrancis.com

and the CRC Press Web site at
http://www.crcpress.com

Contents

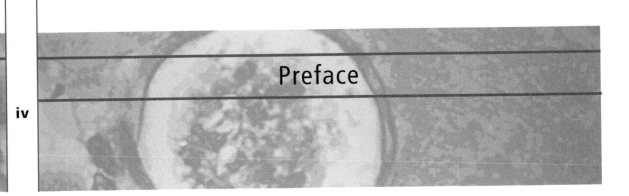

PREFACE TO THE FIRST EDITION

The study of arthropod-borne infectious disease in companion animals is developing rapidly. For example, new species and subspecies of *Babesia* affecting dogs and cats are being characterized as this book is being written. In addition, it is highly likely that the role of arthropods in the transmission of other important canine and feline diseases will be confirmed. This is particularly the case with the haemoplasmas (previously *Haemobartonella* species) of dogs and cats, where investigation of transmission by *Ctenocephalides felis* (the cat flea) is the subject of current intensive research.

With this background, we set out to produce a text that would collect together the important information related to the arthropod-borne infectious diseases of companion animals. Our objectives in producing this book were:

- To provide veterinary surgeons with comprehensive information on clinical presentation, pathogenesis, diagnosis, treatment, control and zoonotic implications of the major arthropod-transmitted diseases of dogs and cats.
- To provide additional information in the same text on relevant aspects of the biology of the arthropod vectors and their wildlife host species. It is hoped this will encourage greater understanding of the challenges required in controlling these infections as well as an appreciation of the biological complexities involved in their maintenance.
- To provide additional information in the same text on the immunological interactions between arthropod-borne pathogens, their vectors and the companion animal hosts. Immune–mediated disease is a hallmark of infection with this specific group of pathogens, and it is hoped that this book will provide veterinary surgeons with a basis for understanding and interpreting the clinical and laboratory evidence for this in cases with suspected arthropod-borne disease. In addition, appreciation of this complex interaction provides a platform for understanding both the difficulties involved in the development of traditional vaccines for this group of infections and the development of novel immunomodulatory approaches to treatment.
- To provide more detailed information in the same text on the expanding array of diagnostic techniques routinely available to veterinary surgeons dealing with these diseases. Arthropod-transmitted diseases provide a real diagnostic challenge. Many tests are available for the same disease, using different technologies and with differing sensitivities and specificities. Tests for exposure to infection, such as antibody-based serology, provide different information from those designed to identify active infection (PCR-based methods). Both sets of information may be useful in difficult cases and this book has been written to enable veterinary practitioners to better understand the laboratory basis for the results they receive.

Arthropod-borne Infectious Diseases of the Dog and Cat is a project that has arisen from the clinical, laboratory diagnostic and research interests of the editors in this rapidly developing field of veterinary medicine. Over a number of years we have met and collaborated with many veterinarians and scientists active in this field who have become valued colleagues and friends. Many of these have contributed the chapters, illustrations or data that form this book. To these contributors we are exceedingly grateful for your excellent reviews and prompt responses to questions or proofreading. Your enthusiasm and rigorous scientific input has helped us to produce a text of which we can all be proud.

We must also acknowledge the superb support from Manson Publishing for this project. The book was born from early discussions with Jill Northcott and we are grateful for her support and gentle cajoling throughout. Michael Manson has been characteristically supportive and it has been a pleasure to work with him. We are very pleased to be able to thank the production team headed by Paul Bennett, and the expert and detailed copyediting provided by Peter Beynon. The hand-drawn sketches produced by individual contributors have been expertly rendered into a uniform style by Cactus Design and Illustration.

We hope this book will prove an informative and practical resource to practising veterinarians who deal with this fascinating group of diseases.

Susan Shaw and Michael Day
September 2005

PREFACE TO SECOND EDITION

Fifteen years ago the United Kingdom relaxed quarantine regulations and introduced the Pet Travel Scheme, allowing increased movement of pet animals to and from other European countries. At that time, the scheme focused on preventing the incursion of canine rabies and non-endemic ecto- and endoparasites into the UK with a range of preventive measures for travelling animals that have since been considerably modified. As the scheme was being established, Susan Shaw and I recognized the potential for travelling pets to encounter a wide range of arthropod-borne infectious diseases that were endemic in southern European countries. We predicted that UK veterinarians would need to recognize and manage cases of these infections in travelling pets and prepare for a future when such infectious agents, and the arthropods that carry them, may become endemic in northern Europe.

With start-up funding from Merial Animal Health, we established the Acarus Laboratory at the University of Bristol to provide rapid molecular diagnosis for these infectious agents and to undertake UK-wide surveillance to monitor the incursion of these pathogens and to document the prevalence of existing endemic infectious agents. At the same time we lobbied for national surveillance and provided continuing education for vet-

erinary practitioners, who were entirely unfamiliar with this group of diseases. The first edition of this book, published in 2005, was a further means of providing this education to the veterinary community.

Fifteen years later, many of our predictions have been proven correct. The UK Pet Travel Scheme now allows an average of 100,000 animals to travel into or out of the UK each year. We have documented many hundreds of animals returning from travel with diseases such as leishmaniosis, babesiosis and monocytic ehrlichiosis. Previously unknown arthropod vectors such as *Rhipicephalus sanguineus* are identified in the field in the UK and autochthonous cases of leishmaniosis and babesiosis in untravelled dogs are reported.

But these changes are now occurring on a much wider global scale. Substantial international movement of pet animals now involves not just travel of individual owned pets, but large scale importation of animals for commercial sale (sometimes illegally) or rehoming. In the latter case, 'rescue' associations will collect free-roaming dogs from southern or eastern European or Asian countries and fly them over long distances to North America or northern Europe. The number of such animal movements is often astounding. In parallel, predictions concerning climate change, incursion of the human population into areas of the natural environment and establishment of vectors and microparasitic infections in non-traditional areas have all occurred on a global scale.

Since publication of the first edition of this book there has also been a rediscovery of the importance of the 'One Health' approach to disease surveillance and control worldwide. The arthropod-borne infections, which involve people, pets, wildlife and the natural environment, are perfect candidates for a One Health approach to scientific investigation, clinical diagnosis and management and the development of control strategies. Accordingly, this edition places particular emphasis on One Health and zoonotic aspects of the diseases under discussion.

I was delighted that many of the contributors to the first edition so readily agreed to update their chapters for this second edition, but I also welcome a number of new chapter authors who provide a new perspective on the diseases discussed. The fundamental structure of this book remains unchanged, but there is a new chapter on haemoplasma infections and a substantially revised and expanded chapter on rare (and particularly viral) arthropod-borne diseases of dogs and cats. Since publication of the first edition, Susan Shaw has retired, but I am grateful that she inspired me to take an interest in this field and know that she will be pleased to see this second edition of the book.

This second edition comes under the Taylor and Francis imprint, but is the seventh book I have worked on with Commissioning Editor Jill Northcott and as ever, I am grateful for her support and enthusiasm. I am pleased to acknowledge the copyediting skills of Peter Beynon and the expertise of the production team led by Kate Nardoni.

We have much still to learn about these arthropod-borne diseases as their prevalence and geographical range expands and new species of the organisms are identified. There remains a need for practicing veterinarians to keep up-to-date in this area and I hope that this book will fulfill that role.

Michael J. Day
January 2016

Dedication

To Christopher and Natalie

and

In memory of my father

Joseph Frank Day (1937–2014)

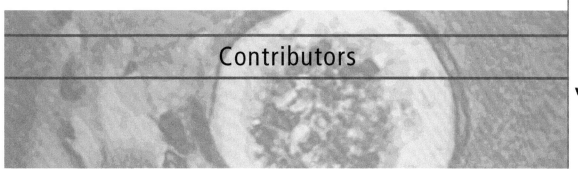

Contributors

Gad Baneth DVM, PhD, DipECVCP
Koret School of Veterinary Medicine
Hebrew University of Jerusalem
Rehovot, Israel

Emi Barker BSc(Hons), BVSc(Hons), PhD, MRCVS
School of Veterinary Sciences
University of Bristol
Langford, United Kingdom

Casey Barton Behravesh MS, DVM, DrPH,
    DipACVPM
Centers for Disease Control and Prevention
Atlanta, Georgia, USA

Richard J. Birtles BSc(Hons), PhD
School of Environment and Life Sciences
University of Salford
Salford, United Kingdom

Anneli Björsdorff DVM, PhD
AniCura
Danderyd, Sweden

Kevin Bown BSc(Hons) MRes, PhD
School of Environment and Life Sciences
University of Salford
Salford, United Kingdom

Michael J. Day BSc, BVMS(Hons), PhD, DSc,
    DiplECVP, FASM, FRCPath, FRCVS
School of Veterinary Sciences
University of Bristol
Langford, United Kingdom

Gerhard Dobler MD
Department of Virology and Rickettsiology
Bundeswehr Institute of Microbiology
Munich, Germany

Luca Ferasin DVM, PhD, CertVC, PGCert(HE),
    DipECVIM-CA, GPCert(B&PS), MRCVS
CVS Referrals
Lumbry Park Veterinary Specialists
Alton
Hampshire, United Kingdom

Shimon Harrus DVM, PhD, DipECVCP
Koret School of Veterinary Medicine
Hebrew University of Jerusalem
Rehovot, Israel

Peter J. Irwin BVetMed, PhD, FANZCVS, MRCVS
College of Veterinary Medicine
School of Veterinary and Life Sciences
Murdoch University
Murdoch, Western Australia

Michael Leschnik DVM, PD
Department for Small Animals and Horses
Veterinary University Vienna
Vienna, Austria

Robert F. Massung PhD
Centers for Disease Control and Prevention
Atlanta, Georgia, USA

Iain Peters BVMS(Hons), PhD, MRCVS
Torrance Diamond Diagnostic Services
Exeter, United Kingdom

Martin Pfeffer DVM, Dr med vet, DiplECVPH
Institut für Tierhygiene und Öffentliches
Veterinärwesen
Veterinärmedizinische Fakultät
Universität Leipzig
Leipzig, Germany

Xavier Roura DVM, PhD, DipECVIM-CA
Servei de Medicina Interna
Hospital Clínic Veterinari
Universitat Autònoma de Barcelona
Bellaterra, Spain

Laia Solano-Gallego DVM, PhD, DipECVCP
Departament de Medicina i Cirurgia Animal
Facultat de Veterinària
Universitat Autònoma de Barcelona
Bellaterra, Spain

Reinhard K. Straubinger DVM, Dr med vet, PhD
Institute for Infectious Diseases and Zoonoses
Faculty of Veterinary Medicine
Ludwig-Maximilian-University of Munich
Munich, Germany

Séverine Tasker BSc, BVSc(Hons), PhD, DSAM,
    DipECVIM-CA, FHEA, MRCVS
Acarus Laboratories
Langford Veterinary Services
School of Veterinary Sciences
University of Bristol
Langford, United Kingdom

Luigi Venco DVM, SCPA, DipEVPC
Pavia, Italy

Nancy A. Vincent-Johnson DVM, MS, DipACVIM,
    DipACVPM
Fort Belvoir Veterinary Center
United States Army Public Health Command
District-Fort Belvoir
Fort Belvoir, Virginia, USA

Richard Wall BSc, MBA, PhD
School of Biological Sciences
University of Bristol
Bristol, United Kingdom

Trevor Waner BVSc, PhD, DipECLAM
Israel Institute for Biological Research
Ness Ziona, Israel

ALP	alkaline phosphatase	LIA	line immunoassay
ALT	alanine aminotransferase	LPS	lipopolysaccharide
ANA	antinuclear antibody	MAMP	microbe-associated molecular pattern
APC	antigen presenting cell	MERS	Middle East respiratory syndrome
APTT	activated partial thromboplastin time	MHC	major histocompatability complex
ATIII	antithrombin III	MLST	multilocus sequence typing
BUN	blood urea nitrogen	NK	natural killer (cell)
CK	creatine kinase	NSAID	non-steroidal anti-inflammatory drug
CME	canine monocytic ehrlichiosis	OspA/B/C	outer surface protein A/B/C
CNS	central nervous system	PACAP	pituitary adenylate cyclase-activating
ConA	concanavalin A		polypeptide
CRP	C-reactive protein	PAMPs	pathogen-associated molecular patterns
CSD	cat scratch disease	PBL	peripheral blood lymphocyte
DEC	diethylcarbamazine citrate	PCR	polymerase chain reaction
DIC	disseminated intravascular coagulation	PCV	packed cell volume
DNA	deoxyribonucleic acid	PDGF	platelet-derived growth factor
DTH	delayed type hypersensitivity	PFGE	pulsed field gel electrophoresis
EEE	eastern equine encephalitis	PGE_2	prostaglandin E_2
ELISA	enzyme-linked immunosorbent assay	PLN	protein losing nephropathy
EM	erythema migrans	PT	prothrombin time
FeLV	feline leukaemia virus	PTE	pulmonary thromboembolism
FIV	feline immunodeficiency virus	qPCR	quantitative polymerase chain reaction
H5N1/7	highly-pathogenic avian influenza	RH	relative humidity
	(haemagglutinin 5 and neuraminidase 1,	RIM	rapid immunomigration
	clade 7)	RMSF	Rocky Mountain spotted fever
HAI	*Hepatazoon americanum* infection	RNA	ribonucleic acid
HARD	heartworm-associated respiratory	R_0	basic reproductive rate
	disease	RVFV	Rift Valley fever virus
HCI	*Hepatazoon canis* infection	SARS	severe acute respiratory syndrome
HIV	human immunodeficiency virus	SFG	spotted fever group
HME	human monocytic ehrlichiosis	SGE	salivary gland extract
HWD	heartworm disease	SPF	specific pathogen-free
IFAT	immunofluorescent antibody test	TBE	tick-borne encephalitis
IFN	interferon	TBEV	tick-borne encephalitis virus
Ig	immunoglobulin (IgA, IgG, etc)	TCP	trimethoprim-sulphadiazine,
IL	interleukin		clindamycin and pyrimethamine
kDa	kilodaltons	TGF	transforming growth factor
LAMP	loop-mediated isothermal amplification	Th	T helper (cell)

TLR	Toll-like receptor	VlsE	Variable major protein-like sequence, expressed (a surface lipoprotein of *Borrelia burgdorferi* expressed by the vlsE gene)
TNT	tumour necrosis factor		
TP	total protein		
Treg	regulatory T cell		
TS	total solids	WBC	white blood cell
UPC	urine protein:creatinine (ratio)	WNV	West Nile virus
VEE	Venezuelan equine encephalitis	WS	Warthin–Starry (stain)
		WSP	*Wolbachia* surface protein

Introduction: Companion Animal Arthropod-borne Diseases and 'One Health'

Michael J. Day

In the First Edition of this book (2005), the concluding section of each chapter presented information on the zoonotic potential and public health significance of the organism under discussion. That brief was given to chapter authors because of the recognition that so many of the pathogens discussed in the book were zoonoses. At the time, new research and the application of molecular diagnostics was rapidly uncovering the fact that many arthropod-borne diseases are shared between man and animals.

In the decade since publication of the First Edition there has been a global shift in understanding and appreciating the significance of zoonotic infectious disease and the fact that new human infections often emerge or re-emerge from animals. One only has to look towards the recent global disease threats of highly-pathogenic avian influenza (H5N1 and H7N9), severe acute respiratory syndrome coronavirus, Middle East respiratory syndrome coronavirus and Ebola virus disease, to appreciate how readily animal reservoirs of infection can extend to affect the human population.

In parallel with these recent infectious disease outbreaks has been the re-emergence of the concept of 'One Health' – providing a paradigm with which to consider the overlap between human and animal disease and how these issues might best be tackled by collaboration between human and veterinary medicine. There is no single and universally accepted definition of One Health and the One Health model is an evolving concept. One Health is nothing new and there is a rich history of comparative anatomy, physiology, pathology and medicine, and of zoonotic infectious disease research, over the millennia (Day, 2011). The modern rediscovery of the concept is often attributed to the veterinary epidemiologist Calvin Schwabe (1927–2006), who coined the term 'One Medicine' and argued for closer links between human medical and veterinary science (Schwabe, 1969). Modern One Health began with a focus on diseases shared between man and animals, but more recently extended to incorporate the concept of 'environmental health' with understanding that changes in an ecosystem can directly impact on human and animal wellbeing. There is now discussion of the 'One Health Triad', which links together human health, animal health (including domestic production animals, wildlife, and more recently, companion animals) and environmental health (**Figure 1**).

Many of the diseases that are discussed in this book have a One Health dimension. There are vast numbers of small companion animals (primarily dogs and cats) throughout

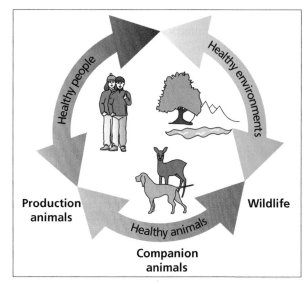

Fig. 1 The 'One Health Triad' encapsulates the continuum between human and animal health and the fact that both of these are impacted by the health of the shared environment. In the context of One Health, animal health covers farmed production animals, wildlife and companion animals. The diseases described in this book cover all three elements including the arthropod vectors within the environment and the way in which these interact with human and animal populations for the transmission of zoonotic infectious disease.

the world, living as either owned pets or working animals or as 'free roaming' populations that might be 'community owned' or truly 'stray'. These animals have integral roles in human society and share an intrinsically close relationship with people, often living in close association in the indoor environment. However, at the same time, companion animals that are permitted free outdoor access come into close contact with wildlife species and with arthropods that live in their environment. These features of the companion animal lifestyle create a risk for human health, when the animal might bring infection into the home and transmit it directly to people, bring infected arthropods into the home that might subsequently attach to their human carers, or simply act as a reservoir of vector-transmitted infection within the community.

There is no better example of a zoonotic arthropod-borne infection of One Health significance than canine zoonotic visceral leishmaniosis (see Chapter 9). This form of leishmaniosis involves transmission of the *Leishmania* spp. pathogen from a canine reservoir to susceptible humans via the bite of phlebotomine sand flies. The World Health Organisation estimates that 200,000 to 400,000 new cases of this disease occur globally each year and that 90% of these cases occur in only six countries: Bangladesh, Brazil, Ethiopia, India, South Sudan and Sudan (WHO, 2012; http://www.who.int/leishmaniasis/en/). This is a disease of poor communities, particularly of children, that is linked to malnutrition, human immunodeficiency virus infection and other immune compromise. The disease has an 'environmental health' aspect as it often focuses on communities that are displaced into endemic areas by human activities such as deforestation and urbanization.

The key to control of human visceral leishmaniosis is control of the infection in the canine reservoir and control of the vector population. However, implementing effective control measures is practically challenging and often politically sensitive. Chemical control of sand fly populations by spraying insecticides has been of limited success and may further harm the environment. A range of control measures have been evaluated for the canine reservoir including culling of seropositive dogs (with attendant animal welfare concerns) or the use of sand fly repellents and vaccines in the dog population. Although there have been some reported local successes with combinations of these approaches, this disease is far from controlled in endemic countries (Palatnik-de-Sousa and Day, 2011).

The solution to control of diseases such as visceral leishmaniosis lies firmly with the One Health approach. Multidisciplinary research groups should be supported to work on effective disease surveillance strategies and the development of more effective therapeutic and preventive (insecticidal and vaccine) approaches. Similarly, combined field teams of human physicians, veterinarians and public health officers are required to work in a coordinated fashion to identify and treat human cases and implement strategies for sand fly control and control of the canine reservoir. Embedding such One Health programmes in turn requires political will and appropriate resourcing, together with the training of One Health teams and education and 'buy-in' of the affected communities.

Although leishmaniosis provides a classical example for the potential for a One Health approach, this is applicable to many of the diseases discussed throughout this book, for example borreliosis, bartonellosis, ehrlichiosis, anaplasmosis, rickettsiosis and a spectrum of other diseases transmitted by ticks, flies, mosquitoes, fleas and bugs. Many of these diseases, of great human significance, are under-researched and the absence of any coordinated form of global infectious disease surveillance in companion animals (Day *et al.*, 2012) means that we have little idea of the true prevalence of the infections.

To that end, the content of this book now carries a real One Health focus, with expanded discussions of new and emerging zoonoses and the engagement of new chapter authors representing human medical science and governmental public health institutions. It is hoped that the content of the book will have broad One Health value to a wider audience than just the practicing veterinarian.

REFERENCES

Day MJ (2011) One Health: the importance of companion animal vector-borne diseases. *Parasites and Vectors* **4**:49.

Day MJ, Breitschwerdt E, Cleaveland S *et al.* (2012) Surveillance of zoonotic infectious diseases transmitted by small companion animals. *Emerging Infectious Diseases* (Internet) DOI: 10.3201/eid1812.120664.

Patatnik-de-Sousa CB, Day MJ (2011) One Health: the global challenge of epidemic and endemic leishmaniasis. *Parasites and Vectors* **4**:197.

Schwabe CW (1969) *Veterinary Medicine and Human Health*, 2nd edn. Williams & Wilkins, Baltimore.

Chapter 1

Arthropod Vectors of Infectious Disease: Biology and Control

Richard Wall

INTRODUCTION

The blood-feeding behaviour of a wide range of arthropods makes them important vectors of pathogens in cats and dogs. They act as vectors in one of two ways, either mechanically or biologically. In mechanical transmission, the arthropod acquires the pathogen on its mouthparts or feet and deposits it in other locations, where it may infect a new host. In biological transmission, the pathogen is normally transmitted from host to host through the body of the arthropod vector. This chapter discusses the biology of the haematophagous arthropods most relevant to transmission of disease in companion animals.

TICKS

Ticks are relatively large, obligate blood-feeding ectoparasites, closely related to mites. They form a relatively small order of only about 800 species in the subclass Acari. The order can be broadly divided into 'hard' and 'soft' ticks, based on the possession of a dorsal scutum in the Ixodidae (the 'hard' ticks, **Figure 1.1**), which is absent in the Argasidae (the 'soft' ticks). Within the Ixodidae, species of the genera *Rhipicephalus*, *Ixodes* and *Dermacentor* are of particular importance as vectors of disease for dogs and cats, since they may transmit a range of viral, bacterial and protozoan pathogens. The Argasidae are parasites primarily of birds, bats and reptiles and will not be discussed here.

Hard ticks are usually relatively large and long-lived. During this time they feed periodically, taking large blood meals, with long intervals off the host between each meal. Since a large proportion of the life cycle of most hard tick species occurs off the host, the habitat in which they live is of particular importance. It must

include sufficient host numbers to sustain the tick population and have a high humidity to allow the ticks to maintain their water balance.

The major tick species known to be of importance in transmitting disease to dogs and cats are listed in **Table 1.1**. Although many ixodid ticks are not host-specific, they are not indiscriminate in the hosts they parasitize. A few show an extremely wide host range, but most occur on a limited range of hosts, which they parasitize with varying intensities.

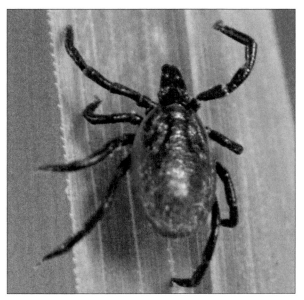

Fig. 1.1 Nymphal hard tick, *Ixodes ricinus*, in dorsal view. Ixodid ticks are relatively large, ranging between 2 and 20 mm in length. The body of the unfed tick is divided into only two sections, the anterior gnathosoma, which bears the mouthparts (the chelicerae), and a posterior idiosoma, which bears the legs. Ticks do not possess antennae and when eyes are present they are simple and are located dorsally at the sides of the scutum.

Table 1.1 **Main tick species known to transmit pathogens to dogs and cats.**

FAMILY	SUBFAMILY	GENUS	KEY SPECIES	DISTRIBUTION
Ixodidae	Ixodinae (Prostriata)	*Ixodes*	*Ixodes ricinus* (sheep, deer tick)	Europe
			Ixodes hexagonus (hedgehog tick)	Europe and north-west Africa
			Ixodes scapularis (black-legged tick)	Eastern North America
			Ixodes pacificus (Western black-legged tick)	Western North America
			Ixodes persulcatus (taiga tick)	North Eastern Europe and Northern Asia
	Rhipicephalinae (Metastriata)	*Dermacentor*	*Dermacentor variabilis* (American dog tick)	North America
			Dermacentor andersoni (Rocky Mountain wood tick)	North America
			Dermacentor reticulatus	Europe
		Rhipicephalus	*Rhipicephalus sanguineus* (brown dog tick)	Worldwide
	Haemaphysalinae (Metastriata)	*Haemaphysalis*	*Haemaphysalis leachi*	Southern Africa
			Haemaphysalis bispinosa	Middle East, Africa, Asia
			Haemaphysalis longicornis	Middle East, Africa, Asia, Oceania
	Ambylomminae (Metastriata)	*Amblyomma*	*Ambylomma americanum* (lone star tick)	North America
			Ambylomma maculatum (Gulf coast tick)	North America
			Ambylomma variegatum (tropical bont tick)	Africa

The brown dog tick *Rhipicephalus sanguineus* is one of the most widely distributed species of tick found worldwide (**Figure 1.2**). Its primary host is the dog and all life-cycle stages may feed on this host. They often infest kennels and domestic premises, where feeding activity may occur all year round. In the northern hemisphere, a particularly important group of ticks is the 'ricinus-persulcatus complex', which includes the North American black-legged tick *I. scapularis*, the European sheep tick *I. ricinus* and the northern Palaearctic taiga tick *Ixodes persulcatus*, which occurs from the Baltic Sea to Japan. *Ixodes ricinus* is usually the most common species of tick infesting dogs and cats throughout much of northern Europe and Asia. It is found commonly in pastures and mixed woodland, where the larval and nymphal stages feed primarily on small mammals and ground-nesting birds and the adult stages on deer or domestic livestock. Its range is believed to be increasing with warmer wetter winters, and feeding on dogs and cats may occur over extended periods of the year. However, the hedgehog tick, *I. hexagonus*, may be the tick found most commonly on cats in peri-urban environments throughout Europe and in north-west Africa. *Dermacentor* species are also frequently encountered in North America and southern and central Europe. Dogs are the preferred hosts of adult *D. variabilis* (American dog tick) while larvae and nymphs feed largely on small rodents.

Morphology

Ixodid ticks are relatively large (2–20 mm in length). The mouthparts are composed of a pair of four-segmented palps (simple sensory organs), which aid host location. Between the palps lies a pair of heavily sclerotized, segmented appendages called chelicerae, housed in cheliceral sheaths (**Figure 1.3**). At the end of each chelicera are a number of tooth-like digits. The chelicerae are capable of moving back and forth and the tooth-like digits are used to cut and pierce the skin of the host animal during feeding. Below the chelicerae is the median hypostome, which emerges from the base of the palps (the basis capituli) and extends anteriorly and ventrally. The hypostome does not move, but is armed with rows of backwardly directed, ventral teeth. The hypostome is thrust into the hole cut by the chelicerae and the teeth are used to attach the tick securely to its host. As the hypostome is inserted, the palps are spread flat onto the surface of the host's skin.

During feeding, hard ticks may remain attached to their host for several days, while they engorge with blood (**Figure 1.4**). For ticks with long mouthparts, attachment by the chelicerae and hypostome is sufficient to anchor the tick in place. However, for ticks with short mouthparts, attachment is maintained during feeding by salivary secretions that harden around the mouthparts and effectively cement the tick in place.

In the Ixodidae, sexual dimorphism is well developed, the dorsal scutum being small in the female and almost covering the whole of the dorsal surface in the male. This allows female ticks to increase in size substantially when they engorge during feeding. Some of the larger species of *Amblyomma* can increase from just under 10 mm to over 25 mm in length and increase

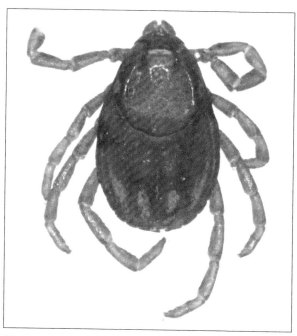

Fig. 1.2 The brown dog tick *Rhipicephalus sanguineus*. Adult female in dorsal view.

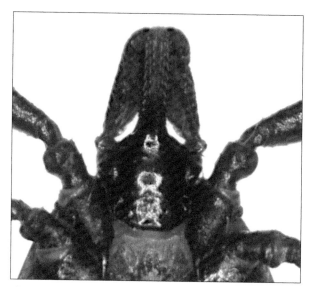

Fig. 1.3 The gnathosoma of the tick *Ixodes ricinus*, showing the ventral teeth of the hypostome flanked by the segmented palps.

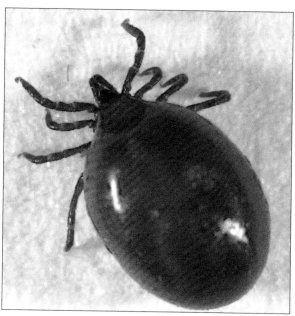

Fig. 1.4 A fully engorged *Ixodes ricinus* nymph.

from about 0.04 g to over 4 g in weight during feeding. Males are not able to engorge to the same degree as females and may take more frequent, smaller meals.

Life cycle

The life cycle of ixodid ticks involves four stages: egg, six-legged larva, eight-legged nymph and eight-legged adult (**Figure 1.5**). During passage through these stages the larvae, nymphs and adults take a number of blood meals. Tick parasitism probably evolved through close association with nest-dwelling (nidiculous) hosts until mechanisms developed that allowed them to remain permanently on their host or to locate and relocate hosts at intervals in the open environment.

Most, though not all, non-nidiculous hard ticks adopt a 'sit and wait' strategy rather than actively searching for hosts. To obtain a blood meal, they climb to the tips of vegetation, usually to a height appropriate for their host. This behaviour is described as 'questing'. Ticks identify a potential host via chemoreceptors on the tarsi of their first pair of legs, using cues such as carbon dioxide and other semiochemicals emitted by the host. Following contact, they transfer to the host and move over the skin surface to find their preferred attachment sites.

For most ixodid ticks, living in an environment where there is a relatively plentiful supply of host animals and in habitats where conditions are suitable

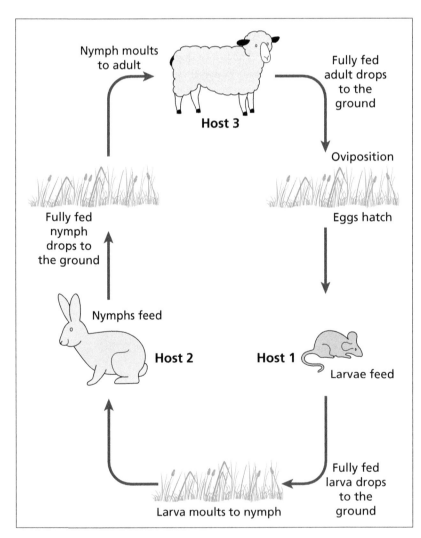

Fig. 1.5 The three-host feeding strategy of an ixodid tick. On finding a suitable host, usually a small mammal or bird, the larvae of ixodid ticks begin to feed. Blood feeding typically takes between 4 and 6 days. On completion of feeding, the larvae drop to the ground where they moult to become nymphs. After another interval, the nymphs begin to quest for a second host and after feeding, drop to the ground and moult to become adults. Finally, after a further interval, adults begin to quest and, on their final host, females mate and engorge. After the final blood meal, adult females drop to the ground where they lay large batches of several thousand eggs over a period of days or weeks. Adult males may remain unattached on the host animal and attempt to mate with as many females as possible.

for good survival during the off-host phase, a three-host life cycle has been adopted. For example, the deer tick *Ixodes scapularis* is a vector of the spirochaetes of *Borrelia burgdorferi* in North America. Larval *I. scapularis* become infected after feeding on small rodents, particularly the white-footed mouse. Bacteria are then transmitted from larval to nymphal and adult stages (transstadial transmission). The preferred host for adult ticks is the white-tailed deer. Therefore, Lyme borreliosis is generally confined to locations where the vector tick, the disease reservoir (the white-footed mouse) and the preferred host (the white-tailed deer) are abundant.

For the relatively small number of ixodid ticks (about 50 species) that inhabit areas where hosts are scarce and lengthy seasonal periods of unfavourable climate occur (e.g. *Rhipicephalus bursa* or *Dermacentor albipictus*), two- and one-host feeding strategies have evolved, respectively.

For many non-nidiculous ticks, the ancestral nest-dwelling habit is reflected in their selective environmental requirements, particularly for high relative humidity. For example, *I. ricinus* begins to quest when temperatures rise above a critical threshold of about 7°C, but requires a humidity above 80% to survive and feed. These environmental constraints restrict feeding activity to relatively short periods of the year during spring and autumn. Outside these periods, ticks remain quiescent, sheltering within the vegetation. Clearly, since tick densities and geographical and temporal activity ranges are strongly determined by microclimate, these may be greatly extended by climate change, particularly mild wet winters.

Vectorial potential

Almost all the ticks of importance as vectors of disease in cats and dogs are three-host species, and it is this movement between different types of vertebrate hosts, and the fact that they are not strictly host-specific in their feeding preferences, that make ticks such important disease vectors. Wild animals are particularly important as reservoirs of pathogens through a wild animal/tick/domestic animal cycle of contact (see Chapter 2). Several other factors contribute to the vectorial capacity of ticks. These include: secure attachment to their host; lengthy feeding periods allowing large numbers of pathogens to be ingested and transmitted; high rates of reproduction; and the transmission of pathogens between tick life cycle stages (transstadial transmis-

sion) and between generations via the egg (transovarial transmission) (see Chapter 2). Infection of a host with tick-transmitted pathogens may be aided by salivary anticoagulants and other active compounds that modulate host cutaneous immunity and inflammation, while at the same time enhancing vasodilation in order to bring more blood to the feeding site (see Chapter 3). The salivary fluid is the principal avenue for disease transmission in the hard ticks.

FLEAS

Fleas (order Siphonaptera) are small, wingless, obligate, blood-feeding insects. The order is relatively small, with about 2,500 described species of which approximately 90% occur on mammals and only 10% on birds. On cats and dogs, *Ctenocephalides felis* and *Ctenocephalides canis* are the two species of major importance worldwide. However, in most geographical areas, even on dogs, *C. felis* predominates.

Morphology and life cycle

Adult fleas are highly modified for an ectoparasitic life and are structurally very different from most other insects (**Figure 1.6**). In contrast to lice or ticks, the flea body is laterally compressed. Adults are wingless and usually between 1 mm and 6 mm in length, with females being larger than males. The head is sessile on the prothorax and the body is covered with backwardly directed setae and, in many cases, with combs (also known as ctenidia). The thorax bears three pairs of legs, the third of which is particularly well developed for jumping. The mouthparts are modified for piercing, with a salivary canal for injecting saliva into the wound and a food canal along which blood is drawn. Both sexes are blood feeders.

At 24°C and 78% relative humidity (RH), and with a plentiful food supply, under most household conditions *C. felis* will complete its developmental cycle in 3–5 weeks (**Figure 1.7**). However, under adverse conditions this can be extended to as long as 190 days. The eggs cannot withstand major variations in temperature and will not survive below 50% RH. At 70% RH and 35°C, 50% of *C. felis* eggs hatch within 1.5 days. At 70% RH and 15°C, it takes 6 days for 50% of eggs to hatch. The duration of the three larval stages is about 1 week at 24°C and 75% RH, but in unfavourable conditions

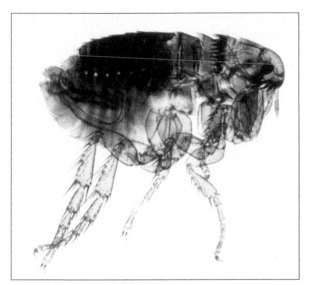

Fig. 1.6 Adult male *Ctenocephalides canis*. The body colour may vary from light brown to black. The body is divided into head, thorax and abdomen, which are armed with spines that are directed backward. The head is high, narrow and cuneate. Eyes are absent in some species of nest flea, but if present, they are usually simple and found on the head in front of the antennae. The shape of the abdomen may be used to distinguish the sexes. In female fleas, both ventral and dorsal surfaces are rounded. In the male flea, the dorsal surface is relatively flatter and the ventral surface greatly curved.

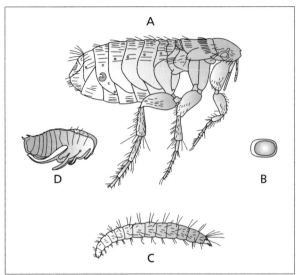

Fig. 1.7 Life cycle of a typical *Ctenocephalides* flea. (A) Adult. Within 24–48 hours of the first blood meal, adult females begin to oviposit. The eggs may be deposited on the host, but will fall to the ground within a few hours. Timing of oviposition may contribute to the concentration of flea eggs at the resting sites used by the host. In the laboratory, an adult female *C. felis* can produce an average of about 30 eggs per day over a life of about 50–100 days. However, on a cat or dog, the average life span is substantially less than this. (B) Egg. Flea eggs are about 0.5 mm in length, pearly white and oval. (C) Larvae. Flea larvae are white and maggot-like with a distinct brownish head and covered with short hairs. Larvae grow in length from about 1.5 mm on hatching to 4–10 mm when fully grown. They have limited powers of movement (probably less than 20 cm before pupation) and are negatively phototactic and positively geotactic. In the domestic environment this behaviour often takes them to the base of carpets. Outdoors, they move into shaded areas under bushes, trees, and leaves. Adult flea faeces are the primary food source for all three larval stages. (D) Pupa. When fully developed, the mature third-stage larva spins a thin, silk cocoon within which the larva pupates. Fragments of detritus, soil and dust adhere to the cocoon, giving it some degree of camouflage and protection from insecticides.

the larval cycle can take up to 200 days. Larvae will only survive at temperatures between 13°C and 35°C and mortality is high below 50% RH. The duration of the pupal stage is about 8–9 days at 24°C and 78% RH.

When fully developed, adults emerge from the pupal cuticle, but may remain within the cocoon for up to 12 months at low temperatures. Emergence may be extremely rapid under optimal conditions and is triggered by mechanical pressure, changes in light, vibrations, elevated carbon dioxide and heat. As adult fleas generally do not actively search for hosts, and hosts may only return to the lair or bedding at infrequent intervals, the ability to remain within the cocoon for extended periods is essential. The air currents created by warm, mobile objects in close proximity induce adult cat fleas to jump. Once on their host, *C. felis* adults feed almost immediately and tend to become permanent residents.

Within 36 hours of adult emergence, most females will have found hosts and mated. Egg laying begins 24–48 hours after the first blood meal.

Vectorial potential

Fleas feed by piercing the skin of the host and inserting the tip of the labrum–epipharynx to extract capillary blood. A female *C. felis* feeds to repletion in 10 minutes, imbibing 7 µl of blood and doubling in weight. Flea feeding is more frequent at higher temperatures as a result of accelerated physiological activity and increased rate of water loss. Fleas are vectors of a range of viruses and bacteria and pathogen transmission is enhanced by their promiscuous feeding habits. Most species of flea are host-preferential rather than host-specific and will try to feed on any available animal. For example, *C. felis* has been found on over 50 different host species. Other factors that contribute to the potential of *C. felis* as a vector include transovarial transmission of some pathogens (*Rickettsia* species) and the transmission of pathogens such as *Bartonella henselae* through adult flea faeces (see Chapters 11 and 13). Cat fleas also act as intermediate hosts for the common tapeworm of dogs and cats, *Dipylidium caninum*, and for the subcutaneous filarioid *Acanthocheilonema reconditum*, infesting dogs worldwide. Both helminths may occasionally be found in humans, particularly young children who, when playing with pets may inadvertently ingest infected fleas.

MOSQUITOES

The mosquitoes, family Culicidae, are a diverse family of true flies (Diptera), containing over 3,500 species, although there is considerable debate about the ranking of some genera. The family occurs worldwide from the Tropics to the Arctic and is divided into three subfamilies: Anophelinae, Culicinae and the primitive Toxorhynchitinae. There are more than 2,500 species of Culicinae, of which the main genera are *Aedes*, containing over 900 species, and *Culex*, with nearly 750 species.

Morphology and life cycle

Mosquitoes are small, slender flies, 2–10 mm in length. Adults of the Culicidae have scales on their wings and body. The wings are long and narrow with a fringe of narrow scales along the posterior border of the wing. There is a long, forwardly directed proboscis, which is longer than the head and thorax combined. Anopheline and culicine mosquitoes can be readily differentiated on morphological and behavioural characteristics (**Figure 1.8**).

Mosquitoes lay their eggs on the surface of water on damp ground, usually at night. They typically deposit batches of 100–150 eggs per oviposition. The larvae of all species are aquatic and they occur in a wide variety of habitats such as the edge of permanent pools, puddles, flooded tree holes or even temporary water-filled containers. Mosquito larvae require between 3 and 20 days to pass through four stadia. The final larval stage moults to become a pupa and this stage may last between 1 and 7 days. Mating normally occurs within 24 hours of emergence and is completed in flight. Mosquitoes feed on nectar and plant juices, but females need a blood meal to develop their ovaries and must feed between each egg batch. Longevity is highly variable and species-specific, but on average, females live for 2–3 weeks, while the male lifespan is shorter.

Mosquitoes are nocturnal or crepuscular feeders, with a wide host range. Host location is achieved using a range of olfactory and visual cues, orientation to wind direction and body warmth. Mosquitoes typically require 4 days to digest a blood meal and produce eggs. Oviposition begins as soon as a suitable site is located. Adult mosquitoes are strong fliers, anopheline species in particular.

Vectorial potential

Most mosquitoes require a blood meal for ovarian development. The source of the blood meal is a major factor in determining the potential of a species to be a nuisance pest and/or vector of disease. When mosquitoes feed, both the mandibles and the maxillae puncture the skin. Saliva passes down the salivary canal in the hypopharynx, while blood passes up the food canal formed by the elongated labrum. Blood feeding takes only a few minutes.

Some pathogens can be transmitted mechanically by mosquitoes, the principal disease example being the myxoma virus that is spread among rabbits primarily by mosquitoes in Australia (although in Europe, the principal vector of myxomatosis is the flea *Spilopsyllus cuniculi*) (see Chapter 2). Mosquitoes also act as biological vectors for a range of viral, nematode and protozoan pathogens. Mosquito vectors can be relatively long lived and may overwinter, allowing pathogen survival from one season to another. When competent mosquitoes feed on the blood of a viraemic vertebrate host, virions are ingested with the blood meal and enter the midgut epithelial cells, within which they replicate. After spreading to the haemocoele, they then disperse to a variety of tissues, particularly the salivary glands, fat bodies, ovaries and nerves. Salivary transmission of the virus occurs when the infected mosquito next feeds on an appropriate host. In some mosquitoes, transovarial transmission of viruses also occurs. Mosquitoes are also vectors of the canine heartworm *Dirofilaria immitis* (see Chapter 5).

A number of basic feeding patterns have been recognized among mosquitoes: different mosquito species have different blood feeding preferences; some will feed only on certain hosts while others are less discriminat-ing and will feed on a variety of hosts depending on their relative abundance. *Culex quinquefasciatus*, for example, frequently feed on dogs but less frequently on cats. This host species preference might explain why dogs are more commonly infected with heartworm than cats.

SAND FLIES

The Psychodidae is large family of true flies (Diptera) containing over 800 species. Within this family, the subfamily Phlebotominae includes biting species known as sand flies. They are widely distributed in the Tropics, Subtropics and around the Mediterranean. There are two genera of Phlebotominae of veterinary importance: in the Old World, *Phlebotomus*, and in the New World, *Lutzomyia*. Sand flies transmit the important zoonotic protozoal infection leishmaniosis in dogs and cats.

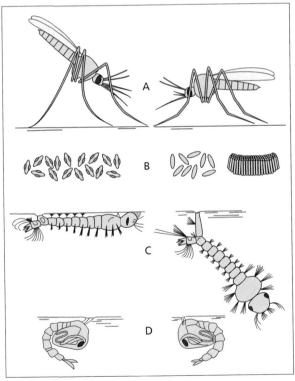

Fig. 1.8 Life-cycle features distinguishing anopheline and culicine mosquitoes. (A) Adults. Living anopheline adults can readily be distinguished from culicines, such as *Aedes* and *Culex*, when resting on a flat surface. On landing, anopheline mosquitoes rest with the proboscis, head, thorax and abdomen in one straight line at an acute angle to the surface. The culicine adult rests with its body slightly angled and its abdomen directed towards the surface. The palps of female anopheline mosquitoes are as long and straight as the proboscis, while in female culicine mosquitoes the palps are usually only about one-quarter of the length of the proboscis. The abdomen of *Anopheles* bears hairs but not scales. (B) Eggs. The eggs of anopheline mosquitoes possess characteristic lateral floats that prevent them from sinking and maintain their orientation in the water. Most species of *Aedes* lay their eggs on moist substrates, where they await adequate water to stimulate hatching. *Culex* form batches of eggs into a raft on the water surface. (C) Larvae. The larvae of *Anopheles* lie parallel to the water surface and breathe through a pair of spiracles at the posterior end of the abdomen. In contrast, larvae of Culicinae hang suspended from the water surface by a prominent posterior breathing siphon with spiracles at its tip. Culicine and *Aedes* larvae feed by filtering out microorganisms from the water using mouth brushes. Anopheline larvae collect particles from the air–water interface. (D) Pupae. Mosquito pupae usually remain at the water surface, but when disturbed can be highly mobile. They do not feed during this phase and breathe by means of respiratory siphons. Adult mosquitoes emerge from the pupal case and crawl from the water to harden their cuticle and inflate their wings.

Morphology and life cycle

Phlebotomine sand flies are narrow bodied and up to 5 mm in length with narrow hairy bodies and long antennae (**Figure 1.9**). They breed in humid, terrestrial habitats. Females lay 50–100 eggs per egg batch in small cracks or holes in damp ground, leaf litter and around the roots of forest trees. The larvae pass through four stadia before pupation and they feed on organic debris (faeces and decaying plant material). The life cycle is slow and takes at least 7–10 weeks, with many Palaearctic species having only two generations per year. Adult sand flies feed on nectar, sap, honeydew and fruit juices and live for 2–6 weeks. Only adult females are blood feeders. Adults often accumulate in refugia where the microclimate is suitable for breeding (e.g. rodent burrows and caves), with females blood feeding on the mammals in close vicinity. They have very limited powers of flight, moving in characteristic short hops, and have a range of perhaps only 100–200 metres.

Vectorial potential

When blood feeding, the toothed mandibles cut the skin while the maxillae hold the mouthparts in place in the wound. Blood is sucked from a subcutaneous pool and up a food canal formed by the labium above and the hypopharynx below. The salivary duct is formed by the underside of the hypopharynx. Blood feeding is limited to areas of exposed, less densely haired areas of skin, such as the ears, eyelids, nose, feet and tail. The feeding activity of most species occurs during dusk or even darkness, although some will bite during daylight. Most sand flies have a broad host range.

Sand flies are important as vectors of canine and feline leishmaniosis (see Chapter 9). *Leishmania* amastigotes are ingested with a blood meal when sand flies feed on an infected host, and they develop extracellularly in the mid- and hindgut. After 3 days, they transform into promastigotes and migrate into the foregut, where multiplication occurs. Infective promastigotes are regurgitated from the mouthparts, foregut and midgut into the dermis of a new host during feeding. This process is assisted by blockage of the foregut caused by congregated parasites, which prevents the fly from feeding effectively, thus ensuring repeated feeding attempts on multiple hosts. Infection is assisted by the presence of vasodilatory enzymes and immunomodulatory chemicals in the fly saliva (see Chapter 3).

In drier areas, phlebotomines may be found aggregating in the burrows of rodents, where females feed on the mammalian occupants or on hosts in the close vicinity, and lay their eggs. This habit, coupled with the short flight range that is characteristic of the subfamily, leads to local concentrations of phlebotomines and the diseases they transmit, and contributes to the focality in disease distribution.

TABANID AND MUSCID FLIES

The Tabanidae and Muscidae are large and important families of true flies (Diptera). More than 4,000 species of tabanids have been described and most species of veterinary importance belong to one of three genera: *Tabanus* (horse flies, greenheads), *Chrysops* (deer flies) and *Haematopota* (clegs). The family Muscidae contains several species (*Musca domestica*, *M. sorbens*, *M. autumnalis* and *M. vetustissima*) that may be important mechanical vectors of disease and some that are also blood feeding (*Haematobia irritans*). The family also includes the stable fly *Stomoxys calcitrans*, which is of importance as a biting

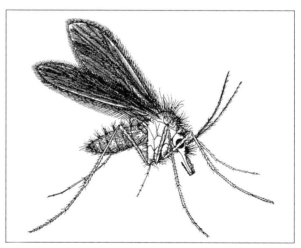

Fig. 1.9 Adult female sand fly, *Phlebotomus papatasi* (reproduced from Smart, 1943). Phlebotomines are densely hairy in appearance with large black eyes and long legs. The wings are narrow, long, hairy and held erect over the thorax when at rest. The antennae are long, 16-segmented, filamentous and covered in fine setae. The thorax is strongly humped. The larvae are elongate, legless and up to 5 mm in length, with a distinct head carrying eyespots and toothed mandibles.

fly of many mammalian hosts, including dogs. The stable fly is now found worldwide, after being introduced into North America from Europe during the 1700s. *Stomoxys niger* and *S. sitiens* may replace *S. calcitrans* as important blood feeding pests in Afrotropical and Oriental regions.

Morphology and life cycles

All the Tabanidae are large (6–30 mm), robust flies (**Figure 1.10**). The head is much broader than long and the eyes are particularly well developed. The adults are strong fliers and are usually diurnal. Both sexes feed on nectar and, in most species, females are also blood feeders on a wide range of hosts. The tabanids are painful and persistent biters.

Tabanid eggs are laid in large masses of 200–1,000 eggs on or near water, and hatch after 4–7 days. The first-stage larvae move to mud or wet soil and quickly moult. The larvae of *Chrysops* may feed on decaying vegetable debris, while those of *Haematopota* and *Tabanus* are carnivorous; therefore, the latter species are often found at relatively low population densities. Most larvae require periods of several months to several years to complete development, during which time they pass through between six and 13 stadia. Pupation takes place close to, or within, dryer soil and requires 2–3 weeks. The life cycle length varies from 10–42 weeks. Most temperate species have only a single generation per year and adults live for 2–4 weeks.

Both sexes of *S. calcitrans* are persistent and strong fliers and are active by day. Female adults are 5–7 mm in length. The body is usually grey, with seven circular black spots on the abdomen and four dark longitudinal stripes on the thorax. Stable flies have piercing and sucking mouthparts, with short maxillary palps, and both sexes are blood feeders. After multiple blood meals, adult females lay eggs in wet straw, garden debris, old stable bedding or manure. Eggs hatch in 5–10 days, depending on temperature. The cream-coloured, saprophagous larvae pass through three stadia and then pupariate. The life cycle length varies from 3–7 weeks, depending on temperature.

Vectorial potential

Tabanid mouthparts are short and strong for slashing, rasping and sponging. They are important mechanical vectors of several viral, bacterial, protozoan and nematode pathogens. When a female tabanid feeds, saliva containing an anticoagulant is pumped into the wound, before blood is sucked up into the food canal. When feeding ceases, the labia of the mouthparts trap a small quantity of blood. Pathogens in this blood may be protected for an hour or more and successfully transmitted to a new host at the next meal. Mechanical transmission is made more likely by the painful nature of tabanid bites. Biting flies are more likely to be dislodged by the host before blood feeding is complete and they will attempt to feed again rapidly, increasing the chance of live pathogen transmission. Tabanids are primarily important as vectors of disease to livestock and humans, but they may play a role in the transmission of *Trypanosoma evansi* to dogs in some areas, leading to death in the absence of treatment.

Stable flies also inflict frequent, painful bites and remain on their hosts only when feeding. They will occasionally follow potential hosts for considerable distances and will follow them indoors. Stable flies are known mechanically to transmit a number of pathogens, such as *Trypanosoma evansi* (causing 'surra' of equines and dogs), and are also suspected of transmitting arboviruses, bacteria, protozoa and nematodes.

TRUE BUGS

The order Hemiptera, known as the true bugs, includes roughly 90,000 insect species. They all have piercing

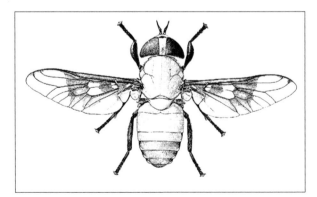

Fig. 1.10 A tabanid, *Tabanus latipes* (reproduced from Castellani and Chalmers, 1913). The body is generally dark in colour, although this can be variable, ranging from dull brown to black or grey. Some species may even be brilliant yellow, green or metallic blue. However, the body also usually carries a pattern of stripes or pale patches and the thorax and abdomen are covered with fine hairs.

and sucking mouthparts and two pairs of wings. Most of the species feed only on plant juices. However, species of the family Ruduviidae, particularly the subfamily Triatominae (known generally as kissing bugs), are of medical and veterinary significance as all species can transmit the protozoan *Trypanosoma cruzi*, the causative agent of Chagas' disease. There are at least 140 species of Triatominae, classified into 17 genera.

Morphology and life cycle

Adult triatomines are generally large insects with broad abdomens. They have long, thin, four-segmented antennae. The forewings have a hardened basal area and a membranous distal portion (**Figure 1.11**). The hind wings are entirely membranous and are folded beneath the forewings. Adult bugs are secretive, hiding in cracks and crevices in buildings and natural habitats. Eggs are laid in groups or loosely on a substrate and they hatch within 10–30 days. There are usually five stadia before the insects reach maturity, the nymphs being similar in appearance to adults, but not possessing wings and being capable of moulting to the next stage after only one blood meal. Depending on temperature, the life cycle may be completed in 3–6 months but usually requires 1–2 years.

Vectorial potential

Feeding is initiated by chemical and physical cues. Carbon dioxide causes increased activity and heat will stimulate probing. When probing is initiated, the rostrum is swung forward and the mandibular stylets are used to cut through the skin and then anchor the mouthparts. The maxillary stylets probe for a blood vessel and saliva containing an anticoagulant passes down the salivary canal while blood is pumped up the food canal. Feeding may take between 3 and 30 minutes. After engorging, the rostrum is removed from the host and the bug defecates, after which it crawls away to find shelter.

The saliva injected with the bites of triatomines contains proteins that can induce mild to severe allergic responses, including anaphylactic reactions that can be fatal. However, the bugs are of greatest medical importance as vectors of Chagas' disease, caused by the protozoan parasite *Trypanosoma cruzi*. If the bug feeds on a host infected with *T. cruzi*, amastigotes or trypomastigotes may be ingested. In the vector the parasite reproduces asexually and metacyclic trypomastigotes develop in its hindgut. The next time the bug feeds, metacyclic trypomastigotes are voided in its faeces and are rubbed or scratched into the bite wound or mucous membranes of the eye, nose or mouth. The interval between feeding and defecation is critical in determining the effectiveness of disease transmission.

The main wild hosts of *T. cruzi* are opossums, marsupials of the genus *Didelphys*, which are widely distributed from Argentina to the USA and have a high incidence of infection. When opossums become established near

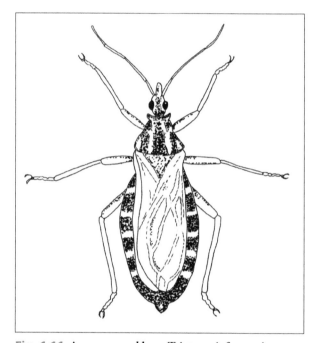

Fig. 1.11 A cone-nosed bug, *Triatoma infestans*, in dorsal view. Triatomine bugs are generally between 20 cm and 30 cm in length. Most species are dark in colour, but are often characteristically marked along the abdomen, pronotum or at the base of the wings, with contrasting splashes of yellow, orange or red. They possess an elongated head with large eyes and four-segmented antennae. The segmented rostrum is formed by the labium, which encloses the stylet-like mouthparts, composed by the modified maxillae and mandibles used to pierce the skin of the host. When the bug is not feeding the rostrum is folded back under the head. An adult bug can take up to three times its own weight in blood. They feed roughly every 5–10 days, although they can survive prolonged periods without blood.

houses, they can infect triatomines that enter houses and infect the residents directly. Infected dogs and cats within the household may become sources of infection for resident triatomines.

CONTROL

When dealing with arthropod-transmitted infections, prevention of arthropod attack is desirable, as even low levels of biting may be sufficient to result in transmission. However, chemicals used for this purpose, particularly when applied to the environment, may be expensive and result in effects on non-target organisms and selection for resistance. Therefore, the choice of product requires detailed consideration of the vector species in question, its behaviour and biology, the mechanism and kinetics of transmission of infection and the level of infectious challenge.

Over the past 10 years, the problems associated with direct treatment of the environment have encouraged increased development of products for topical or systemic administration to small companion animals. These include a number of newer generation insecticidal and acaricidal chemicals, such as fipronil, imidacloprid, nitenpyram and selemectin, as well as reformulations of existing compounds such as amitraz and the pyrethroids permethrin and deltamethrin. Many of the newer products are highly arthropod specific, resulting in increased mammalian safety. In addition, they have prolonged residual activity, thus decreasing the frequency of administration. Products combining ectoparasiticides with insect development inhibitors, such as methoprene and lufenuron, are now available for on-animal use. Formulations for on-animal use are varied, although many of the newer drugs are 'spot-on' preparations. Others include sprays, dips, collars, shampoos, foams and powders, as well as oral preparations. Environmental treatments suitable for domestic premises include traditional insecticides (e.g. organophosphates, carbamates and pyrethrins), either alone or in combination with insect growth regulators, and biological control using nematodes.

Although there are several management strategies available for control of arthropods on dogs and cats, control of arthropod vectors in wildlife reservoirs still remains a major challenge.

Tick control

Animals should be inspected for ticks daily, particularly during the spring and summer. On cats and dogs, the majority of adult ticks attach to the front of the body, particularly the ears, face, neck and interdigital areas. However, there may be variation between tick species in this respect. Larvae and nymphs may also be found along the dorsum. Attached ticks should be removed from cats and dogs using purpose-designed, tick-removing tools. Jerking, twisting or crushing ticks during removal should be avoided. They should not be handled without gloves and, once removed, should be disposed of carefully.

Where practicable, contact between pets and known areas of high tick density should be limited at times of year when tick activity is known to be high. There are several acaricides developed for use on dogs and cats, and those that kill or repel ticks before or soon after they attach are particularly valuable. Environmental treatment with organophosphates or pyrethroids in domestic premises may be useful under some circumstances. However, since off-host life cycle stages are often in highly inaccessible locations, environmental treatment is usually of only limited efficacy.

Flea control

For optimal control of flea-transmitted infections, the adults already infesting dogs and cats should be killed immediately and reinfestation from the environment prevented. A wide range of products is available (**Table 1.2**). Many of the new chemical products with excellent long-acting flea adulticidal activity also have contact ovicidal and/or larvicidal activity. In addition, combination with insect growth regulators (e.g. chitin synthesis inhibitors, juvenile hormone analogues) applied directly to the animal not only increases ovicidal and/or larvicidal activity, but also delivers it effectively to the sleeping areas most likely to be infested, without unnecessarily contaminating the environment. Insect growth regulators do not kill adult fleas and are not suitable by themselves for controlling flea-transmitted diseases unless used in a completely closed environment. Frequent vacuuming can help to reduce environmental infestation and pet bedding should be washed at high temperatures.

Table 1.2 Insecticides, acaricides and insect growth regulators used in control of arthropod infestations of dogs and cats.

ACTIVE INGREDIENT	PRODUCT EXAMPLES	ACTION ON ARTHROPOD VECTORS	APPLICATION
Amitraz (triazapentadiene)	Mitaban (Zoetis), Preventic (Virbac), Taktic (MSD Animal Health) and various generic brands	Neurotoxin and repellent; insecticide and acaricide. It interferes with octopamine receptors of the CNS and inhibits monoamine oxidases and prostaglandin synthesis. It may also act as a synergist	Collar or topical pour-on
Carbamates (e.g. carbaryl, propoxur, bendiocarb)	Various	Neurotoxins; cholinesterase inhibitors; general adulticides	Topical or environmental preparations
Pyriproxifen (insect growth inhibitor)	Various	Juvenile hormone and juvenile hormone analogues. Flea larvicide	Environmental preparations, collars, spot-ons
Methoprene (insect growth inhibitor)	Staykil (Ceva Animal Health) (methoprene combined with permethrin)	Insect growth inhibitor. Flea larvicide (with permethrin providing adulticide)	Environmental preparation
Lufenuron (benzoyl phenylurea – insect growth inhibitor)	Program (Elanco Animal Health)	Chitin synthesis inhibitor. Flea ovicide and some larvicidal activity	Oral or depot injection
Fipronil (phenylpyrazole)	Frontline, Frontline Combo (Merial) (a combination of fiprinil and methoprene); Certifect (Merial) (a combination of fiprinil, amitraz, and methoprene)	Neurotoxin; inhibits GABA-mediated receptors in the arthropod CNS; flea adulticide, acaricide. When formulated with methoprene, flea larvicide	Topical spot-on, spray
Imidocloprid (chloronicotinyl, pyridylmethylamine)	Advantage, Advantix for dogs (Bayer)	Neurotoxin; inhibits nicotinergic-mediated receptors. Flea adulticide. When formulated with permethrin will kill and repel ticks and flies in dogs	Topical spot-on
Isoxazoline (afoxalaner, fluralaner)	NexGard (Merial), Bravecto (MSD Animal Health)	Fixation on GABA and glutamate receptors of chloride ion channels of the synapses; mortality of adult fleas and ticks	Oral
Natural botanical products (eucalyptus oil, pennyroyal oil, tea tree oil, citrus oil and D-limonene, rotenone)	Various	Insecticidal or insect repellent properties. However, precise efficacy unknown. Neurotoxity after ingestion at high concentrations. Do not use in cats	Topical
Nitempyram (neonicotinoid, pyridylmethylamine)	Capstar (Elanco Animal Health)	Neurotoxin; binds and inhibits insect specific nicotinic acetylcholine receptors; rapid acting flea adulticide	Oral
Organophosphates (e.g. malathion, ronnel, chlorpyrifos, fenthion, dichlorvos, cythioate, diazanon, propetamphos, phosmet)	Various	Neurotoxins; cholinesterase inhibitors; general adulticides	Topical or systemic formulations; plus environmental preparations
Pyrethroids (e.g. permethrin, deltamethrin, others)	Various	Synthetic insecticides derived from pyrethrins; interfere with sodium activation gate of the nerve cells; tick, flea, fly adulticide and repellent. Do not use in cats	Topical or environmental preparations. Impregnated collars
Dinotefuran (neonicetinoid)	Vectra 3D (Ceva Animal Health) (dinotefuran combined with pyriproxyfen and permethrin)	Kills adult fleas, ticks and sand flies. Dinotefuran acts on nicotinic acetylcholine receptors, permethrin interferes with nerve sodium channels. Pyriproxyfen is an insect growth regulator that prevents fertile egg production and development of juvenile stages	Spot-on
Selamectin (macroycliclactone)	Stronghold, Revolution (Zoetis)	Neurotoxin; binds to glutamate-gated chloride channels in the arthropod CNS; flea adulticide and larvicide. Some acaricidal activity	Topical spot-on

CNS, central nervous system; GABA, gamma-aminobutyric acid.

Fly control

The most effective method to prevent fly bites and transmission of infection is to ensure that pets avoid areas of high fly density and are kept indoors when fly activity is highest.

Approaches to achieving long-term fly control often require environmental modification to remove breeding sites for larvae insects. These may include drainage of wetlands for mosquito control. However, such approaches are usually beyond the scope of the pet owner and are usually slow to effect interruption of disease transmission. Hence, adult control, which aims to kill the infective active females, should be the frontline approach.

Flies spend a limited time on their hosts and are difficult to control using insecticides unless these have rapid killing or repellent activity. Permethrin and deltamethrin are the only insecticides with sufficient repellent activity and rapidity of action to make them suitable for the control of sand fly biting in dogs (**Table 1.2**). Neither insecticide is suitable for cats.

The environmental use of residual insecticides is difficult for insects that do not have readily identified breeding or resting sites. Tabanid and many muscid larvae are generally inaccessible to insecticides. Most adult insect vectors are relatively strong fliers and can move several miles from where they developed as larvae. Hence, successful control of larvae in one site may not result in significant reductions in adult fly numbers, biting activity or disease transmission. In some countries, public control agencies are responsible for controlling mosquito and other vector numbers. In areas where mosquito and other fly populations are problematic, the domestic environment may be protected by fine mesh window and door screens, draining standing water or treating it with chemical insecticides or the microbial insecticide produced by *Bacillus thuringiensis* subspecies *israelensis*. The use of any insecticide product should be combined with good sanitation practices that reduce breeding sites.

Triatomine control

Bugs shelter in cracks and crevices of human and animal habitations. Fewer recesses in which bugs can shelter makes it more difficult for them to establish and remain undetected. The application of residual insecticides to the bugs daytime resting places in bedrooms and animal shelters, previously using the organochlorine insecticide benzene hexachloride and, more recently, synthetic pyrethroids, has proved highly effective, with the latter giving much greater residual activity on mud walls than other insecticides. This is often enough to eliminate existing populations of the bugs within a house, although reintroductions are possible.

FURTHER READING

Dantas-Torres F (2008) The brown dog tick, *Rhipicephalus sanguineus* (Latreille, 1806) (Acari: Ixodidae): from taxonomy to control. *Veterinary Parasitology* **152**:173–185.

Dryden MW, Rust MK (1994) The cat flea: biology, ecology and control. *Veterinary Parasitology* **52**:1–19.

Estrada-Pena A, Venzal JM, Sanchez Acedo C (2006) The tick *Ixodes ricinus*: distribution and climate preferences in the western Palaearctic. *Medical and Veterinary Entomology* **20**:189–197.

Jennett AL, Smith FD, Wall R (2013) Tick infestation risk for dogs in a peri-urban park. *Parasites and Vectors* **6**:358.

Jongejan F, Uilenberg G (2004) The global importance of ticks. *Parasitology* **129**:S3–S14.

Needham GR, Teal PD (1991) Off-host physiological ecology of ixodid ticks. *Annual Review of Entomology* **36**:659–681.

Russell RC, Otranto D, Wall RL (2014) *The Encylopedia of Medical and Veterinary Entomology*. CABI, Wallingford.

Rust MK, Dryden MW (1997) The biology, ecology and management of the cat flea. *Annual Review of Entomology* **42**:451–473.

INTRODUCTION

As interest in emerging microparasitic infections of man and domestic animals, such as *Borrelia burgdorferi*, *Anaplasma phagocytophilum* and *Bartonella* species, has grown in recent decades, the key role of wildlife in their maintenance has led to increased interest in the ecology of these agents in their natural hosts. While much is still unknown, it is apparent that complex interactions between hosts, vectors and microparasites (i.e. bacteria, viruses and protozoa) have evolved to enable the continued existence of such agents in natural systems. This chapter will highlight a number of wildlife species important in the maintenance of arthropod-borne infections, and some of the key ecological adaptations involved.

THE IMPORTANCE OF WILDLIFE IN THE MAINTENANCE OF ARTHROPOD-BORNE INFECTIONS

The concept of reservoir hosts

Wild animals have been implicated in the epidemiology of many arthropod-borne infections and, as more research into emerging diseases takes place, more wildlife reservoirs will be identified. Several of the infections discussed in detail elsewhere in this book are maintained in wildlife hosts, and infection and disease in humans and domesticated animals occurs only 'accidentally' as a result of being bitten by a vector. These accidental hosts play little role in maintaining the microparasite in nature. Those species deemed essential for maintaining the infection within its natural ecological system are termed reservoir hosts. Such hosts must be susceptible to infection and allow the microparasite to reach the stage of development required for it to be transmitted. Infection can persist within populations of reservoir hosts in the absence of host species other than arthropod vectors, and

infection in accidental host species usually results from contact, either directly or indirectly (i.e. via an arthropod vector), with a reservoir host. For example, dogs and cats can become infected with *B. burgdorferi* if fed on by an infected tick that has, in turn, fed on an infected rodent during an earlier developmental stage, but dogs and cats play no significant role in the overall epidemiology of the infection. In other cases, dogs and cats themselves may be reservoir hosts for an infection. For example, both wild and domestic species of cat appear to be the sole reservoir host for *Bartonella henselae* and *Bartonella clarridgeiae*, while dogs appear to fill this role for *Bartonella vinsonii* subspecies *berkhoffii*.

For many of the infections described in later chapters there is more than one reservoir species involved in maintaining the microparasite in nature, and the number of species recognized as reservoirs continues to increase. For example, while rodents have long been identified as reservoirs of numerous arthropod-borne infections, until recently relatively little was known about the role of shrews, despite them often sharing habitat and ectoparasites with rodents. Recent studies have suggested that shrews may play at least as important a role as rodents in maintaining *B. burgdorferi* and other tick-borne infections in both the USA and Europe. This highlights the fact that as continued ecological and epidemiological studies are conducted, the list of potential reservoir hosts will increase.

Infection in reservoir and accidental hosts

A difference often commented on between the behaviour of arthropod-borne parasites in reservoir hosts and accidental hosts is in the pathogenesis of the infection and resultant disease. Many reservoir hosts show few clinical signs of infection. For example, there is little evidence of clinical disease in rodents with bartonellosis, babesiosis or granulocytic anaplasmosis. In addition, while a laboratory study previously reported clinical signs in juvenile white-footed mice (*Peromyscus leucopus*) infected with *B. burgdorferi*, more recent field-based studies have demonstrated that no ill-effects of infection could be detected at the population level, with survival of infected mice being similar to that of those free from infection. However, more subtle signs of infection in reservoir hosts have been reported, with cowpox virus having a significant effect on the fecundity of its wild rodent reservoir. Such signs can only be detected through intensive study of wild systems. In general, while the selection pressures on hosts and parasites may often lead to the co-evolution of traits resulting in relatively subtle disease, no such selection occurs during infection of accidental hosts. Therefore, although some accidental host species can have inapparent infections (in which case they will probably not be noticed), in others the same agent, expressing genes that have evolved for survival in reservoir hosts, may cause obvious disease. If these diseased, accidental hosts happen to be domesticated animals or humans, then the causative agent will be much studied as a 'pathogen', even though the occurrence of disease in such hosts might be considered accidental.

The co-evolution of reservoir hosts and agents can lead to diverse ecological and pathogenic properties among apparently closely related agents. For example, while it is often thought that *B. burgdorferi* (see Chapter 10) has a broad range of reservoir host species, which includes rodents, lagomorphs, insectivores, birds and even reptiles, there is strong evidence for ecologically important relationships between a particular host species and the species of *Borrelia* for which it acts as reservoir. *Borrelia afzelii*, for example, is primarily associated with rodents and *Borrelia garinii* with birds. Studies suggest that the host ranges of these different species of *Borrelia* are determined, at least in part, by differences in their sensitivity to host complement. While *B. afzelii* is resistant to rodent complement and can thus survive and be acquired by a feeding tick such as *Ixodes ricinus*, it is sensitive to the complement of hosts such as birds. As such, a tick infected with *B. afzelii* by feeding on a rodent in one instar may lose that infection if it feeds on a bird during the next instar. These slight differences in phenotype, which enable closely related agents to each exploit their own ecological niches, can lead to differences in behaviour and, therefore, pathogenicity in accidental hosts. Within the species that make up the *B. burgdorferi* complex, only some appear to be associated with specific clinical syndromes in dogs, cats and humans. For example, Lyme arthritis is associated with *B. burgdorferi* sensu stricto infection, neuroborreliosis with *B. garinii* and *B. afzelii* is associated with acrodermatitis chronica atophicans. The pathogenic status of other *Borrelia* species such as *Borrelia valaisiana* remains uncertain (see Chapter 10).

Co-infection

It should be noted that wildlife species can also be important reservoir hosts for many different microparasites, so vectors feeding on them can acquire multiple infections and consequently transmit these to accidental hosts such as humans and companion animals. Wild rodents in the USA may be infected concurrently with *B. burgdorferi*, *Babesia microti*, *Anaplasma phagocytophilum* and various *Bartonella* species, and similar findings have been reported in Europe. Recent studies have reported that interactions exist between the community of microparasites that infects field voles (*Microtus agrestis*) in northern England. Individuals infected with *B. microti* were significantly less likely to be infected with *Bartonella* species and vice versa. Conversely, being infected with *B. microti* appeared to increase susceptibility to infection with *A. phagocytophilum*. What is not clear is the pathological effect of co-infections compared with single infections. However, in domesticated animals, sheep are known to suffer more serious disease when infected with both louping-ill virus and *A. phagocytophilum*, so co-infections in cats and dogs may lead to more severe disease. In addition, in rodent communities, different rodent species may differ in their role as hosts to the various microparasites. For example, bank voles (*Clethrionomys glareolus* [**Figure 2.1**]) and wood mice (*Apodemus sylvaticus* [**Figure 2.2**]) in the UK are both reservoirs for the same community of *Bartonella* species at relatively high prevalences (up to 70%), but bank voles are significantly more likely to be infected with *A. phagocytophilum* than are wood mice, and each rodent species is infected with its own specific trypanosome. The mechanisms by which these differences occur are unclear, but if hosts living in close proximity and exposed to similar microparasites differ in their response to such infections, it seems obvious that such microparasites may invoke vastly different responses in accidental hosts.

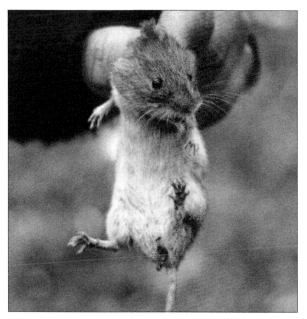

Fig. 2.1 Throughout the world, wild rodents such as this bank vole (*Clethrionomys glareolus*) are important reservoir hosts for a multitude of vector-borne infections. This species alone is a reservoir for *Borrelia burgdorferi*, *Anaplasma phagocytophilum*, *Babesia microti*, various *Bartonella* species and tick-borne encephalitis virus.

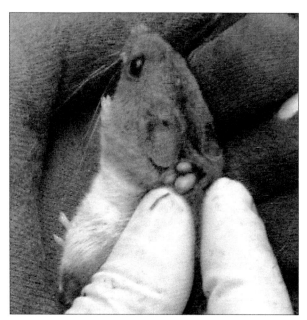

Fig. 2.2 A wood mouse (*Apodemus sylvaticus*) infested with adult *Ixodes trianguliceps* ticks.

Hosts not regarded as being reservoirs for an infection can still be vitally important in the epidemiology of that infection. The possible 'sterilizing' effect on ticks infected with certain *Borrelia* species when they feed on some hosts has been mentioned already, and this can reduce transmission of the parasite amongst a community of tick hosts. In contrast, many deer species appear to be poor hosts for *B. burgdorferi* spirochaetes, as their complement has borreliacidal activity and transmission to and from ticks feeding on deer does not occur. Yet deer can still be a vital component of the epidemiology of borreliosis, as they feed large numbers of adult ticks and thus contribute to the size of subsequent tick populations, the earlier instars of which feed on infected and infectious hosts such as mice (**Box 2.1**).

Box 2.1 The complex ecology of Lyme disease.

A possible network of events has been described for Lyme disease in the eastern USA that illustrates the potential complexity of interactions that drive the dynamics of infections in wildlife and can lead to outbreaks of disease in other hosts. The main host of *Borrelia burgdorferi* sensu stricto in the area is the white-footed mouse *Peromyscus leucopus*. Mouse population dynamics depend on the amount of food available, in particular acorn crop sizes in the large oak woodlands. A particularly large acorn yield (which itself depends on a number of environmental factors) leads to greater survival and fecundity of mice, with a consequent population explosion the following year. The ready availability of acorns also attracts deer to the same areas, and the deer harbour large numbers of adult ticks. These ticks lay their eggs, which hatch into larvae the following year, just in time to feed on the now greatly expanded mouse population. All of these factors combine to produce an explosion of *Borrelia*-infected nymphs and larvae and consequent outbreaks of Lyme disease in humans.

It has even been suggested that the emergence of human Lyme disease in the eastern USA might be a delayed consequence of the extinction of the passenger pigeon (*Ectopistes migratorius*) a century ago. Flocks of passenger pigeons are known to have migrated annually to areas with large crops of acorns, and there is some contemporary evidence that this effectively suppressed mouse populations and deer immigration. This in turn may have reduced the risk of Lyme disease to accidental hosts such as humans.

These examples highlight the important effects biodiversity can have on arthropod-borne infections. Increases in the abundance of less competent hosts can reduce the overall prevalence of infection in vectors – the 'dilution effect' – although this may be offset by increases in the vector population size. As such, while the risk of acquiring infection from a bite may fall, the risk of being bitten in the first instance may rise.

HOW ARE ARTHROPOD-BORNE INFECTIONS MAINTAINED BY WILDLIFE?

Basic epidemiology of infectious diseases

For any parasitic infection to persist, it is essential that, on average, each infection results in at least one additional infection of another individual host. The number of new (or 'secondary') infections occurring as a result of each original (or 'primary') infection is termed the basic reproductive rate (R_0). Therefore, in mathematical terms, for a microparasite to be maintained in a population, R_0 must be >1. If R_0 falls below one, then, over time, that microparasite will disappear from the population. Infection of incidental hosts such as cats and dogs may not lead to infection of another individual, due to physiological or ecological differences between themselves and reservoir hosts or as a result of veterinary treatment. Consequently, many accidental hosts are 'dead-end' hosts.

Mechanisms of persistence in wildlife populations

There are a number of obstacles to R_0 remaining greater than one. Passage of an infection from one host to another depends on a variety of factors. First, an infected host must encounter a competent vector, which must subsequently find and feed on another suitable host, and thus the distribution and behaviour of vectors are crucial to understanding infection dynamics.

Distribution of vectors in the environment

The distribution of parasites in nature is not usually random, but is aggregated (clumped) within the host population. This is generally true for all macroparasites, including nematodes, cestodes, insects and arachnids. This aggregation of parasites within a host population results in a situation where many of the individuals will be free from parasites, while a small proportion of individuals will be heavily parasitized. In fact, many host–parasite relationships have been shown to conform to the '20/80 rule', whereby 20% of the host population are burdened with 80% of the parasites. Two independent studies of the relationship between *I. ricinus* and rodent hosts reported that 20% of the rodents were infested with approximately 80% of the tick larvae and the majority of nymphs. Such an aggregated distribution has been shown to be essential for the maintenance

of tick-borne encephalitis virus (TBEV) by enabling co-feeding transmission (**Box 2.2**) and by increasing R_0 by three or four.

There are a number of causes for aggregation of ticks in host populations, one of which is the manner in which female ticks lay eggs. Female ixodid ticks such as *I. ricinus* and *Ixodes scapularis* lay a single, large egg mass after processing their final blood meal. Such egg masses can comprise several thousand eggs. If eggs from such masses hatch successfully, then within a relatively small area, several thousand questing larvae can be found. Any host in the area is thus likely to acquire a large number of larvae, while those hosts travelling in areas where egg masses are absent are unlikely to come into contact with larvae at all.

The foraging behaviour of ticks is another potential mechanism leading to their aggregation on hosts. Ticks use a number of cues to locate hosts including carbon dioxide and ammonia, pheromones and body temperature. In cases where pheromones released by feeding

---

Box 2.2 Co-feeding transmission between ticks.

Within the past decade or so, the traditional view that arthropods could only acquire infections by feeding on hosts that were parasitaemic, or through transovarial transmission, has been shown to be incorrect. Co-feeding enables microparasite transmission between ticks in the absence of a host parasitaemia. This phenomenon, first reported for Thogoto virus, has since been demonstrated to be an important route of transmission for *Borrelia burgdorferi*, TBE group flaviviruses and possibly *Anaplasma phagocytophilum*. Co-feeding transmission increases the chances of transmission of microparasites such as TBEV, where the infected hosts are only infective to ticks for a few days or where parasitaemia never reaches infective levels. As ticks typically feed for between 4 days and 2 weeks, the period over which naïve ticks can acquire infection by feeding alongside infected ticks is greatly extended. Indeed, non-viraemic co-feeding transmission of TBEV may be essential for its persistence, and this is further aided by the high number of ticks found on individual hosts.

As well as increasing the period over which transmission can occur, co-feeding transmission also enables ticks to acquire infection while feeding on hosts that are immune to the microparasite infection. When rodents are challenged with TBEV, they produce an immune response that clears the viraemia and protects them against further challenge. However, despite this apparent immunity, transmission can still occur between infected and naïve ticks via dendritic cells that take up the virus and then migrate to the feeding sites of other ticks. This enables immune wild rodents to continue to act as vectors of TBEV between ticks feeding on them.

females attract adult males to a host, it is obvious that this can result in aggregation of numbers of ticks on a host.

In addition to vector biology, there are several host-related factors that can influence parasite distribution within a population. One of the most important of these is host gender. Males of many species carry a higher parasite burden than females, one reason being that they have a larger territory. For example, male field voles (*Microtus agrestis*) have home ranges about twice the size as those of females. As a result, the chance of encountering parasites in the environment is much greater.

Another possible way in which gender differences can affect parasite distribution is through the immunomodulatory effects of sex hormones and the consequent ability of the host to eliminate parasites. Experimental studies performed with male sand lizards (*Lacerta agilis*) implanted with testosterone showed that implanted males acquire heavier tick burdens than untreated males. This was postulated to be due to the immunosuppressive effects of testosterone. A further example can be found in bank voles. Bank voles are frequently exposed to ticks and they can develop a density-dependent immunity that results in both reduced attachment of ticks and significantly reduced feeding success of those ticks that attach successfully. However, testosterone can impair this acquired immunity in male bank voles. In addition, *B. microti* infections in bank voles given testosterone implants produce a more severe parasitaemia of longer duration than those in control animals. It is therefore apparent that certain groups within a host population, such as reproductively active males, may be of greater significance in the perpetuation of arthropod-borne infections than others.

The importance to microparasite transmission of cohorts determined by age and gender within a population is demonstrated by the following example. In a study of adult yellow-necked mice (*Apodemus flavicollis*), although only 26% of the individuals captured were males, they made up a significantly greater proportion of the population involved in transmission of TBEV. Therefore, in terms of disease control, targeting this group would be much more efficient than targeting the population as a whole.

In addition to determining the spatial distribution of vectors, host factors can sometimes determine their temporal distribution. An example is the intricate relationship that exists between *Spilopsyllus cuniculi* fleas

and rabbits. Hormones released by female rabbits in late pregnancy are essential for the maturation of *Spilopsyllus* flea eggs, thus ensuring that emergence of the next generation of adult fleas coincides with the presence of newborn rabbits. In addition, growth hormone produced by newborn rabbits stimulates increased flea mating and feeding, thus maximizing productivity. Once the production of growth hormone declines, the fleas return to the mother and their reproduction halts.

An example of hosts determining both the spatial and temporal distribution of vectors has already been mentioned. Deer in North America, attracted to areas where the acorn crop is high, bring with them the adult ticks that will produce the larvae to feed on the following year's population of mice.

Environmental factors such as climate can also have a dramatic effect on parasite development and survival. For example, the distribution of TBEV can be predicted using satellite-derived data on environmental conditions. In rodents, which are generally regarded as the most important mammalian host for TBEV, detectable viraemia is rare and, when it does occur, is very short-lived. As a result, the transmission of TBEV relies heavily on infected nymphs feeding in synchrony with naïve larval ticks to enable non-systemic co-feeding transmission (**Box 2.3**) to occur. This happens where summers are warm enough to allow rapid development of eggs, but also where autumns cool down quickly enough to force emerging larvae to overwinter without feeding. This results in both nymphs and larvae starting to quest at the same time the following spring. This phenomenon is susceptible to climatic changes, and it has been suggested that under the predicted warmer climatic conditions, the synchrony between larvae and nymphs may diminish or disappear in some regions, perhaps resulting in the loss of TBEV from areas where it is currently endemic, whilst facilitating its spread into other regions as the synchrony between larvae and nymphs would occur.

Vector competence and microparasite acquisition

Once a vector has acquired infection, it must then feed on another competent host for the infection to perpetuate. Vector competence for some infections is less restricted than for others. Much depends on whether the mode of transmission is merely mechani-

---

Box 2.3 Are enzootic infections of epidemiological interest?

Identifying a wildlife species as a reservoir host of a particular infection is only the first step in determining its epidemiological importance. Rodents have long been recognized as competent hosts for multiple tick-borne infections, but in the UK their role in the epidemiology of such infections has been questioned as studies have indicated that they feed on relatively few nymphs or adult *Ixodes ricinus* – the potentially infectious stages. A study of field voles (*Microtus agrestis*) in northern England (**Figures 2.3a, b**) showed that they were infected with both *Anaplasma phagocytophilum* and *Babesia microti*, and two species of tick: the generalist *I. ricinus* and the small mammal specific *Ixodes trianguliceps*. Investigations into the potential for enzootic infections transmitted between small mammals by *I. trianguliceps* to escape into larger mammals, including domesticated animals and humans, via *I. ricinus* suggested that this did not occur. Instead, it appeared that two distinct ecological cycles co-existed: one comprised of small mammals and *I. triangulceps* and the other large mammals (deer) and *I. ricinus*. Genetic analysis of the strains of *A. phagocytophilum* demonstrated that the strain present in small mammals and *I. trainaguliceps* did not appear in either deer or questing *I. ricinus*, and vice-versa. Similarly, no *B. microti* was detected in questing *I. ricinus*, and detailed genetic analyses of *B. microti* strains indicates that only a small cluster of strains are associated with human infections, while many others are restricted to their wildlife host. These results suggest that when identifying potential reservoir hosts for infectious diseases, it is important to ascertain the genotype of the agent as they may be of limited epidemiological significance.

Box 2.4 Myxomatosis – a disease in a reservoir host?

Rabbit myxomatosis illustrates an aspect of the relationship between host, agent and vector that is often misunderstood – that of the role sometimes played by disease. It is a common misconception that endemic infectious agents and their hosts will always co-evolve such that disease no longer occurs. Myxoma virus is endemic in rabbits of the genus *Sylvilagus* in southern USA and Central and South America, and in these hosts, with which it is assumed to have co-evolved over thousands of years, it causes little disease. Although such low pathogenicity in natural reservoir hosts is often the case, it is by no means a foregone conclusion. In susceptible European rabbits (*Oryctolagus cuniculus*), myxomatosis is a severe disease that often ends in the death of the host, and the co-evolution of myxoma virus and European rabbits, albeit over only half a century, provides an interesting model for study. When first introduced into rabbit populations in both Europe and Australia, there was certainly no selection against highly pathogenic strains of virus – in fact quite the opposite. Immediately after introduction, highly virulent strains of virus were selectively advantaged. Increased virulence was associated with a greater area of infected skin on which fleas and mosquitoes could feed and higher densities of virus in that tissue (and therefore on the vectors' mouthparts). Both factors combined to increase transmission. The virus strains with the highest R_0 were those with the highest virulence and pathogenicity – and the result for rabbit populations was catastrophic. However, as the number of susceptible rabbits plunged, acquired immunity and the selection of innately more resistant lines of rabbits reduced the population susceptible to infection and, therefore, the frequency of contact between infectious and susceptible hosts. At this stage, viral strains causing longer periods of infection had a selective advantage over more pathogenic strains, as they had a greater chance of being transmitted before the host died. Although this may at first sight appear to support the contention that co-evolution always leads to reduced pathogenicity, it remains the case that within any individual susceptible rabbit, or small population of susceptible rabbits, the more transmissible strains of myxoma virus (in this case, the more virulent and pathogenic strains) will always outcompete the less transmissible, less pathogenic strains.

The relationship between myxoma virus and wild rabbit populations today appears to be fairly stable – the rabbit population in the UK is currently about 40% of that in the 1950s – with smaller populations of rabbits existing in dynamic equilibrium with moderately virulent viruses.

The important point is that selection pressure acted to maximize R_0, requiring an evolutionary 'trade-off' between infectious period and pathogenicity, the balance of which will depend on the life histories of the parasite and its host in any particular environment.

---

cal, where the vector acts as little more than a hypodermic needle, or biological, where the microparasite interacts in a more fundamental way (e.g. by replicating in the vector). Infections such as myxomatosis in rabbits persist as a result of mechanical transmission (**Box 2.4**) (**Figure 2.4**). In Australia and much of Europe the principal vectors appear to be mosquitoes, while in the UK, myxoma virus is primarily transmitted by fleas. In both situations the vector acquires the virus by feeding through infected skin. The virus survives on the mouthparts of the vector and is transmitted to a naïve host. As there is no biological interaction with the vector, viral survival depends on its ability to persist in the environment. Myxoma virus is a particularly robust virus, as are many poxviruses. It remains infective for many months both in the environment and on the mouthparts of the flea, while the mammalian host remains infectious for only a few weeks. Not all arthropod-borne infections

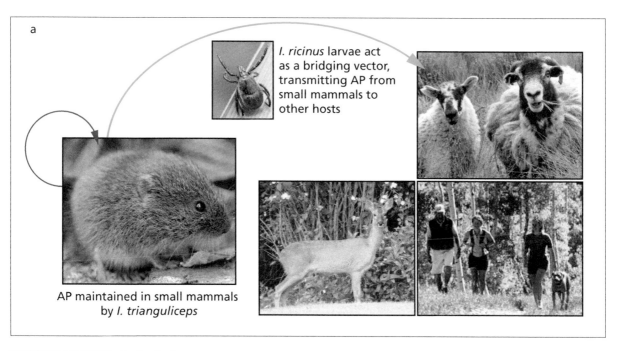

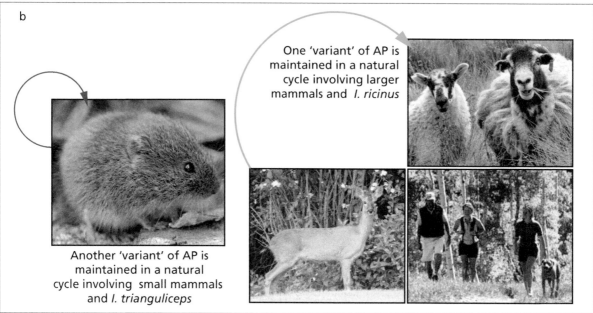

Figs. 2.3a, b One hypothesis regarding how rodents could play an important role in the epidemiology of tick-borne infections is through enzootic infections escaping via a bridge vector. A study of field voles (*Microtus agrestis*) showed that instead two distinct cycles exist, with rodents being of limited epidemiological significance. AP, *Anaplasma phagocytophilum*.

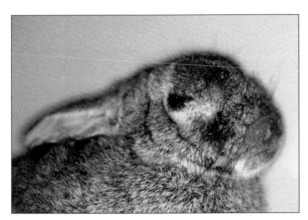

Fig. 2.4 **A rabbit showing clinical signs associated with myxomatosis. Infection in reservoir hosts is usually thought to be asymptomatic, but this is an obvious exception and an interesting study in the co-evolution of host and pathogen.**

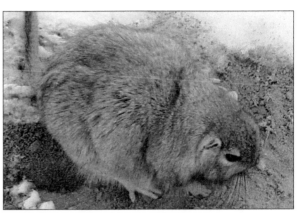

Fig. 2.5 **Giant gerbils (*Rhombomys opimus*) in Kazakhstan are important reservoir hosts for plague. Infection in other species occurs as a result of increases in the abundance of these giant gerbils. (Courtesy M. Begon)**

are transmitted in a merely mechanical manner. In some cases transmission may be reliant on interactions between the vector and the microparasite. For example, when some species of flea feed on rodents infected with the plague bacillus (*Yersinia pestis*), the bacilli colonize the flea's proventriculus, where they replicate (**Figure 2.5**). Eventually, perhaps after feeding on several other rodents, the accumulation of bacteria at this site obstructs the flea's intestinal tract. Although the infected flea continues to feed despite the obstruction, ingested blood is regurgitated back into the vertebrate host, taking with it many bacteria.

Tick-borne infections differ fundamentally from those that are insect-borne because of differences in their feeding behaviour. The period between feeding on different individual hosts is greatly extended for many tick-borne infections. While most insects, particularly flies and mosquitoes, may feed on a number of hosts within a very short period, the life cycle of ticks prohibits such events. Hard ticks generally feed on three different hosts before completing their life cycle, and usually only on a single host during each instar, while the period between feeds can be several months. Recent studies on the tick *I. ricinus* suggest that questing nymphs and adults can survive for up to 12 months post moult, and that generally there is only one cohort of ticks recruited into the population each year. In such a situation, it is

obvious that for a microparasite to persist within a population, it must be able to survive within the tick for several months and, as such, transmission of tick-borne infections is almost invariably biological rather than mechanical. After feeding, excretion of waste products from the tick is rapid, and those microparasites unable to infect the tissues of the tick will also be excreted. The ability of microparasites to survive the moult and diapause that ticks undergo after each blood meal is termed trans-stadial transmission. *B. burgdorferi* spirochaetes survive in the midgut of the tick, where they remain until the tick feeds on another host. At this stage they migrate to the tick salivary glands, from where they can potentially infect the vertebrate host. The environment within a tick is vastly different to that within a mammal or bird, but one way in which spirochaetes overcome this is by expressing different proteins, depending on their environment. While in the midgut of a resting tick, they primarily express outer surface protein (Osp) A (OspA). If resident in a feeding tick, they downregulate OspA and upregulate OspC as they migrate to the salivary glands. Spirochaetes continue to express OspC during the initial stages of infection in the host. Conversely, when uninfected ticks acquire spirochaetes the bacteria upregulate OspA, which appears to be important in binding the spirochaete to the midgut wall (see Chapter 10).

Some tick-borne infections are also transmitted transovarially and, in such cases, vertebrates may be more important as hosts for the vector rather than as hosts to the infectious agent. Transmission of *Rickettsia rickettsii* (a member of the spotted fever group) from adult female *Dermacentor variabilis* to eggs and subsequently larvae can approach 100% efficiency under laboratory conditions, although figures of 30–50% appear to be more representative of those seen in nature. There is also some evidence that infection with *R. rickettsii* can have a detrimental effect on the ticks themselves. Despite this, it appears that transovarial transmission may be more important in perpetuating infection in nature than the acquisition of the organism from rickettsaemic hosts, as rickettsaemia in mammalian hosts is generally short lived.

CONCLUSION

This chapter has introduced some of the concepts, often still being debated, about the ecological mechanisms that enable microparasites to persist in wild animal populations, and it has also provided explanations for some of the differences in the epidemiology and pathogenicity of arthropod-borne infections in wildlife compared with domestic animals and humans. It is vital to understand the ecology of arthropod-borne infections in their reservoir hosts if we are to control these infections in accidental hosts such as domestic animals and human beings.

FURTHER READING

Bown KJ, Lambin X, Ogden NH *et al.* (2009) Delineating *Anaplasma phagocytophilum* ecotypes in coexisting, discrete enzootic cycles. *Emerging Infectious Diseases* **15**:1948–1954.

Brisson D, Dykhuizen DE, Ostfeld RS (2008) Conspicuous impacts of inconspicuous hosts on the Lyme disease epidemic. *Proceedings of the Royal Society B: Biological Sciences* **275**:227–235.

Telfer S, Lambin X, Birtles R *et al.* (2010) Species interactions in a parasite community drive infection risk in a wildlife population. *Science* **300**:243–246.

Michael J. Day

INTRODUCTION

The transmission of infectious agents by haemophagous arthropods involves a unique three-way interaction between arthropod, microorganism and the host immune system. The aim of the arthropod in this inter-

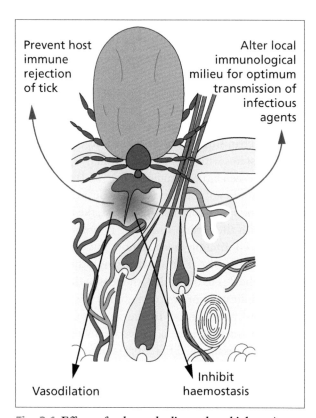

Fig. 3.1 **Effects of arthropod saliva on host biology. As part of the feeding process, haemophagous arthropods inject saliva into the host dermal microenvironment. Arthropod saliva mediates a range of local effects including vasodilation, inhibition of haemostasis and inhibition of host inflammatory and immune responses. In the case of ticks, there is also salivary transmission of infectious agents.**

action is to obtain a blood meal, using basic mechanisms that are relatively conserved between arthropod species. These include penetration of the host epidermal barrier and the secretion of a range of vasoactive and anticoagulant molecules that encourage local blood flow and permit uptake of the uncoagulated blood meal. Additionally, there is modulation of the local cutaneous immune and inflammatory responses by potent arthropod-derived molecules that are injected into the feeding site. This modulation may extend to influencing the immune response in regional lymphoid tissue and the systemic immune system and acting to prevent rejection of the arthropod, particularly those that require prolonged attachment to the host (i.e. ticks).

This manipulation of the host dermal microenvironment by infected arthropods also provides an advantage to microorganisms by creating an optimum environment for their transmission and the establishment of infection (**Figure 3.1**). This is exemplified by the persistence of infectious agents at the site of injection by ticks, which permits the infection of naïve ticks in the absence of systemic infection of the host ('saliva-activated transmission') (**Figure 3.2**). Additionally, the presence of organisms within an arthropod may modify its behaviour. For example, *Borrelia*-infected ticks have altered questing behaviour, which provides them with an advantage in terms of acquiring their target host. In contrast, *Leishmania*-infected sand flies also have modified feeding behaviour, but here the advantage is to the microorganism rather than the arthropod. The plug of *Leishmania* parasites within the proventriculus interferes with the intake of blood, making it necessary for the sandfly to probe the host dermis more frequently.

Arthropod-borne infectious agents must also migrate through the body of the arthropod, typically involving movement through the midgut, haemolymph, salivary gland and, in some cases, ovary. During this migration, the microparasites must evade the arthropod immune

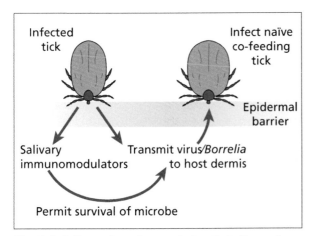

Fig. 3.2 **Saliva-activated transmission. In 'saliva-activated transmission' an arthropod injects an infectious agent into the host dermis. This agent persists at this location, likely due to inhibition of the host immune response by salivary molecules. For example, the saliva of some ticks inhibits the anti-viral effects of interferon and permits local replication of tick-transmitted virus. The persistent microbe may be taken up by uninfected arthropods that take a blood meal from the site, and this occurs in the absence of systemic viral infection. This mechanism has also been demonstrated for transmission of *Borrelia* that may be taken up by uninfected ticks prior to systemic spread of infection.**

response so that they might be transmitted successfully to a new target host. Ticks, for example, have an innate immune system that comprises of antimicrobial peptides (e.g. defensins and tick-specific microplusin/hebraein, 5.3 kDa family proteins), lysozymes, a complement-like system and phagocytic haemocytes. The microparasites may also subvert gene expression in the arthropod host in order to ensure their survival and transmission. For example, *Borrelia burgdorferi* sensu lato bacteria upregulate expression of the *salp15* gene in *Ixodes scapularis* ticks, leading to increased quantities of salp15 protein in the tick salivary glands during feeding. The *Borrelia* bind to salp15 (via their outer surface protein [OSP]-C) when transmitted and the protein confers protection from host antibody- and complement-mediated killing (specifically by inhibiting formation of the membrane attack complex of the terminal complement pathway) in addition to inhibit-

ing host dendritic cell and T-cell responses. In the latter case, salp15 binds specifically to the CD4 molecule on T helper (Th) cells and downregulates their function. In contrast, although salp15 is also bound by OSP-C from *Borrelia garinii* and *Borrelia afzelii*, these organisms are not protected from antibody-mediated killing in the host. Similarly, *Anaplasma phagocytophilum* upregulates *salp16* gene expression and utilizes this protein to survive within *I. scapularis* and to infect the tick salivary glands. *A. phagocytophilum* also utilizes a secreted tick protein (P11) to infect haemocytes, enabling it to move from the midgut to the salivary glands in haemolymph. Such interactions are likely a result of the prolonged co-evolution of arthropods and the microorganisms that they carry.

The infectious agents transmitted by arthropods produce disease by a complex pathogenesis that may in part involve secondary immune-mediated phenomena. Both arthropod and microorganism may be involved in manipulating the host immune system to induce these sequelae to infection.

Unravelling of these complex pathways provides an insight into potential stages at which immunological control of the organism or the vector may be achieved. These mechanisms have been defined largely in experimental systems with a range of tick and fly species, but there have been limited studies in dogs and there are no reported studies of the interaction of ticks or flies with the immune system of cats. In contrast, the interaction of fleas with the canine and feline immune system is an area of continuing investigation, but these studies address the nature of salivary allergens rather than the ability of the flea to transmit pathogens to the host.

The application of new technology (i.e. transcriptomics and proteomics) to the study of the host–arthropod–microbe interface is now providing further insights. For example, differential gene expression has been studied in the salivary glands of *Ixodes ricinus* ticks that were infected or not infected with the bacterium *Bartonella henselae*. Bacterial infection was associated with upregulation of 819 transcripts and downregulation of 517 transcripts in infected ticks. The most highly upregulated gene was that encoding the molecule IrSPI, a serine protease inhibitor, and when this gene was 'silenced' there was reduced tick feeding and a lower number of bacteria within the salivary gland of infected ticks. A proteomic study of the salivary glands of *I. ricinus* ticks infected with various strains of *Borrelia burgdorferi* sensu lato revealed upregulation of a number of proteins, dependent on the strain of bacteria. These proteins were often involved in protein synthesis and processing.

This chapter will focus on relatively well characterized interactions of the mammalian immune system with ticks and sand flies, and the microorganisms transmitted by these arthropods. The potential for vaccination as a means of control of arthropod infestation and disease transmission will be addressed. Finally, the interaction of arthropod-borne microbes with the host immune system and the induction of secondary immune-mediated disease as part of the pathogenesis of infection will be discussed.

THE TICK–HOST INTERFACE: TICK MODULATION OF HOST BIOLOGY

Ticks have evolved specialized mechanisms that make them particularly effective haemophagous parasites, and the majority of these mechanisms are related to the secretion of a range of salivary proteins. The composition of tick salivary proteins has been studied biochemically. There is broad conservation in the range of molecules (by molecular weight) over several tick species and specific molecules are induced in the early stages of feeding. In several tick species, clear differences in the composition of male and female tick saliva have been demonstrated. In fed *Rhipicephalus appendiculatus*, specific novel proteins appear in haemolymph and then in saliva, suggesting that some inducible salivary antigens are obtained from haemolymph in this tick.

Tick cement

The action of tick mouthparts and deposition of 'cement' creates a firm attachment of tick to host that permits prolonged feeding and transmission of infectious agents. A 90 kDa salivary protein that is conserved amongst tick species and secreted maximally during the first 2 days of feeding has been suggested to be a cement component. A 29 kDa protein from *Haemaphysalis longicornis* has been cloned and sequenced and it has been proposed that this is also a cement component. Immunization of rabbits with the recombinant 29 kDa protein confers protection. A recombinant version of a cement protein (64TRP) from *R. appendiculatus* has been used as a vaccine to inhibit transmission of tick-borne encephalitis virus in a murine model. 64TRP is expressed in the salivary glands of feeding ticks and there may be cross-reactivity between 64TRP and a host dermal protein.

Salivary anticoagulants

A continual flow of blood is required from the tick attachment site into the tick gut. This is achieved by the production of a range of anticoagulant salivary molecules that are injected into the feeding site. For example, apyrase is an inhibitor of adenosine diphosphate-induced platelet aggregation produced by many haemophagous parasites. *Amblyomma americanum* saliva inhibits factor Xa and thrombin, and saliva from *R. appendiculatus* contains an anticoagulant that increases in concentration throughout feeding. Two anticoagulants have been characterized in the saliva of *I. ricinus*: an antithromboplastin (ixodin) and a thrombin inhibitor (ixin). A serine protease inhibitor from *I. scapularis* (IxscS-1E1) is inhibitory of thrombin and trypsin, and a recombinant version of the molecule has been shown to inhibit platelet activation and reduce the activated partial prothrombin time and thrombin time *in vitro*.

Salivary osmoregulation and control of secretion

In addition to producing cement and anticoagulant molecules, the tick salivary gland also functions in osmoregulation. Excess fluid from an ingested blood meal is re-secreted to the host via tick saliva, and in free-living ticks the salivary gland functions in absorption of water vapour from the air. Tick salivary tissue undergoes hypertrophy and duct dilation during feeding and secretion is under neurological control, specifically via the interaction of dopamine with dopamine receptors expressed in the salivary tissue. The amount of dopamine in the salivary glands of *I. scapularis* ticks increases progressively up to the fifth day of feeding, when rapid engorgement begins.

Salivary toxins

The salivary glands of a range of tick species secrete potent neurotoxins that interfere with the function of the neuromuscular synapse. This results in ascending motor paresis ('tick paralysis') and death may follow respiratory paralysis. A good example is the Australian tick *Ixodes holocyclus*, which produces the toxin holocyclin that may affect both dogs and cats.

Salivary anti-inflammatory and wound healing molecules

Anti-inflammatory factors are also secreted into the host dermal microenvironment. These contribute to the ability of the tick to maintain prolonged attachment and, coincidentally, provide an optimum milieu for the transmission and establishment of infectious agents. Tick saliva contains prostaglandin E_2 (PGE_2). This interacts with a PGE_2 receptor within the tick salivary gland, leading to secretion of further bioactive salivary proteins that may facilitate acquisition of a blood meal. Additionally, tick-derived PGE_2 may have effector functions when delivered to host tissue including local vasodilation (enhancing delivery of the blood meal to the tick), inhibition of macrophage production of pro-inflammatory cytokines (e.g. tumour necrosis factor [TNF]-α) and impairment of fibroblast migration (for wound healing). These effects may be mediated by the production of further PGE_2 by the host macrophages. Ticks cannot synthesize the prostaglandin precursor arachidonic acid, and must acquire this from the host. $PGF_{2\alpha}$, PGD_2 and PGB_2 have also been identified in saliva from ticks fed arachidonic acid.

I. scapularis saliva contains anti-angiogenic activity as measured *in vitro* by impairment of microvascular endothelial cell proliferation and chick aorta vascular 'sprouting'. This would suggest that tick saliva is inhibitory of angiogenesis-dependent wound healing and tissue repair, which is advantageous to the prolonged period of tick feeding.

The saliva of *I. scapularis* also has a kininase activity mediated by dipeptidyl carboxypeptidase. This inhibits bradykinin, therefore reducing local pain and inflammation and the likelihood of the host grooming-out the tick. The saliva of *R. appendiculatus* contains histamine-binding proteins that may compete with host histamine receptors for histamine and, therefore, reduce local inflammation. A novel, low molecular weight, anti-complement protein (isac) from the saliva of *I. scapularis* inhibits the alternative pathway of the complement cascade and inhibits generation of chemotactic C3a. In contrast, saliva from *Dermacentor andersoni* activates complement C5 to produce chemotactic effects. The effect of tick saliva on the production of chemokines has also been examined. Salivary gland extract (SGE) from *R. appendiculatus* has inhibitory effects against human CXCL8, CCL2, CCU, CCL5 and CCL11 *in vitro*. The salivary chemokine-binding proteins produced by ticks have been termed 'evasins' and their function has been characterized. Evasin-1 binds to CCL3, CCL4 and CCL18, evasin-3 binds to CXCL8 and CXCL1, and evasin-4 binds to CCL5 and CCL11.

Tick saliva also modulates the acute neutrophilic inflammatory response following tick attachment and transmission of microparasites. Neutrophilic infiltration does not affect the survival of *B. burgdorferi* sensu stricto after transmission via *I. ricinus*, and this modulatory mechanism involves inhibition of neutrophil reactive oxygen species rather than impairing the ability of neutrophils to form extracellular 'NETs' (neutrophil extracellular traps of extruded DNA).

The early host inflammatory response to attachment of *I. scapularis* nymphs to murine skin has been examined by gene expression microarray of biopsy samples collected 1, 3, 6 and 12 hours post attachment. At 1 and 3 hours there was no tissue cellular infiltration, but upregulation of genes related to post-translational modification. At 6 and 12 hours there was a neutrophilic inflammatory response, accompanied by upregulation of genes related to cytoskeletal rearrangements, cell division, inflammation and chemotaxis, with downregulation of genes associated with formation of extracellular matrix and cellular signalling.

The anti-inflammatory effects of tick saliva are summarized in **Figure 3.3**.

Salivary immunomodulatory factors

The host immune response engendered by tick attachment fits readily within the concept of functionally diverse CD4+ T lymphocyte populations that mediate different aspects of immunity. This model states that distinct subsets of CD4+ T lymphocytes mediate humoral and cell-mediated immune responses. Th2 CD4+ T lymphocytes produce the cytokines interleukin (IL)-4, IL-5, IL-6, IL-9 and IL-13 enabling them to provide T-cell 'help' for B-cell activation, differentiation into plasma cells and antibody production. In contrast, Th1 CD4+ T cells produce IL-2 and interferon (IFN)-γ allowing them to 'help' the cellular (cytotoxic) action of CD8+ cytotoxic T cells, macrophages and natural killer (NK) cells. Th17 cells produce the signature cytokines IL-17 and IL-22, allowing them to regulate cellular inflammatory responses in infectious and immune-mediated diseases (**Figure 3.4**). This model explains why immune responses may become polarized towards a dominant humoral or cell-mediated response ('immune deviation').

These T-cell subsets have a common precursor (a naïve CD4+ T cell that produces a mixed cytokine profile), which requires particular activation signals to drive differentiation towards the mature Th1, Th17 or Th2 phenotype. These signals are largely derived from the antigen-presenting cell (APC) that activates the antigen-specific T lymphocyte. The nature of the APC signalling is determined by the binding of conserved molecular sequences (often derived from microbes) known as 'pathogen-associated molecular patterns' (PAMPs) or 'microbe-associated molecular patterns', with one of a series of 'pattern recognition receptors' expressed by the APC either on the surface membrane

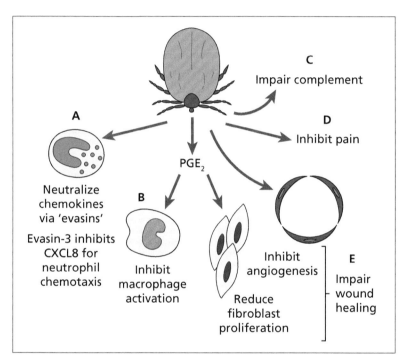

Fig. 3.3 Summary of the anti-inflammatory effects of tick saliva. These include: **(A)** neutralization of chemokines by salivary 'evasins' leading to reduced recruitment of inflammatory cells; **(B)** inhibition of macrophage activation and pro-inflammatory cytokine production by salivary PGE$_2$; **(C)** inhibition of the complement pathways; **(D)** inhibition of pain pathways (e.g. by bradykinin inhibition); and **(E)** inhibition of wound healing by salivary anti-angiogenic factors and reduced fibroblast proliferation mediated by PGE$_2$.

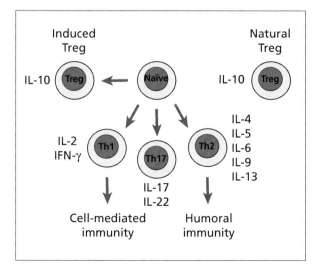

Fig. 3.4 Functional dichotomy of helper T lymphocytes. Functional subpopulations of CD4+ T lymphocytes are derived from a common naïve T cell precursor. These cells are defined by the profile of cytokines that each selectively produces. Th1 cells are responsible for cell-mediated immunity through production of IFN-γ. Th2 cells mediate humoral immunity, providing B-cell help for production of IgE, IgA and IgG via production of a panel of interleukins. Th17 cells (producing IL-17 and IL-22) are important in a range of cellular immune and inflammatory responses. All of these effector immune responses are in turn controlled (suppressed) by induced T regulatory cells (Tregs) and a distinct population of natural Tregs controls the occurrence of deleterious autoimmune responses.

or within the cytoplasm. For example, many bacterial sequences will induce the APC to secrete IL-12 and IL-18, which drives the development of a Th1-dominated immune response (**Figure 3.5**).

In addition to differentiating towards an 'effector' T cell, promoting and amplifying an immune response, the naïve precursor T cell might be directed towards a cell with downregulatory phenotype (a regulatory T cell or Treg). Treg cells suppress immune responses by virtue of the production of cytokines such as IL-10 or transforming growth factor (TGF)-β. Treg cells may be induced during the course of an active immune response to foreign antigen (an induced Treg) or may be present continually within the body in order to control effector T cells that might promote a deleterious autoimmune response (natural Tregs). However, not all regulation is mediated via IL-10 production from classical Treg cells. It appears that there is 'plasticity' in the function of Th1 and Th2 cells, which means that these too can become a source of IL-10 and have some immunoregulatory function. It is thought that the simultaneous production of IFN-γ and IL-10 by Th1

cells might underlie the chronic non-healing nature of many arthropod-borne infections. This has been shown in experimental models of leishmaniosis (**Figure 3.6**) and an investigation of cytokine gene expression in the skin of infected dogs has shown increased IFN-γ and TNF-α mRNA in asymptomatic infected dogs compared with control animals and an association between the level of cutaneous parasitism and increasing expression of IL-10 and TGF-β genes. These findings imply a strong Th1 response containing infection in the asymptomatic dogs, and in dogs with high infectious potential a cutaneous milieu dominated by regulatory cytokines permits survival of the organisms.

The immunomodulatory effects of tick saliva may be manifest as an altered balance in the nature of the T-cell response engendered by tick-derived or microbe-derived antigens. This altered balance may be determined by the effects of tick saliva on the APC signalling of T cells and is best detected by assessing the profile of cytokines produced by the activated T cells. These properties of tick saliva have been demonstrated by incorporation of *I. ricinus* SGE into *in-vitro* cell culture

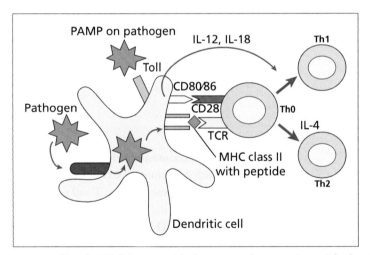

Fig. 3.5 Induction of the adaptive immune response to pathogens. Induction of Th1, Th2, Th17 or Treg immune responses depends largely on signals delivered to the naïve T cell precursor by the dendritic antigen presenting cell (APC). The naïve T cell requires three separate stimulatory signals in order to be activated. Initially, a conserved motif expressed by the infectious agent (the 'pathogen-associated molecular pattern' or PAMP) binds to a surface 'pattern recognition receptor' (PRR) such as the Toll-like receptor (TLR) shown. These antigens derived from pathogens are taken up and processed by the APC into peptide fragments that associate with class II molecules of the major histocompatibility complex (MHC). This complex of MHC class II and peptide is expressed on the APC membrane, where it can be recognized by the T-cell receptor (TCR) of the naïve T cell, providing 'signal 1' for T-cell activation. Activation of the dendritic cell also leads to enhanced expression of co-stimulatory molecules (e.g. CD80/86 shown), which bind to ligands on the naïve T-cell membrane, providing 'signal 2' for T-cell activation. Finally, the activated dendritic cell produces specific cytokines (e.g. IL-12 and IL-18 shown) that bind to cytokine receptors on the naïve T cell, providing 'signal 3' for its activation and also determining which functional subset that T cell will become (a Th1 cell in the example shown). In this way, through the activation of specific PRRs, the nature of the infecting pathogen should drive the most appropriate host protective (adaptive) immune response designed to counteract that pathogen.

systems. A range of other immunomodulatory effects of *I. ricinus* SGE has also been shown, including reduction of cytotoxic function by activated murine NK cells and reduction of the ability of lipopolysaccharide (LPS)-stimulated macrophages to produce nitric oxide.

Recent studies have investigated the effect of tick salivary proteins on host dendritic APC function. Inclusion of *I. ricinus* saliva into co-cultures of splenic dendritic cells from C3H/HeN mice and *Borrelia afzelii* led to reduction in phagocytosis of the bacteria by the dendritic cells, reduced cytokine production by the dendritic cells (including IL-6, IL-10, IL-12 and TNF-α) and reduced ability of the dendritic cells to activate CD4⁺ T cells. A recombinant salivary gland protein from *R. appendiculatus* (Japanin; a 17.7 kDa N-glycoslyated lipocalin) has been shown to alter dendritic cell expression of membrane co-stimulatory molecules, to alter their secretion of pro-inflammatory, anti-inflammatory and T-cell polarizing cytokines and to inhibit their differentiation from monocytes. The molecular pathways affected by tick saliva are those that are activated following engagement of dendritic cell PAMPs such as Toll-like receptor (TLR)-2 and TLR-4. When dendritic cells are stimulated by TLR-2 ligands in the presence of saliva from *Rhipicephalus sanguineus*, the dendritic cells take on a regulatory phenotype, characterized by secretion of IL-10 and reduced secretion of IL-12 and TNF-α. Similarly, in the presence of *I. ricinus* saliva, dendritic cell stimulation by ligation of

CD40, TLR-3, TLR-7 or TLR-9 results in impaired maturation and antigen presentation, with preferential induction of Th2 responses over Th1 and Th17 activation. *In-vivo* administration of *I. ricinus* saliva reduces the migration of dendritic cells from skin to draining lymph nodes and reduces the ability of dendritic cells taken from those nodes to activate T cells *in vitro*.

Other studies have confirmed the immunomodulatory capacity of saliva from *R. sanguineus*. When lymph node cultures were established from tick-infested mice and stimulated with the mitogen concanavalin A (ConA), there was reduced proliferation (relative to uninfested controls) and a distinct Th2 and Treg cytokine profile, with elevated IL-4, IL-10 and TGF-β, and reduced IL-2 and IFN-γ production. *R. sanguineus* saliva also inhibits ConA and antigen-driven proliferation and IL-2 production of murine splenic T cells.

In experimental rodent systems the immunomodulatory effects of tick saliva may be dependent on the strain of mouse used in the study. For example, exposure of C3H/HeJ mice to *B. burgdorferi*-infected *I. scapularis* results in CD4⁺ T-cell proliferation and preferential Th2 immunity (raised IL-4, reduced IL-2, IFN-γ), but these effects are not marked in Balb/c mice. These observations may underlie the susceptibility of C3H mice to borreliosis. In this experimental model, administration of recombinant Th1 cytokines to mice infested with *Borrelia*-infected *I. scapularis* led to a switch from Th2 to Th1 immunity. The effect of repeated infestation with

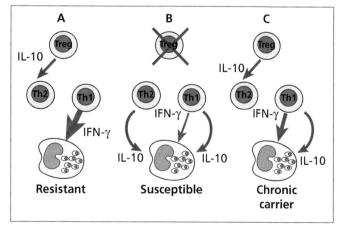

Fig. 3.6 **T-cell activity in leishmaniosis with varying clinical outcome. (A) In a resistant animal the response is dominated by Th1 cells producing large quantities of IFN-γ, which signals infected macrophages to destroy the intracellular amastigotes. At the same time, the action of Th2 cells is inhibited by Tregs producing IL-10. (B) In a susceptible animal there is a weak Th1 response. Tregs no longer inhibit Th2 cells. The cytokine milieu is dominated by IL-10 produced by 'plasticity' in the Th1 and Th2 populations and the infection continues unchecked. (C) In a chronic carrier animal (an infected reservoir not showing clinical disease), Tregs inhibit Th2 cells via IL-10 production, but sterilization of the infection does not occur because the Th1 cells produce both IFN-γ and IL-10. (After Trinchieri G (2007)** *Journal of Experimental Medicine* **204:239–243.)**

uninfected *I. scapularis* on cytokine production by C3H/HeN and Balb/c mice has also been compared. Neither strain of mouse became resistant to *I. scapularis* after four cycles of infestation, but in both strains there was polarization of the cytokine profile to a Th2 phenotype.

The immunosuppressive action of tick saliva has also been documented with *in-vitro* studies of human cells. Saliva from fed *Dermacentor reticulatus* inhibits human NK cell function, but saliva from unfed ticks does not. Similar but less potent inhibition of NK cells is mediated by SGE from *Amblyomma variegatum* and *Haemaphysalis inermis*, but does not occur with SGE from *I. ricinus* or *R. appendiculatus*. SGE from *R. appendiculatus* reduces cytokine mRNA expression (IFN-γ, IL-1, IL-5, IL-6, IL-7, IL-8 and TNF-α) by LPS-stimulated human peripheral blood lymphocytes (PBLs), and SGE from a range of ixodid ticks can neutralize IL-8 (also called CSCL8) and inhibit the neutrophil chemotaxis induced by this chemokine. Similarly, cattle infested with *Rhipicephalus (Boophilus) microplus* have altered *in-vivo* immune function (reduced proportion of T cells in the blood and reduced antibody response to immunization with ovalbumin), and *R. microplus* saliva can suppress the *in-vitro* response of bovine PBLs to the mitogen phytohaemagglutinin. Experimental infestation of sheep with *Amblyomma variegatum* can influence the clinical course of *Dermatophilus congolensis* infection at a separate skin site. Co-infected sheep have chronic, non-healing dermatophilosis, with chronic mononuclear cell infiltration of the dermis.

There have been limited studies of the interaction of tick saliva with the canine immune system. A series of studies from Japan have shown that infestation of dogs with *R. sanguineus* causes suppression of antibody production, neutrophil function and the response of blood lymphocytes to mitogens, and that *R. sanguineus* SGE can mimic these effects *in vitro*, suppressing both T and B lymphocyte subpopulations.

Some studies have addressed the molecular weight of the tick salivary immunosuppressive proteins by fractionation of saliva before inclusion in the *in-vitro* systems described. The immunosuppressive activity of *R. sanguineus* saliva is mediated by proteins of <10 kDa. Saliva from *Ixodes dammini* has an immunosuppressive activity at >5 kDa and saliva from *Dermacentor andersoni* has two immunosuppressive components of molecular weights 36–43 and <3 kDa.

The effects of tick saliva on the host immune system are summarized in **Figure 3.7**.

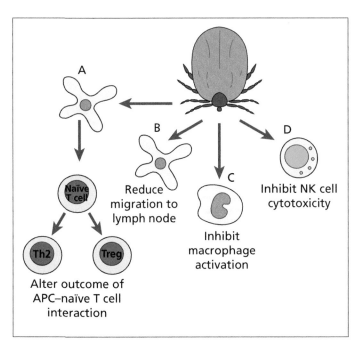

Fig. 3.7 A model for the immunomodulatory effects of tick saliva. Salivary immunoregulatory molecules may: (A) alter the outcome of the interaction between dendritic antigen presenting cell (APC) and the naïve T cell, promoting Th2 or T regulatory cell (Treg) immunity over a protective Th1 response; (B) reduce migration of APCs from the site of tick attachment to the regional draining lymph node; (C) inhibit the activation of macrophages; and (D) inhibit the activity of natural killer (NK) cells.

THE SAND FLY–HOST INTERFACE: SAND FLY MODULATION OF HOST BIOLOGY

In contrast to ticks, the interaction between host and haemophagous flies is relatively transient. Despite this, these insects also inject their hosts with powerful vasoactive, anticoagulant and immunomodulatory substances. The latter may not necessarily benefit an individual parasite, but they will ensure that the host does not develop protective immunity and that it remains susceptible to the entire parasite population over a period of time. This section will focus on the sand fly vectors of leishmaniosis, as they are the most relevant to companion animal disease.

Salivary anticoagulants

The protein content of saliva is far greater in female sand flies and it increases over the first 3 days after emergence, which correlates with the fact that these flies do not usually bite hosts until after that time. Sand fly saliva has potent anticoagulant activity mediated by apyrase. SGE from the New World sand fly *Lutzomyia longipalpis* contains the powerful vasodilatory polypeptide maxadilan, while the saliva of Old World sand flies (e.g. *Phlebotomus papatasi*) mediates vasodilation via adenosine and 5'-AMP. The saliva of *L. longipalpis* also contains hyaluronidase, which may aid dispersal of other salivary molecules and of *Leishmania* within the host dermis.

Salivary immunomodulatory molecules

The saliva of the sand fly has potent immunoregulatory activity, which is thought to underlie the ability of the saliva markedly to exacerbate *Leishmania* infection. SGE from *P. papatasi* causes a switch from a Th1 to Th2 response in mice infected with *Leishmania major* (e.g. increased IL-4 and reduced IFN-γ in lymph nodes draining sites of experimental infection in the presence of SGE), and is inhibitory of macrophage function *in vitro*. These effects may be mediated by adenosine and 5'-AMP.

SGE from *L. longipalpis* inhibits presentation of *Leishmania* antigens by macrophages and thus suppresses antigen-specific lymphocyte proliferative responses and delayed type hypersensitivity (DTH). Macrophages co-cultured with *L. longipalpis* SGE were refractory to activation by IFN-γ and unable to produce nitric oxide, hydrogen peroxide or proinflammatory cytokines (e.g. TNF-α) – all necessary for destruction of the intracellular amastigotes. These effects are mediated by maxadilan, which has dual action as a vasodilator. Maxadilan has homology with mammalian pituitary adenylate cyclase-activating polypeptide and utilizes the receptor for this molecule that is expressed by macrophages. In an experimental murine model of *L. major* infection, the increased infectivity caused by sand fly saliva was shown to be due to maxadilan. The immunomodulatory effects of sand fly saliva may cause *in-vitro* 'bystander suppression' of other immune responses.

HOST IMMUNE RESPONSE TO ARTHROPODS

This section discusses the protective host immune response to arthropods, as opposed to the ability of the arthropod to manipulate host immunity, as has been described above. In general terms it appears that both humoral and cell-mediated immune responses are made to arthropod salivary proteins. The cutaneous immune response to tick attachment has been characterized in a number of species (**Figure 3.8**). More is known about humoral immune responses than cellular responses, as these are more readily monitored. Several human epidemiological studies have shown that tick-exposed humans make anti-tick antibody responses, and these may correlate with the seroprevalence of infectious diseases in the same patients. For example, in a study of a Californian population, a significant correlation between seropositivity for *B. burgdorferi* sensu lato and *I. pacificus* was reported. Similarly, antibody to a 24 kDa protein of *R. sanguineus* has been identified in the serum of dogs following two experimental infestations.

A series of studies has examined the comparative immune response to *R. sanguineus* made by dogs and guinea pigs. In these experiments, dogs were unable to develop resistance to infestation, while guinea pigs did become resistant. In one study, histopathological changes at tick attachment sites in each species were examined between 4 and 96 hours of attachment in primary, secondary or tertiary infestations. Although both species responded with a mononuclear cell infiltrate, the major difference was that dogs also responded with a neutrophilic infiltrate, while guinea pigs had a predominant eosinophil infiltrate, suggesting that this underlies resistance in the guinea pig. However, this

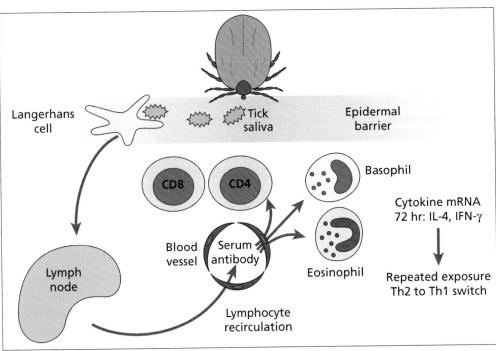

Fig. 3.8 The host immune response to arthropods. The infested host will mount an immune response to arthropods, and repeated exposure can induce resistance in some individuals. In the case of ticks, the immune response will predominantly be directed against the injected salivary antigens. These will be captured by dendritic antigen presenting cells in the epidermis (Langerhans cells) or dermis, and carried to the regional draining lymph nodes where activation of antigen-specific T and B lymphocytes occurs. Serum antibody specific for the salivary antigens will be induced. Antigen-specific T cells will be recruited back to the site of tick exposure via the interaction of lymphocyte homing receptors and the vascular addressins expressed by the endothelium of vessels in the tick attachment site. Locally produced cytokines and chemokines will recruit other leucocytes, chiefly eosinophils and basophils, to this dermal location. The nature of the dermal immune response will initially (up to 72 hours) reflect the immunomodulatory properties of the tick saliva (Th2 dominated), with mRNA encoding both IL-4 and IFN-γ found at the attachment sites. With time the cytokine profile will switch and the site will become Th1-dominated and CD8+ T cells will be recruited.

study is at odds with the commonly accepted description of the histopathology of tick attachment sites in the dog, which includes a granulomatous inflammation and an eosinophil response (**Figure 3.9**). This may in part reflect the kinetics of the host response, as most skin biopsies collected in a clinical setting will be from tick bite reactions of greater than 96 hours duration. Other factors that may account for this discrepancy include the species and strain of tick, and whether the tick is infected with microorganisms.

In a similar study, the intradermal skin test response to an *R. sanguineus* extract was compared in naïve and infested, and naïve and infested guinea pigs. Infested dogs developed a strong immediate reaction, but infested guinea pigs had both immediate and delayed reactions. Control animals had no significant

response. This provides evidence that cell-mediated immunity is one factor important for tick elimination and that this may be lacking in *R. sanguineus*-infested dogs. Resistance to *I. scapularis* has also been studied in the dog using a repeat infestation model. Tick performance parameters decreased with increasing exposure, suggesting the development of a protective immune response.

The immune response at the cutaneous site of tick attachment and in the regional draining lymph node has been investigated in sheep exposed to primary and secondary infestations with *Hyaloma anatolicum anatolicum* ticks. At both 72 hours and 8 days after attachment, there were increases in CD1+ and major histocompatibility complex (MHC) class II+ APCs and CD8+ T cells and T cells expressing the γδ T-cell receptor, within

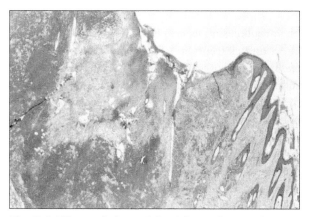

Fig. 3.9 Histopathology of the tick attachment site. Skin biopsy from a tick attachment site on a dog. There is a central region of ulceration and necrosis that correlates with the site of attachment and production of the salivary cement substance. This is surrounded by a heavy infiltration of mixed mononuclear cells (including macrophages, lymphocytes and plasma cells) and eosinophils in this relatively chronic lesion. (Haematoxylin and eosin stain)

the skin and draining lymph nodes. A recent study has investigated the cutaneous response to experimental challenge with *R. microplus* of resistant and susceptible cattle. Skin biopsy samples taken at 0, 24 and 48 hours post infestation were subjected to gene expression microarray analysis to search for differentially expressed genes. At 48 hours post infestation, skin from resistant cattle showed upregulation of genes encoding molecules involved in the complement and coagulation cascades, antigen presentation, cellular activation, differentiation and migration, oxidative stress and leukotriene synthesis. Parallel studies in this model system have examined cellular recruitment into tissue and the role of vascular endothelial adhesion molecules in this process. Resistant cattle have more basophils and eosinophils at tick attachment sites compared with susceptible animals and with a low-level infestation, resistant cattle have less expression of intercellular adhesion molecule-1, vascular cell adhesion molecule-1 and P-selectin than susceptible animals. Resistant cattle also had greater expression of E-selectin, which mediates the influx of memory T cells into the skin.

The immune response to the salivary proteins of sand fly saliva has been studied in experimental models and it is clear that strong antibody and DTH responses can be made following the bite of uninfected sand flies, injection with SGE or with recombinant salivary proteins. However, despite numerous studies of the immune response to *Leishmania* in infected dogs, there have been few investigations of the cutaneous response to sand fly saliva or the nature of the cutaneous lesions that might develop following the bite of these flies.

VACCINATION AGAINST ARTHROPODS

Vaccination against ticks

Vaccination strategies have been devised to limit tick infestation and, therefore, the transmission of tick-borne microbes. Additionally, there has been much research into the development of vaccines for the individual microbial agents themselves (e.g. *Borrelia*, *Babesia* and *Leishmania*). Detailed discussion of the latter is beyond the scope of this review, but will be covered in the individual chapters of this book.

Tick salivary cDNA libraries have been created and molecules of immunological relevance have been identified by screening the libraries expressed in vector systems with sera from immune animals. For example, a feeding-induced gene from *I. scapularis* (*salp 16*) was cloned in this manner and recombinant salp 16 produced. Although *I. scapularis*-infested guinea pigs made high-titred serum antibody to salp 16, vaccination with the recombinant molecule did not protect from infestation.

Although there have been numerous such studies of candidate tick vaccines, only one type of recombinant product has been produced commercially (TickGARD®, Hoechst Animal Health, Australia; Gavac™, Heber Biotec, Cuba). These vaccines for bovine *R. microplus* infestation contain the recombinant antigen Bm86 and induce antibodies in immunized cattle that mediate lysis of tick gut cells when the antibodies are ingested in a blood meal. The reduced tick burden and fecundity produced as a result allows decreased frequency of acaricide application to vaccinated animals. Some strains of *R. microplus* are resistant to Bm86 vaccine, but may be susceptible to a preparation containing the Bm95 recombinant antigen. Some tick-derived molecules may induce cross-protection against other tick species that carry homologous antigenic epitopes, and the Bm86 vaccine offers such cross-protection against at least two other tick species.

Rabbits vaccinated with a 20 amino acid synthetic peptide derived from the PO protein of *R. sanguineus* show reduced tick survival and fecundity when challenged with ticks. The PO protein is involved in the assembly of the 60S ribosomal subunit and the vaccinal peptide comes from a region of the molecule that is most dissimilar to the equivalent host protein. The efficacy of vaccinating naïve dogs with salivary gland or midgut extracts of *R. sanguineus* before repeat experimental challenge 7 and 21 days after the final vaccination has also been investigated. During these challenges there was reduced tick attachment (for both salivary and midgut vaccines), feeding period and engorgement weight (greatest with salivary vaccine) and fecundity (greatest with midgut vaccine). The observed greater efficacy of the gut extract may reflect the fact that the host is normally exposed to salivary antigens, and the tick may have developed means of suppressing the host response to such antigens during co-evolution. Moreover, a control group repeatedly exposed to *R. sanguineus* also showed transient reductions in these tick performance parameters, suggesting that dogs can develop spontaneous immunity to *R. sanguineus*. Immunization of dogs with gut extract of *R. sanguineus* in Freund's adjuvant was more effective than this extract adjuvanted in saponin, evidence for the importance of cell-mediated immunity in resistance of dogs to these ticks.

A similar study has been reported in cattle with *Hyalomma marginatum* extracts, but in this instance immunity induced by repeat infestation or salivary extract vaccination was superior to immunity induced by vaccination with an intestinal extract of the tick. Vaccination of cattle with SGE of *Hyalomma anatolicum* in Freund's incomplete adjuvant can be enhanced by incorporation of the additional adjuvant effect of *Ascaris suis* extract into the vaccine. The *A. suis* extract enhances IgE responses and produces a greater immediate hypersensitivity skin test reaction in immunized calves.

Recent attention has focused on the possibility of developing vaccines targeting universally conserved molecules in arthropod vectors. Akirins are a family of evolutionarily conserved proteins in insects and vertebrates that function as transcription factors for nuclear factor kappa B-dependent gene expression. The tick orthologue of akirin is subolesin and insects and ticks have only a single akirin/subolesin gene, making this

an appropriate vaccine target. An experimental recombinant subolesin vaccine given to cattle had significant effect on tick fecundity after challenge with *R. microplus* larvae and other vaccination trials have shown that subolesin vaccine can reduce the fecundity of a range of hard and soft tick species, mosquitoes, sand flies, poultry red mites and sea lice.

An ideal vaccine might protect against both tick infestation and the transmission of microparasites. A study examining the vaccine potential of several molecules involved in the tick–microparasite interaction (including subolesin) has shown that a number of these candidates reduced infestation and fecundity of *R. microplus* ticks on cattle and also reduced the DNA copies of *Babesia bigemina* and *Anaplasma marginale* within feeding ticks. Other experimental studies have shown similar reduction in tick infection with *A. phagocytophilum* and *B. burgdorferi* sensu lato after subolesin vaccination.

Vaccination against sand flies

Vaccination against other arthropods has also been investigated as a potential control measure for the microbial infections they transmit. Mice infected experimentally with *Leishmania major* develop significantly more severe disease when co-injected with entire SGE or with synthetic maxadilan from *L. longipalpis*, suggesting that this latter molecule is responsible for the disease exacerbation caused by sand fly saliva. Vaccination with synthetic maxadilan induces a Th1 immune response and serum antibody specific for the molecule, and protects mice from experimental infection with *L. major*. The Old World sand fly *P. papatasi* does not produce maxadilan, but pre-exposure to the bite of uninfected *Phlebotomus* confers resistance to infection with *L. major* with a strong DTH response, suggesting a similar effect with an alternative candidate protein. One study characterized nine salivary proteins from *P. papatasi* and demonstrated that a recombinant form of one of these (SP15) was able to induce strong DTH in mice and was protective when used as a vaccine against *L. major*.

An unpublished abstract reported an experimental study in dogs co-injected with *Leishmania* and sand fly SGE. Relative to controls that received only *Leishmania*, the test dogs developed clinical leishmaniosis several months earlier, which correlated with earlier demonstration of *Leishmania*-specific T-cell proliferative responses and IL-4 production. The investigators suggested that this 'early onset' model of canine leishmaniosis would permit more rapid assessment of *Leishmania* vaccines in the dog model.

Immune-mediated sequelae to arthropod-transmitted infectious disease

The arthropod-transmitted pathogens that are the subject of this book have a complex pathogenesis within the host. In broad terms, many of the clinical disease manifestations in leishmaniosis, babesiosis, ehrlichiosis, anaplasmosis, borreliosis, rickettsiosis, bartonellosis and hepatozoonosis are related to the interaction of the infectious agent with the host immune system. These clinical manifestations will be discussed in other chapters. It is suggested that the initial interaction of arthropod products with the host immune system may redirect host immunity to a state that is optimum for subsequent immune-mediated disease related to the microbe (**Figure 3.10**). In this respect, if arthropod salivary molecules are able to subvert the host immune system and create a 'switch' to Th2 (humoral) immunity, the likelihood is that if an infectious agent is superimposed on the immune system in this state, there will be humoral immune-mediated sequelae. For example:

- Hyperglobulinaemia via polyclonal or monoclonal B-cell activation (e.g. in leishmaniosis or monocytic ehrlichiosis).
- Induction of autoantibody (e.g. anti-erythrocyte in babesiosis, anti-platelet in ehrlichiosis and rickettsiosis, both autoantibodies and antinuclear antibody in leishmaniosis) or induction of cross-reactive antibody by molecular mimicry between autoantigen and epitopes of the infectious agent (e.g. cross-reactivity of antibodies to neuroaxonal proteins and flagellin from *Borrelia*).
- Formation of circulating immune complexes of antibody and microbial or self antigen that may potentially lodge in capillary beds and cause local tissue pathology (e.g. uveitis, polyarthritis, vasculitis and glomerulonephritis that may occur in leishmaniosis).
- Granulomatous inflammatory aggregates of parasitized macrophages that are unable effectively to kill the intracellular microbe (e.g. dermal

lesions in leishmaniosis). In this respect, the chronic non-healing nature of infections such as leishmaniosis may involve Th1 cells producing both IFN-γ and IL-10, with the IL-10 preventing complete sterilization of the infection and permitting persistence of intracellular amastigotes (see **Figure 3.6**).

Such effects may be further complicated when there is multiple co-infection with arthropod-transmitted infectious agents. This model of dominant Th2 immunity is not all-encompassing, as Th1 (cell-mediated) effects do comprise part of the pathogenesis of such infections; for example, the mononuclear cell synovitis that occurs in borreliosis is T-cell mediated and the specificity of these T cells has been characterized.

In evolutionary terms, the balance between an organism producing tissue infection and secondary immune-mediated pathology is described as the 'trade-off hypothesis'. The parasite must maximize its 'fitness' by increasing its rate of transmission from the infected host to new hosts (via the arthropod vector in this instance), while ensuring that it does not kill its host due to immune-mediated tissue damage. The parasite must therefore maintain an intermediate level of virulence in order to achieve these aims.

CONCLUSIONS

The attachment of an infected arthropod to a mammalian host creates a severe challenge to the host immune system. Host immunity to arthropods and arthropod-transmitted infectious agents is based on a cell-mediated (Th1) response, but arthropod salivary molecules are able to subvert host immunity to a dominant Th2 (humoral) form. This permits prolonged feeding by individual arthropods (ticks) or populations (sand flies) and transmission of infectious agents into an environment in which the host preferentially generates humoral immunity to the organism. This latter effect may underlie the range of immunopathogenic mechanisms that characterize arthropod-borne infections. Chronicity of infection may also be mediated by a partial switch of effector Th1 cells to a regulatory phenotype involving production of IL-10.

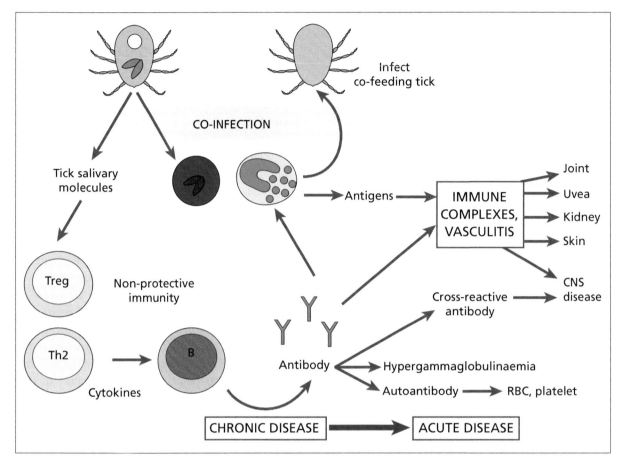

Fig. 3.10 Summary of the interaction between arthropod, infectious agent and the host immune system. Injection of arthropod salivary molecules results in redirection of the host immune system to a Th2 or Treg phenotype, both locally within the dermis and within the regional draining lymph node. In rodent model systems this effect may also involve the systemic immune system. Salivary immunomodulation permits prolonged or repeated exposure to the arthropod and allows transmission of the arthropod-borne infectious agent (or agents in co-infections) and establishment of infection in the absence of a protective (Th1) immune response. Uninfected arthropods co-feeding at the site may acquire infection ('saliva-activated transmission'). The infectious agent may spread from the site of inoculation to produce parasitaemia and acute infectious disease. The bias towards Th2 immunity may also underlie the chronic, secondary, immune-mediated sequelae to infection. These include excessive polyclonal B-cell activation (hypergammaglobulinaemia), the formation of circulating immune complexes that may deposit within the microvasculature and the induction of autoantibodies or antibodies that cross-react with microbial and self epitopes. (Redrawn after Shaw SE *et al.* (2001) *Trends in Parasitology* 17:74–80.)

FURTHER READING

Boppana DKV, Wikel SK, Raj DG *et al.* (2010) Cellular infiltration at skin lesions and draining lymph nodes of sheep infested with adult *Hyalomma anatolicum anatolicum* ticks. *Parasitology* **131**:657–667.

Carli E, Tasca S, Trotta M *et al.* (2009) Detection of erythrocyte binding IgM and IgG by flow cytometry in sick dogs with *Babesia canis canis* or *Babesia canis vogeli* infection. *Veterinary Parasitology* **162**:51–57.

Carvalho WA, Domingues R, de Azevedo Prata MC *et al.* (2014) Microarray analysis of tick-infested skin in resistant and susceptible cattle confirms the role of inflammatory pathways in immune activation and larval rejection. *Veterinary Parasitology* **205**:307–317.

Carvalho WA, Franzin AM, Rodriguez Abetepaulo AR *et al.* (2010) Modulation of cutaneous inflammation induced by ticks in contrasting phenotypes of infestation in bovines. *Veterinary Parasitology* **167**:260–273.

Cotte V, Sabatier L, Schnell G *et al.* (2014) Differential expression of *Ixodes ricinus* salivary gland proteins in the presence of the *Borrelia burgdorferi* sensu lato complex. *Journal of Proteomics* **96**:29–43.

Day MJ (2011) The immunopathology of canine vector-borne diseases. *Parasites and Vectors* **4**:48.

de la Fuente J, Moreno-Cid JA, Canales M *et al.* (2011) Targeting arthropod subolesin/akirin for the development of a universal vaccine for control of vector infestations and pathogen transmission. *Veterinary Parasitology* **181**:17–22.

de la Fuente J, Moreno-Cid JA, Galindo RC *et al.* (2013) Subolesin/akirin vaccines for the control of arthropod vectors and vector borne pathogens. *Transboundary and Emerging Diseases* **60**:172–178.

Deruaz M, Frauenschuh A, Alessandri AL *et al.* (2008) Ticks produce highly selective chemokine binding proteins with anti-inflammatory activity. *Journal of Experimental Medicine* **205**:2019–2031.

Ginel PJ, Camacho S, Lucena R (2008) Anti-histone antibodies in dogs with leishmaniasis and glomerulonephritis. *Research in Veterinary Science* **85**:510–514.

Hajdusek O, Sima R, Ayllon N *et al.* (2013) Interaction of the tick immune system with transmitted pathogens. *Frontiers in Cellular and Infection Microbiology* **3**:26.

Heinze DM, Carmical JR, Aronson JF *et al.* (2012) Early immunologic events at the tick–host interface. *PLoS One* **7**:e47301.

Ibelli AMG, Kim TK, Hill CC *et al.* (2014) A blood meal-induced *Ixodes scapularis* tick saliva serpin inhibits trypsin and thrombin, and interferes with platelet aggregation and blood clotting. *International Journal for Parasitology* **44**:369–379.

Kumar B, Nagar G, de la Fuente J *et al.* (2014) Subolesin: a candidate vaccine antigen for the control of cattle tick infestations in Indian situation. *Vaccine* **32**:3488–3494.

Liu XY, de la Fuente J, Cote M *et al.* (2014) IrSPI, a tick serine protease inhibitor involved in tick feeding and *Bartonella henselae* infection. *PLoS Neglected Tropical Diseases* **8**:e2993.

Long GH, Boots M (2011) How can immunopathology shape the evolution of parasite virulence? *Trends in Parasitology* **27**:300–305.

Majtan J, Kouremenou C, Rysnik O *et al.* (2013) Novel immunomodulators from hard ticks selectively reprogramme human dendritic cell responses. *PLoS Pathogens* **9**:e1003450.

Menezes-Souza D, Correa-Oliveira R, Guerra-Sa R *et al.* (2011) Cytokine and transcription factor profiles in the skin of dogs naturally infected by *Leishmania chagasi* presenting distinct cutaneous parasite density and clinical status. *Veterinary Parasitology* **177**:39–49.

Menten-Dedoyart C, Faccinetto C, Golovchenko M *et al.* (2012) Neutrophil extracellular traps entrap and kill *Borrelia burgdorferi* sensu stricto spirochetes and are not affected by *Ixodes ricinus* tick saliva. *Journal of Immunology* **189**:5393–5401.

Merino O, Antunes S, Mosqueda J *et al.* (2013) Vaccination with proteins involved in tick–pathogen interactions reduces vector infestations and pathogen infection. *Vaccine* **31**:5889–5896.

Poole NM, Mamidanna G, Smith RA *et al.* (2013) Prostaglandin E$_2$ in tick saliva regulates host cell migration and cytokine profile. *FASEB Journal* **27**:436.

Rodriguez-Mallon A, Fernandez E, Encinosa PE *et al.* (2012) A novel tick antigen shows high vaccine efficacy against the dog tick, *Rhipicephalus sanguineus*. *Vaccine* **30**:1782–1789.

Skallova A, Lezzi G, Ampenberger F *et al.* (2008) Tick saliva inhibits dendritic cell migration, maturation and function, while promoting development of Th2 responses. *Journal of Immunology* **180**:6186–6192.

Slamova M, Skallova A, Palenikova J *et al.* (2011) Effect of tick saliva on immune interactions between *Borrelia afzelii* and murine dendritic cells. *Parasite Immunology* **33**:654–660.

Sultana H, Neelakanta G, Kantor FS *et al.* (2010) *Anaplasma phagocytophilum* induces actin phosphorylation to selectively regulate gene transcription in *Ixodes scapularis* ticks. *Journal of Experimental Medicine* **207:**1727–1743.

Trinchieri G (2007) Interleukin-10 production by effector T cells: Th1 cells show self control. *Journal of Experimental Medicine* **204:**239–243.

Chapter 4

Laboratory Diagnosis of Arthropod-borne Infections

Iain R. Peters

INTRODUCTION

Diagnosis of the diseases associated with the arthropod-borne pathogens discussed in this book is often challenging. These pathogens are generally difficult (if at all possible) to cultivate *in vitro*, are often present in very low numbers in peripheral blood and may evoke a variable antibody response. The clinical signs associated with infection with these pathogens are often vague and non-specific. The individual organisms are dealt with in detail in later chapters. This chapter gives an overview of the potential range of diagnostic tests used for determining infection with these agents, although some may not be available for routine clinical diagnosis.

MICROSCOPY

In the hands of experienced microscopists, some parasites may be identified on the basis of their morphology (e.g. *Babesia divergens*), their cellular tropisms (e.g. *Ehrlichia canis* selectively infects monocytes; *Anaplasma platys* infects platelets; and *A. phagocytophilum* infects neutrophils), or their staining characteristics in peripheral blood smears (e.g. *Mycoplasma haemofelis*, 'Candidatus M. haemominutum' and 'Candidatus M. turicensis').

This methodology can have a limited sensitivity as sufficient organisms need to be present to allow identification and organism numbers can rapidly fluctuate (e.g. *M. haemofelis* in blood smears). In addition, false-positive results may result from staining artefacts and incorrect identification of other cellular inclusions (e.g. Howell–Jolly bodies). A common problem encountered in pathology laboratories is the interpretation of suboptimally prepared blood smears. A checklist of considerations necessary for optimum smear preparation is shown in **Table 4.1**.

Standard differential stains such as May–Grünwald–Giemsa work well on blood smears for identification

of large protozoan parasites (e.g. *Leishmania* species and *Babesia* species) and the multicellular aggregates (morulae) of *Ehrlichia* species In order to view bacteria such as *Bartonella* or the rickettsias directly, more advanced staining methods such as the Warthin–Starry silver stain can be employed using suitably prepared biopsy material. However, these stains are relatively non-specific and results must be interpreted with caution.

Darkfield microscopy, which utilizes a special condenser to direct light toward an object at an angle rather

Table 4.1 **Making the perfect blood film.**
<ul><li>**Use EDTA as anti-coagulant.** EDTA gives superior preservation of host and parasite cell morphology.</li><li>**Mix blood well (but gently) prior to making the film.**</li><li>**Avoid delay in making the blood film.** Blood films should ideally be made within 1 hour of collecting the blood sample; even if the sample cannot be stained or examined, it is better if the film is prepared as soon as possible.</li><li>**Avoid using too much blood.** The commonest problem. A tiny drop should be applied to the slide using an applicator or pipette tip.</li><li>**Spread the film evenly.** Spread the blood drop using another glass slide. Touch the drop then draw the slide away at an angle of 30–40° in a smooth glide.</li><li>**Air-dry the film as soon as possible.** Water-induced artefacts are reduced by rapid drying of the slide. Waving the slide vigorously, or using a flame or hair drier, are all effective, particularly in humid environments.</li><li>**Keep staining solutions clean.** Stain sediment is a common problem in the diagnosis of haemoplasmas and *Babesia* spp. Stains should be filtered before use. Fresh stain and fixative solutions should be prepared regularly.</li><li>**Use a coverslip.** Using a coverslip greatly enhances the visual image. It may be temporarily mounted with immersion oil.</li></ul>
(Dr P. Irwin, personal communication)

than from below, may be used to visualize motile bacteria, such as *Borrelia* species. Using this method, particles or cells are seen as light objects against a dark background. Darkfield microscopy or phase contrast microscopy may be used on fresh material (e.g. synovial fluid) to observe organisms. Antibodies specific for particular pathogens, linked to fluorescent dyes, can be used in conjunction with a fluorescence microscope to detect organisms in blood smears or tissue sections.

PATHOGEN CULTURE/PROPAGATION

The arthropod-borne pathogens generally have exacting nutritional requirements, reflecting their intracellular or epicellular modes of existence, and are difficult to grow *in vitro* even if the culture conditions are known. In exceptional cases, where growth on synthetic or semi-synthetic media is possible, growth rates are very slow, with an attendant high risk of fungal or bacterial contamination despite rigorous aseptic technique. For example, *Borrelia burgdorferi* and certain *Bartonella* species (e.g. *B. henselae*) can be grown on media. In both cases it can take a month between inoculation with clinical material and identification of visible growth, making culture inappropriate for diagnosis.

Culture has the advantage of allowing analysis of relatively large sample volumes, increasing its overall sensitivity. This is because a single organism in a millilitre of blood could potentially give rise to a colony that can be used as the basis for more advanced tests. Ideally, several replicates of each sample should be inoculated to allow contamination and sensitivity issues to be addressed. In addition, care must be exercised in sample handling and transport to maximize the chance of viable organisms being used in the culture.

IMMUNODIAGNOSTIC TESTS (SEROLOGY)

Immunodiagnostic tests involve the detection of either antibody or antigen within a clinical sample (e.g. serum, whole blood, urine or cerebrospinal fluid). Serology, in the context of this chapter, is the study of serum (or plasma in some applications) antibody responses to infectious agents. Serum (or plasma) should be separated as soon as possible from the blood clot or cell pellet to minimize the chance of haemoglobin contamination, which may interfere with some applica-

tions. Gel tubes provide an efficient means of obtaining a clear, stable serum sample.

Exposure of animals to complex non-self antigens (e.g. bacterial proteins) usually results in the induction of an immune response. This response is characterized by the generation of humoral (antibody) and/or cell-mediated immunity. The nature and scale of the humoral immune response can give valuable information about host exposure to an infectious agent, but is less helpful in assessing active infection or in quantifying the infectious load. Some of the more relevant methods involved in the detection of antibodies with specificities for particular organisms or proteins are described below.

The kinetics of the humoral response to many pathogenic organisms have been described in detail and should be understood if logical conclusions are to be drawn from serological testing. The response to sequential challenge with antigen in terms of antibody class and concentration is illustrated (**Figure 4.1**). The nature of the response is determined by the number of exposures to the antigen. Following the initial exposure, a second or third exposure (or, more realistically, continued exposure) gives rise to more rapid induction of IgG compared with IgM, which predominates in the early stages of infection.

Infection, or 'challenge', with a pathogen to which the animal has had no previous exposure evokes a weak IgM response after 1 week, and a gradually increasing IgG response. Measuring antibody levels in an animal with acute-onset disease, such as babesiosis, would thus give little useful diagnostic information. For more chronic and persistent infections, such as those caused by *Ehrlichia canis*, measuring antibody levels may be more useful clinically, particularly when correlated with the epidemiology of the disease in question. For example, low levels of antibody to *Rickettsia rickettsii* may be incidental in animals that are, or have been, resident in endemic areas, but may be significant in animals that have returned to a non-endemic area after a short visit to an endemic area.

The production of antibodies is an idiosyncratic process, varying in both scale and specificity between animals depending on age, health status and genetic background. The best way of assessing whether seroconversion to a particular pathogen has occurred is to analyze paired samples collected 2–3 weeks apart. A rising antibody titre suggests a recent and, therefore, clinically significant infection, especially if supported by appropriate clinical signs. A potential, alternative method for determining recent infection is to measure antigen-specific IgM concentrations. This is technically more demanding and may give spurious results where high concentrations of IgG are present in a sample. IgM concentrations may be particularly useful in cases where diseases are endemic and a high proportion of the population may have antigen-specific IgG.

Antibodies recognize small (~12 amino acid) regions of antigenic proteins as well as larger structural ('conformational') determinants. Because of the modular way in which biological polymers are 'designed', it is quite often the case that two unrelated proteins will share structural or protein sequence motifs. This leads to the phenomenon of cross-reaction whereby antibodies may recognize molecules other than those that originally generated the immune response. While this is an excellent strategy, in evolutionary terms, for experimental purposes it can be frustrating, leading to false-positive results. For example, if looking for antibodies against the agent of Lyme disease, *Borrelia burgdorferi* sensu stricto, it is important to ensure that exposure to related, non-pathogenic spirochaetes, or to vaccinal antibodies (e.g. to *Leptospira* species), will not be detected by the assay.

A number of the arthropod-borne pathogens specifically target cells involved in the immune response; for example, *Leishmania* species multiply in macrophages and *Ehrlichia canis* has a tropism for monocytes. These organisms frequently dysregulate antibody production, causing the production of large quantities of non-specific IgG, clinically recognized as monoclonal or polyclonal gammopathies. These are mostly non-functional antibodies with respect to the organism, although they may be autoreactive and thus contribute to pathology. However, they may also cause interference in diagnostic serological methods. The presence of gammopathy can be a useful clue when investigating more chronic arthropod-borne infections; indeed, IgG 'spikes' on serum electrophoresis are sometimes the first results to raise suspicion as to the possibility of an infectious agent being responsible for disease. To complicate matters further, certain arthropod-borne pathogens are actively immunosuppressive (e.g. *Anaplasma phagocytophilum*) and infected animals may show spuriously low antibody levels despite active infection.

Despite the caveats described above, antibody-based diagnostic tests are widely used commercially and in practice. Five methods are commonly used for detecting antibodies (antigen) in clinical samples and these are described below.

Enzyme-linked immunosorbent assay

Enzyme-linked immunosorbent assay (ELISA) uses the principle that proteins can be induced to adhere irreversibly to certain plastic surfaces. Immobilized

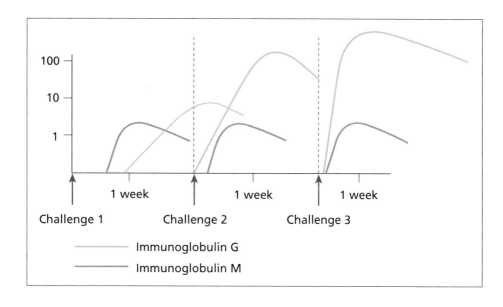

Fig. 4.1 Humoral immune responses to sequential challenge with antigen in terms of antibody class and concentration.

antigen can be used to 'trap' complementary antibodies in a serum sample. The amount of antibody in the sample is determined by using a series of serum dilutions and assessing the limit at which the detection signal is statistically indistinguishable from that of background 'noise'. Binding of this primary serum antibody to the immobilized antigen is detected using a secondary antibody, produced against purified immunoglobulins of the species from which the test serum came, that has been conjugated to an enzyme (usually alkaline phosphatase or horseradish peroxidase). After a series of incubation steps, a visualization reagent is added, which contains a chromogenic substrate for the conjugated enzymes. The reaction is stopped after a set period of time and the last serum dilution resulting in an unequivocally detectable amount of colour is determined spectrophotometrically. The titre of antibody is defined as the inverse of this last detectable dilution (e.g. a serum sample titrating to a dilution of 1 in 2,000 is quoted as having an antibody titre of 2,000). The processes involved are depicted in **Figure 4.2**.

ELISAs have become the preferred format for determining the presence of antibodies against pathogens from which antigens are freely available; that is, for pathogens that are relatively easy to cultivate or from which protein antigens have been identified, cloned and expressed as recombinant proteins. The attraction of ELISA technology is that it can be performed in a microtitre plate format, is easy to automate and produces numerical, objective data. These features make ELISAs ideal for studies where the immune status of large numbers of animals is to be determined, as in vaccine trials or sero-epidemiological surveys. If the appropriate second antibodies are used, IgM or IgG (or both) can be measured in a sample.

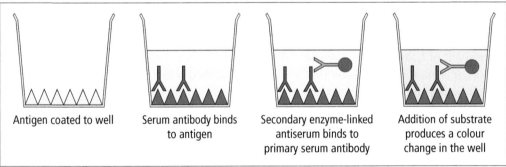

| Antigen coated to well | Serum antibody binds to antigen | Secondary enzyme-linked antiserum binds to primary serum antibody | Addition of substrate produces a colour change in the well |

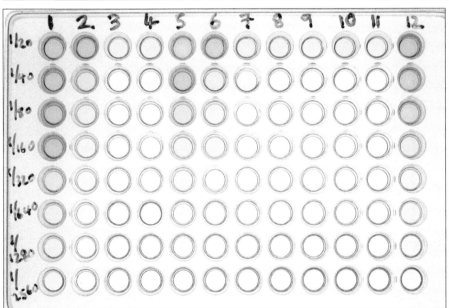

Fig. 4.2 ELISA. Commercial test kits are usually provided with the antigen of interest immobilized onto the plate. Effective washing between steps is essential for reproducible, accurate results. The plate shown compares the antibody levels between a number of cats infected with feline immunodeficiency virus. Individual animals are designated on the top row, with dilutions shown down the side.

The ELISA format can also be used to detect antigen in samples if high affinity antibodies are available with which to coat the plates (the capture antibody) and to detect bound antigen (the visualization antibody). Monoclonal antibodies (or fragments) are generally used in this context. For example, antigen ELISA is a sensitive and specific tool for diagnosing *Dirofilaria immitis* (heartworm) infection. In some instances, multiple pathogens can be tested for simultaneously in a single module.

Immunofluorescent antibody test

Where culture of organisms is difficult, or not advisable due to safety concerns, another serological technique may be used. In immunofluorescent antibody tests (IFATs), organisms may be detected in infected cells or tissues of a patient (direct IFAT) or, more commonly, the presence of serum antigen-specific antibodies may be determined using an infected cell or tissue substrate (indirect IFAT). The robustness of the antibody molecule is used to provide a reagent that can discriminate between closely related protein molecules. In an IFAT, infected cells, usually derived from tissue culture, are fixed onto microscope slides or microtitre plates. A procedure similar to that described for ELISA (see above) is then employed to determine if a serum sample contains antibodies against the particular pathogen (**Figure 4.3**). However, instead of using a chromogenic conjugate, the second antibody is labelled with a dye molecule (e.g. fluorescein or Texas red), which fluoresces under light of a particular wavelength. Samples containing antibodies cause the organisms within infected cells to glow brightly when viewed with a fluorescence microscope. This method has been widely used in studying antibody status to *Leishmania* and *Babesia* species. As with ELISA, the amount of antibody in a sample is determined by limiting dilution and the results are given as a titre.

A recent extension to this methodology has been the determination of antibody status to *Leishmania* using the IFAT methodology combined with flow cytometry. Previously cultured, fixed *Leishmania* promastigotes are incubated with increasing dilutions of test serum and bound antibody is labelled with fluorochrome-labelled anti-canine IgG antibodies. The sample is then analysed by flow cytometry with the percentage of fluorescent promastigotes (those with serum antibody bound) determined. Initial studies have shown the potential for this methodology to both quantify the titre of serum

antibody and differentiate infection from vaccine-derived immunity.

A similar but less sensitive method, the direct IFAT, involves incubating test tissue sections or blood smears with a high affinity, fluorochrome-labelled antibody, often a monoclonal antibody specific for the pathogen in question. This method is used to detect pathogens such as *A. phagocytophilum*, where the number of infected cells may be low. Under fluorescent light, the infected cells are immediately apparent.

Agglutination-based tests

The multivalency of antigen-binding sites on antibody molecules (two for IgG; ten for IgM) allows them to cross-link macromolecular structures (**Figure 4.4**). This cross-linking, or agglutination, is clearly visible because the initial homogeneous suspension of carrier particles (e.g. latex beads or tanned red blood cells) becomes turbid as the individual particles aggregate. This test can be performed on any solid surface and can use inexpensive carriers such as latex beads. The agglutination occurs rapidly at room temperature. Agglutination tests provide a rapid, simple method for detection of pathogen exposure or for determination of post-vaccination titres. Because the test relies

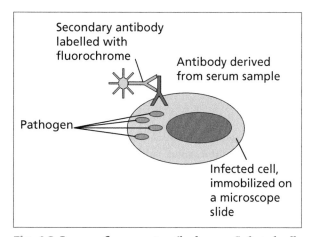

Fig. 4.3 Immunofluorescent antibody assay. Infected cells are immobilized onto an inert substrate. Serum (serially diluted in a number of tests performed in parallel) is then applied. After washing unbound antibodies away, an appropriate purified antibody bound to a fluorescent dye is added. An intense fluorescence is observed in tests containing antibody concentrations above a certain threshold.

on a universal property of antibodies, it can be used for all species suspected of seroconversion to a pathogen. Agglutination tests are also valuable because they can detect antigen or antibody, provided that target material is available to coat the beads.

Rapid immunomigration tests

A number of 'in-practice' tests have been developed that allow rapid determination of an animal's immune status with respect to particular infectious agents. A number of the tests available for arthropod-borne pathogens are variants of the ELISA technique described earlier (e.g. ImmunoComb™ [see **Figure 12.20**] and SNAP™ tests).

The SNAP™ test utilizes antigen (or antibody in the case of *Dirofilaria immitis* antigen detection) immobilized on a membrane to capture antibody (or antigen) in the test sample. The test procedure involves mixing the sample (blood) with a solution containing antigen (or antibody) linked to an enzyme conjugate. The mixture is applied

to the test device and the solution migrates through the membrane and interacts with the immobilized antigen (or antibody). Once the sample has migrated sufficiently, the device is depressed, activating a wash step that removes unbound components and clears the reading window. The chromogenic substrate causes development of a colour spot when the conjugate is present attached to the target antibody (antigen) complexes. In some instances, multiple pathogens can be tested for simultaneously in a single module, such as the SNAP 4Dx™ kit (**Figure 4.5**), which allows simultaneous testing for the presence of antibodies to *A. phagocytophilum, Anaplasma platys, Ehrlichia canis* and *Borrelia burgdorferi* and *Dirofilaria immitis* antigen in a blood sample.

A different method, known as rapid immunomigration (RIM), is used in tests such as the WITNESS™ system. This method is a passive chromatography system where animal serum is added to a membrane containing gold-labelled antigens in solution. Any specific antibodies in the serum bind to the antigen and

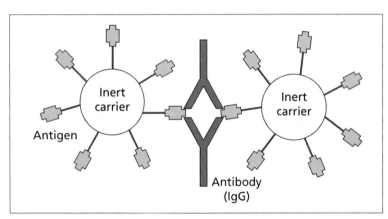

Fig. 4.4 **Agglutination-based assay. Diagrammatic representation of the first stage of the agglutination process. The bivalency of the IgG molecule allows it to cross-link relatively large particles. The cross-linking becomes apparent as the particles cohere and the original solution becomes heterogeneous. This is seen as an increased rate of agglutination of the inert carrier. IgM molecules are pentavalent and are much more efficient 'agglutinins'.**

Fig. 4.5 **An example of a seropositive sample tested with the SNAP 4Dx™ test kit. The sample generates both a blue spot in the positive control position (1) and a second spot identifying seropositivity to *Ehrlichia* (*canis* or *ewingii*) (2). This sample also yielded a positive qPCR result for *Ehrlichia*.**

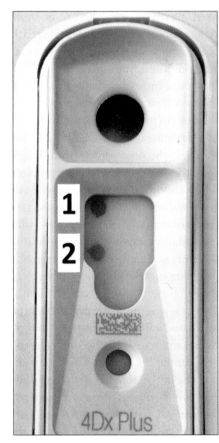

the resultant antibody–antigen complexes move along the test strip until they reach a matrix, which precipitates the complex. Antibody–antigen complexes appear as a pink line in this precipitation zone. The kit comes with appropriate positive and negative controls and is semi-quantitative. In an alternative method, the test kit contains labelled antibodies to a particular antigen, allowing antigen in a sample to be detected. An example is shown in **Figure 4.6**.

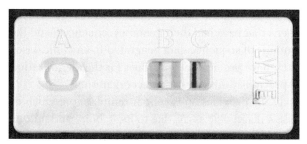

Fig. 4.6 Rapid immunomigration. The slide shows a positive result for *Borrelia* serology. Serum is added to well A; a pink band in window B indicates a positive result. The band in window C is a positive control that shows that the test is functioning correctly.

Immunoblotting ('western blotting' or 'dot blotting')

ELISA, IFAT, agglutination and RIM tests generally employ a complex mixture of antigens such as cellular homogenates to capture reactive antibodies. Therefore, when a positive result is obtained, minimal information is obtained about the antigen–antibody binding events occurring in the test. For example, an animal may have antibodies that non-specifically adhere to a component of the plastic microtitre plate in an ELISA test, and the subsequent reaction would be read as a positive reaction to a pathogen. Alternatively, antibodies to common environmental antigens may cross-react with components of the antigen mixture used in the test of interest, producing false seropositivity. It is possible to circumvent these problems using pathogen-specific recombinant proteins that are also relevant to the disease process.

An alternative method for visualizing antigen-antibody interactions is immunoblotting. A complex mixture of antigens (best applied to proteins) is separated according to molecular weight, using denaturing sodium dodecyl sulphate polyacrylamide gel electrophoresis. The proteins are then transferred and immobilized on an inert membrane (e.g. nitrocellulose or polyvinylidene difluoride). Unoccupied protein-binding sites are then 'blocked' and the membrane is 'probed' with a primary antibody against the antigen(s) of interest, as in ELISAs and IFATs. An enzyme-labelled second antibody is then used to detect binding of primary antibody; addition of a specific substrate solution (giving a precipitate in this case, rather than the soluble ELISA product) then allows visualization of antigenic bands. The molecular weights of these bands can be determined by reference to a mixture of known molecular weight proteins separated on the same gel (**Figure 4.7**). An alternative to chromogenic

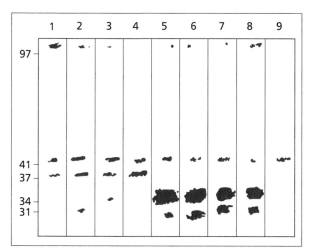

Fig. 4.7 Immunoblot analysis to compare the antibody profiles of dogs that have been naturally infected or vaccinated with *Borrelia burgdorferi* (simplified for clarity); all dogs positive by standard ELISA. Proteins from sonicated *B. burgdorferi* were separated by sodium dodecysulphate polyacrylamide gel electrophoresis then transferred to nitrocellulose. Strips of membrane were then probed with sera from naturally infected (1–4) or vaccinated animals (5–8). Serum from an animal from a Lyme disease-free area was used as a control (9). It can be seen that antibodies to antigens of 97 kDa and 41 kDa are common to both groups of dogs. Antibodies to the 34 kDa and 31 kDa proteins (OspB and OspA repectively) are much more pronounced in the vaccinated animals. The 41 kDa band (flagellin) is shared with other spirochaetes including *Leptospira* species, perhaps explaining the cross-reactive antibody seen in the negative control. In this example, 37 kDa bands appear to be diagnostic for natural infection.

substrates are substrates that emit light that can then be detected on photographic film; this chemiluminescent system is more versatile and can give enhanced sensitivity. The results from clinical samples can be compared with patterns seen in confirmed infections and they add weight to the credibility of ELISA tests. The use of immunoblotting has become established in the diagnosis of Lyme disease, where ELISA results have a significant false-positive rate and where vaccinal antibodies (which are detected by ELISA) can be distinguished from naturally induced antibodies.

MOLECULAR DIAGNOSTIC TESTS

Serology and PCR are two important techniques for the diagnosis of arthropod-borne pathogens in animals with compatible clinical signs. The two methodologies are complementary and appreciation of the differences in the capabilities of the two methodologies allows selection of the most appropriate test(s) (**Box 4.1**).

The genome of a pathogen contains all the information required to produce the proteins and RNA molecules that it requires to successfully propagate itself. Genes that are essential for life often have DNA sequences that are highly similar amongst apparently unrelated organisms. The subtle changes in DNA sequences that occur due to random mutation, and which offer a selective advantage or are selectively neutral over geological time frames, differentiate one pathogen from another and these differences can be exploited to allow differentiation of these organisms. The recent expansion in the number and range of pathogens that have had their genomes sequenced, and the amount of sequence data generated from clinical isolates, have provided new avenues for the identification of previously difficult-to-detect organisms.

DNA provides an excellent template on which to base a diagnostic assay, due to its stability and unique structure. A number of commercially available technologies exist for reliable and reproducible extraction of

---

Box 4.1 Comparison of serology and PCR testing.

The results obtained from the two testing modalities depend on the time at which the sample is taken in the course of the infection and the infection kinetics. An example of these kinetics during an infection with a blood-borne pathogen is shown in **Figure 4.8**. The results of polymerase chain reaction (PCR) and serological testing would vary depending on the time point at which the animal is tested. A blood sample obtained at point A would provide a positive result with PCR, but would be seronegative as this sample has been taken prior to seroconversion. A sample obtained at point B would be both PCR and serologically positive. If the organism was eliminated from the animal at the point at which the first negative blood PCR result was obtained (blue arrow), then samples obtained at points C1 and C2 would be PCR negative, but serology positive. However, if the organism was sequestered elsewhere within the body (e.g. bone marrow) with intermittent release into the systemic circulation (broken red lines), the PCR results could either be positive (C1) or negative (C2), but the animal would remain seropositive throughout.

	SEROLOGY	POLYMERASE CHAIN REACTION
Test detects	Antibody response to pathogen	Nucleic acid (DNA) from pathogen
Advantages	Detects infected and recovered animals Sample (blood) easily obtained	Specific pathogen identification in infected animals Monitoring effectiveness of therapy (qPCR)
Limitations	Clinical signs may be present in animals prior to seroconversion Antibody may persist for months (years) following pathogen elimination Positive result may reflect previous exposure rather than active infection	Negative results do not exclude infection Pathogens may only be present in anatomical locations that are difficult to sample

highly pure nucleic acids from all classes of pathogens in a variety of different sample types, including tissues and blood. This extracted DNA can then be used in any of a number of assays that utilize the nucleotide base-pairing characteristics of DNA to generate a diagnostic signal.

The DNA sequence of a gene characterized from three different, closely related organisms is shown in **Figure 4.9**. It can be seen that sequences consist of areas where the nucleotides are the same between the three species, while at other positions the bases vary. These sequence patterns reflect the fact that the product of the gene (e.g. an enzyme in this case) has areas that are critical and which must be composed of specific amino acids if the enzyme is to function and the organism to survive. Other positions, however, act as scaffolding to maintain the critical regions in the correct spatial orientation. In these areas the DNA and resultant amino acid sequence may be more variable. The degree of sequence conservation therefore varies between different regions of the same molecule. As two organisms evolve from a common ancestor, the nucleotide sequence of the genomes of the two progeny lines will change in a characteristic way. Mutations in non-critical regions of the genome are likely to be passed on to progeny and thus maintained, while the chance of a mutation in a critical region leading to a viable offspring, and thus transmis-

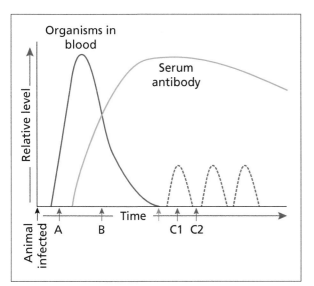

Fig. 4.8 An example of infection of an animal with a blood-borne pathogen. The relative level of organisms in the blood (solid and broken red lines) and serum antibody (green line) are shown against time following infection (black arrow). The point at which the animal is infected is indicated (black arrow) and when the organism first disappears from the blood (blue arrow). Different sampling points are indicated with red arrows and text.

```
Species A  1  5' GGTTAACGAT GTTAACATGA ACGAGTACTG GTACCATTTG AAACCAGACA ACGGCCAGTA 60

Species B  1  5' GGTTAACGAT GTTAACATGA TGCGATTATC CTGGATAATG TCGAGAGTCG TGGGCCTCAA 60

Species C  1  5' GGTTAACGAT GTTAACATGA ATGCGTACTA GTACCATTCA ATTACACACC ACGGCCAGTA 60


Species A  61 GGATCGGTTC GGGTTACCAA CTTAAGGCCT GCCCGGCACG ACACTAATTC CCGGGTTTAA 3' 120

Species B  61 CGTTGCGTAG CGGTGACCGA TGTAAGCCGA GCCCGGATTG ACACTAATTC CCGGGTTTAA 3' 120

Species C  61 CCATCGGTAC TGGTTACCAA TTAAAGGGCT GCCCGGATCG ACACTAATTC CCGGGTTTAA 3' 120
```

Fig. 4.9 An example of DNA sequences encoding a hypothetical gene from three related organisms (A–C). If primers or probes complementary to the sequence region highlighted in blue were used, then they would selectively anneal (hybridize) to the DNA from the target organism but not from the other two, provided suitable reaction conditions were used. Primers or probes complementary to the conserved regions (red) would anneal to DNA from all three species.

sion of this mutation, is much lower. This continuum of point mutation frequency allows discrimination between closely related organisms (which will differ in fast-changing non-critical regions) and more disparate organisms, where rare changes in critical regions will have occurred over a much longer time span.

All the methods described below exploit the fact that related organisms share DNA sequences; the more closely related two organisms are, the more highly conserved the nucleotide sequence of their genomes will be.

Polymerase chain reaction

PCR is a method that involves the amplification of target DNA sequences by repeated cycles of synthetic oligonucleotide primer-driven DNA synthesis. The key to the process is the use of a thermostable DNA polymerase (such as that derived from the hot spring bacterium *Thermus aquaticus*), which is optimally active at elevated temperatures (75–80°C) and maintains its activity when heated to the temperatures required to melt double-stranded DNA (e.g. 95°C). Therefore, newly synthesized double-stranded DNA can be dissociated, by heating, to act as templates for subsequent rounds of primer binding and DNA synthesis while maintaining polymerase enzyme activity **(Figure 4.10)**.

As the technology involved in determining the nucleotide sequences of pathogen genes has developed, a vast array of sequence information has been placed in databases such as GenBank. This information can be used to determine areas of genes that are conserved between species, genera and families of pathogenic organisms, or areas that are specific to individual strains. In parallel with this explosion of information, the commercial synthesis of oligonucleotide probes and the generation of economically priced, rapid DNA extraction kits mean that DNA-based diagnostic methods

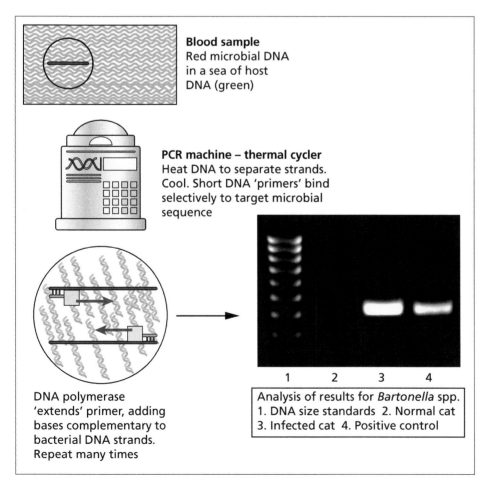

Blood sample
Red microbial DNA in a sea of host DNA (green)

PCR machine – thermal cycler
Heat DNA to separate strands. Cool. Short DNA 'primers' bind selectively to target microbial sequence

DNA polymerase 'extends' primer, adding bases complementary to bacterial DNA strands. Repeat many times

1   2   3   4

Analysis of results for *Bartonella* spp.
1. DNA size standards   2. Normal cat
3. Infected cat   4. Positive control

Fig. 4.10 The polymerase chain reaction process as a diagnostic tool.

have become widely available. In many cases, where microbial culture is impossible, slow or undesirable because of biohazard considerations, PCR is becoming the method of choice in the diagnostic laboratory because of its sensitivity, selectivity and speed.

A number of PCR methodologies are available, but the two most commonly used are conventional (end-point) and real-time (quantitative) PCR (qPCR). The primary difference between these methodologies is in the strategy used to measure the accumulation of the products from the amplification reaction. Conventional PCR measures the products at the end of the thermocycling protocol, while real-time PCR measures the accumulation during the thermocycling protocol using a fluorescent dye or fluorogenic-dye labelled probe **(Figures 4.11, 4.12)**.

A number of different test formats are available for qPCR, but the common factor is that as PCR product is produced, the amount of fluorescence increases proportionately. Fluorescence is monitored throughout the assay and these data are converted into quantitative results reflecting the amount of pathogen in the sample (rather than the qualitative results given by conventional PCR). Therefore, this method has great advantages in assessing pathogen 'load' and responses to treatment.

A number of different thermocycling platforms have been developed, many with the ability to monitor fluo-

Fig. 4.11 Real-time PCR using SYBR green.

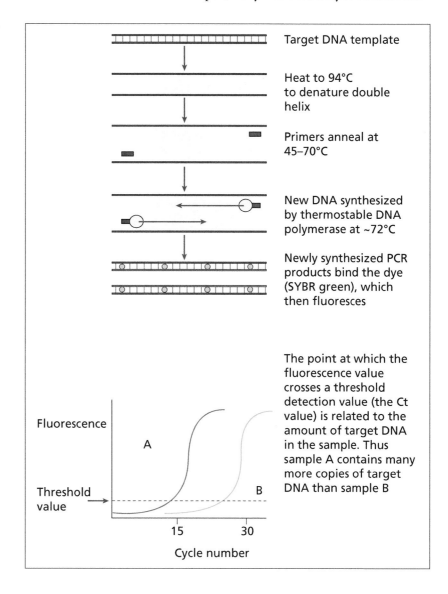

Alternative method 1. 'Taqman' probes. An oligonucleotide with a fluorophore (F) at one end and a quencher (Q) at the other is called a Taqman probe. This binds to the middle of the amplified portion of template DNA. As the DNA polymerase (P) copies the template it degrades the probe, releasing the fluorophore and emitting fluorescence

Alternative method 2. Molecular beacons. A hybridization probe is designed that has a central portion, which is complementary to the desired target. Each end of the probe has nucleotide sequences that are complementary to each other and allow base pairing to occur. The ends of the probe are labelled with a fluorescent reporter dye (R) and a quencher (Q). When the probe is 'zipped up' (no target template) there is no fluorescence, but when a template is available the probe unzips and fluorescence is emitted

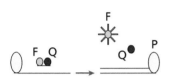

Fig. 4.12 **Real-time PCR using alternative methods to generate a fluorescence signal.**

rescence at a number of different wavelengths and thus multiple fluorescent dyes within a single sample. This gives rise to the potential to develop 'multiplex' assays where a number of different organisms, gene targets or reaction controls can be probed simultaneously. In multiplex systems, labelled probes with different fluorescent dyes are used with distinct, non-overlapping signal spectra. At each cycle during the assay, the machine assesses the fluorescence produced by the binding of each probe independently. This has the potential to increase the speed and reduce the costs of testing for multiple pathogens in a single sample. However, these multiplex assays can be technically difficult and costly to develop and require careful optimization to ensure that the individual reactions work efficiently within the multiplex, such that there is no reduction in assay sensitivity, particularly as infection with multiple agents is possible. A more common application of the multiplex potential of qPCR is the incorporation of an internal control reaction, which ensures the successful extraction and amplification of the DNA from a sample to reduce the chance of false-negative results due to experimental error or PCR inhibitors within the sample.

The major problem with all PCR-based methodologies is their extreme sensitivity. This makes contamination a major concern, and laboratory design should consider the need to keep reagent preparation, DNA extraction from samples, thermal cycling and agarose electrophoresis analysis (where conventional PCR is used) physically separate to minimize the generation of false-positive results.

Probe-based hybridization assays

Although PCR is the most commonly used molecular diagnostic technique, other methodologies have exploited the robust nature and unique structure of DNA to aid pathogen detection and identification. The double helical structure of DNA can be 'unzipped' by heating (as with PCR) or alkali treatment, without damaging the bonds between adjacent nucleotides. This results in two single-stranded molecules that can be immobilized (to stop re-annealing) onto inert supports such as nitrocellulose. These single-stranded molecules can then act as targets for labelled oligonucleotide probes, which are designed to have sequences complementary to a portion of the genome of a particular group of organisms (see **Figure 4.9**). This is the basis for a variety of probe-based blotting/hybridization assays derived from the original method devised by Southern in the 1970s.

Originally, radioactively labelled probes were used and autoradiography was necessary to demonstrate that binding of probe to target had occurred. More recently, enzyme-linked probes have been developed that allow

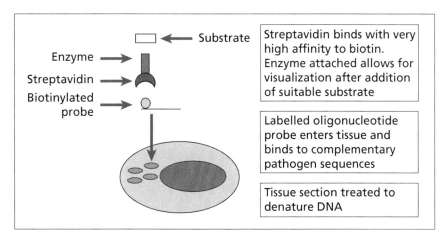

Fig. 4.13 *In-situ* hybridization. Enzyme-labelled oligonucleotide probes can be used to detect the presence of complementary DNA sequences in tissue samples. In this case a biotinylated oligonucleotide is shown.

Streptavidin binds with very high affinity to biotin. Enzyme attached allows for visualization after addition of suitable substrate

Labelled oligonucleotide probe enters tissue and binds to complementary pathogen sequences

Tissue section treated to denature DNA

for chromogenic or chemiluminescent detection of binding events. Fluorescent dyes have also been used to allow visualization of probe binding.

In-situ hybridization of probes (**Figure 4.13**) to bacterial (or viral) DNA has the potential for detecting infections in tissue sections or cytological preparations with sufficient infective load (**Figure 4.14**). This methodology has the advantage of allowing localization of the pathogen to a particular anatomical location and/or cell-type within the host. The usefulness of this technique as a routine laboratory diagnostic tool or in-practice test is limited by the equipment, expertise and time required to perform it and the sensitivity of this type of test, which is likely lower that other techniques (e.g. qPCR).

XENODIAGNOSIS

The difficulty in cultivating many tick-borne organisms can be circumvented by feeding laboratory reared, 'clean', arthropod vectors (e.g. ticks, fleas or flies) on presumptively infected blood. Under optimal environmental conditions, organisms will multiply rapidly in the appropriate vector and can be easily visualized by plain immunofluorescence enhanced microscopy. This amplification method has been used to advantage in the diagnosis of human *Trypanosoma cruzi* infection. Triatomid bug nymphs are allowed to feed on people with presumed chronic Chagas' disease. On engorgement (20–30 minutes), the bugs are removed and kept under controlled conditions for 20–30 days. At this time, motile trypanosomes are detected by darkfield

microscopy in the faeces and body contents of the bug if the person on whom it fed was infected. Although the use of this methodology has largely been replaced by alternative diagnostic methods (e.g. PCR), it is still used in research, particularly in the study of canine leishmaniosis.

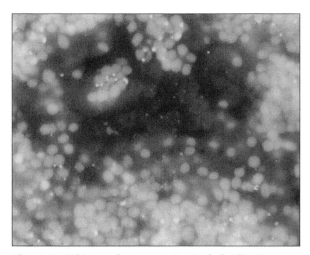

Fig. 4.14 This is a fluorescent *in-situ* hybridization (FISH) image taken from a section of spleen collected from a cat infected with *Mycoplasma haemofelis* (13 days post infection) and incubated with a digoxigenin-labelled probe targeting the 16S rDNA gene of *M. haemofelis*. The binding of the probe was visualized using a fluorescein-labelled anti-digoxigenin antibody. The *M. haemofelis* organisms can be identified on the surface of the red blood cells within the splenic sinusoids.

FURTHER READING

Allison RW, Little SE (2013) Diagnosis of rickettsial diseases in dogs and cats. *Veterinary Clinical Pathology* **42**:127–144.

Andrade RA, Silva Araujo MS, Reis AB *et al.* (2009) Advances in flow cytometric serology for canine visceral leishmaniasis: diagnostic applications when distinct clinical forms, vaccination and other canine pathogens become a challenge. *Veterinary Immunology and Immunopathology* **128**:79–86.

Barth C, Straubinger RK, Muller E *et al.* (2014) Comparison of different diagnostic tools for the detection of *Anaplasma phagocytophilum* in dogs. *Veterinary Clinical Pathology* **43**:180–184.

Chandrashekar R, Mainville CA, Beall MJ *et al.* (2010) Performance of a commercially available in-clinic ELISA for the detection of antibodies against *Anaplasma phagocytophilum*, *Ehrlichia canis*, and *Borrelia burgdorferi* and *Dirofilaria immitis* antigen in dogs. *American Journal of Veterinary Research* **71**:1443–1450.

de Andrade RA, Reis AB, Gontijo CM *et al.* (2007) Clinical value of anti-*Leishmania* (*Leishmania*) *chagasi* IgG titers detected by flow cytometry to distinguish infected from vaccinated dogs. *Veterinary Immunology and Immunopathology* **116**:85–97.

Drazenovich N, Foley J, Brown RN (2006) Use of real-time quantitative PCR targeting the msp2 protein gene to identify cryptic *Anaplasma phagocytophilum* infections in wildlife and domestic animals. *Vector Borne Zoonotic Diseases* **6**:83–90.

Duncan AW, Maggi RG, Breitschwerdt EB (2007) A combined approach for the enhanced detection and isolation of *Bartonella* species in dog blood samples: pre-enrichment liquid culture followed by PCR and subculture onto agar plates. *Journal of Microbiological Methods* **69**:273–281.

Eddlestone SM, Gaunt SD, Neer TM *et al.* (2007) PCR detection of *Anaplasma platys* in blood and tissue of dogs during acute phase of experimental infection. *Experimental Parasitology* **115**:205–210.

Gaunt S, Beall M, Stillman B *et al.* (2010) Experimental infection and co-infection of dogs with *Anaplasma platys* and *Ehrlichia canis*: hematologic, serologic and molecular findings. *Parasites and Vectors* **3**, 33.

Maggi RG, Birkenheuer AJ, Hegarty BC *et al.* (2014) Comparison of serological and molecular panels for diagnosis of vector-borne diseases in dogs. *Parasites and Vectors* **7**:127.

Oliva G, Scalone A, Foglia Manzillo V *et al.* (2006) Incidence and time course of *Leishmania infantum* infections examined by parasitological, serologic, and nested-PCR techniques in a cohort of naive dogs exposed to three consecutive transmission seasons. *Journal of Clinical Microbiology* **44**:1318–1322.

Otranto D, Testini G, Dantas-Torres F *et al.* (2010) Diagnosis of canine vector-borne diseases in young dogs: a longitudinal study. *Journal of Clinical Microbiology* **48**:3316–3324.

Rene-Martellet M, Lebert I, Chene J *et al.* (2015) Diagnosis and incidence risk of clinical canine monocytic ehrlichiosis under field conditions in Southern Europe. *Parasites and Vectors* **8**:3.

Srivastava P, Dayama A, Mehrotra S *et al.* (2010) Diagnosis of visceral leishmaniasis. *Transactions of the Royal Society of Tropical Medicine and Hygiene* **105**:1–6.

Wagner B, Freer H, Rollins A *et al.* (2011) A fluorescent bead-based multiplex assay for the simultaneous detection of antibodies to *B. burgdorferi* outer surface proteins in canine serum. *Veterinary Immunology and Immunopathology* **140**:190–198.

ACKNOWLEDGMENT

In the first edition of this book, this chapter was prepared by Martin Kenny. This revised and updated chapter is based on that original content and Dr Peters acknowledges this earlier work and Dr Kenny as the source of some of the illustrative material used in the chapter.

Chapter 5

Filarial Infections

Luca Ferasin
Luigi Venco

INTRODUCTION

Filarial infections (filariasis) are caused by roundworms (Phylum Nematoda) belonging to the order Spirurida, superfamily Filarioidea (commonly referred to as 'filarids'). There are approximately 200 species of filarial nematodes and some of them can cause severe pathologies in people and animals. These parasites require an arthropod intermediate host, commonly a biting insect, to complete their biological cycle and for transmission. The first larval stages (L1) of these filarial nematodes are known as microfilariae and are found in the bloodstream or in the subcutaneous tissues of the definitive host, from which they may be ingested during arthropod feeding. Adult nematodes may be found in a variety of different organs and tissues, depending on the species of parasite and the type of host. The microfilariae of each species have a characteristic morphology that may be used to diagnose the type of infection.

The primary pathological lesions occurring during filarial infections are caused by the presence of adults in a specific organ or tissue. However, the immune response against the parasites may also play a pivotal role in the pathophysiological mechanisms and, in many circumstances, microfilariae can also cause significant lesions.

Filarial infections are often classified according to the localization of the parasite within the host and the consequent pathological manifestations:

- Lymphatic filariasis (e.g. *Wucheria bancrofti* and *Brugia* species) is caused by the presence of nematodes in the lymphatic vessels.
- Subcutaneous filariasis (e.g. *Dirofilaria repens*, *Onchocerca volvulus*, *Loa loa*, *Dracunculus medinensis*) is caused by the presence of adults in the subcutaneous tissues, which can sometimes be seen migrating through the body.
- Dermal filariasis (filarids belonging to the genus *Cercopithifilaria*, which are transmitted by hard ticks [Ixodidae]), parasitize a range of host species, including dogs in which larvae reside only in the subcutaneous tissues and do not circulate in the bloodstream.
- Serous cavity filariasis (e.g. *Setaria* species, *Mansonella* species) is characterized by the presence of parasites in the pleural or peritoneal cavity.
- Cardiopulmonary filariasis (*Dirofilaria immitis*) is infection of the pulmonary arteries and the right side of the heart.
- Arterial filariasis (*Elaeophora schneideri*) is caused by the presence of adult worms in the systemic arteries.
- Ectopic filariasis is characterized by the incidental localization of a parasite in organs or tissues that are not typical of that particular species (e.g. the presence of *D. immitis* in systemic arteries).

The biology and epidemiology of the filarial parasites affecting dogs and cats are summarized in **Table 5.1**. The most important and geographically widespread filarial disease in the dog and cat is caused by *D. immitis* and is known as heartworm disease (HWD). *D. repens* is also frequently observed in pet animals and represents a more common zoonotic risk than *D. immitis*. *Dipetalonema reconditum* is another filarial nematode commonly found in dogs, but having minimal clinical significance.

Brugiasis (*B. malayi* and *B. pahangi*) is a filarial infection that affects lymph nodes and lymphatic vessels of dogs and cats in confined regions of south-east Asia.

Table 5.1 Biology and epidemiology of the principal agents of filarial infections.

Species	*Dirofilaria immitis*	*Dirofilaria (Nochtiella) repens*	*Dipetalonema reconditum*	*Brugia* spp.
Family	Onchocercidae	Onchocercidae	Setariidae	Onchocercidae
Common name(s) of the disease	Heartworm	Subcutaneous filariasis	Subcutaneous filariasis	Brugian filariasis, elephantiasis
Definitive hosts	Dogs, cats, wild canids and felids, sea lions, ferrets, humans	Dogs, cats, foxes, bears humans	Canids	Humans, felids, dogs, monkeys
Intermediate hosts	Mosquitoes	Mosquitoes	Fleas, ticks, lice	Mosquitoes
Geographical distribution	Tropical, subtropical and warm temperate areas of the world	Southern Europe, Africa, Asia, USA, Canada	USA, Africa, Italy, Spain	India, Malaysia, Southeast Asia
Morphology (adults)	M: 120–160 mm F: 250–300 mm	M: 50–70 mm F: 130–170 mm	M: 13 mm F: 23 mm	M: 20 mm × 200–300 µm F: 50 mm × 200–300 µm
Morphology (microfilariae)	300 × 8–10 µm	360 × 12 µm	270 × 4.5 µm	210 × 6 µm
Site of lesions (adults)	Right ventricle and pulmonary arteries; ectopic sites such as the eye, CNS, systemic arteries, body cavity	Subcutaneous tissues	Connective tissue; ectopic sites such as the body cavity and kidney	Lymph nodes and lymphatic vessels
Site of lesions (microfilariae)	Peripheral blood vessels	Peripheral blood vessels	Peripheral blood vessels	Lymphatic and capillary vessels

CARDIOPULMONARY DIROFILARIASIS (HEARTWORM DISEASE)

Background, aetiology and epidemiology

Dirofilariasis, or HWD, is a filarial infection caused by *Dirofilaria immitis* (**Figures 5.1, 5.2**). The parasite is located primarily in the pulmonary arteries and right side of the heart in dogs and, less commonly, cats and ferrets. The infection can also occur in other species, such as wild canids, California sea lions, harbour seals, wild felids and humans, but these species are normally considered 'aberrant' or 'dead-end' hosts since the parasites rarely undergo final maturation to complete their biological cycle. *D. immitis* has also been described in horses, beavers, bears, raccoons, wolverines, muskrats and red pandas.

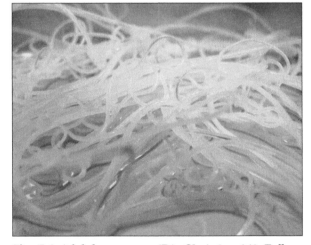

Fig. 5.1 Adult heartworms (*Dirofilaria immitis*). Fully mature adults at 6.5 months after infection reach lengths of 15–18 cm (males) and 25–30 cm (females).

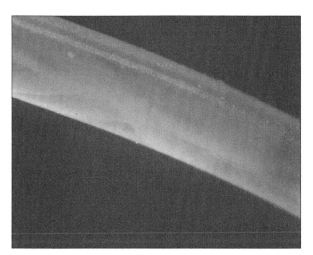

Fig. 5.2 Magnification of the cuticle of an adult heart-worm. Transverse striations can be observed, but longitudinal ridges, which are commonly present in other species of *Dirofilaria* (i.e. *Dirofilaria repens*), are lacking in *Dirofilaria immitis*.

Life cycle

Dirofilariasis is transmitted by a mosquito bite and there are more than 70 mosquito species that can potentially transmit the infection (**Table 5.2**).

Female *D. immitis* adults are viviparous and can release immature larvae (L1 or microfilariae) into the circulation. Microfilariae are ingested by a mosquito during a blood meal. Mosquitoes are not only vectors, but also obligatory intermediate hosts, and infection cannot be transmitted without a sufficient period of larval maturation (from L1 to L3) in the Malpighian tubules of the insect. The maturation period is variable, depending on environmental temperature. Development cannot occur below a threshold temperature of 14°C and the cycle will be temporarily suspended until warmer conditions resume. When the average daily temperature is 30°C the maturation can be completed in 8 days, while it takes approximately 1 month when the environmental temperature is 18°C. As a consequence, transmission of infective larvae is limited to warm seasons and it varies depending on the geographical location.

The infective L3 larvae migrate from the Malpighian tubules to the lumen of the labial sheath in the vector's mouth and, during a later blood meal on an appropri-ate host, the L3 larvae will exit the labium, enter the bite wound and penetrate local connective tissues. After approximately 1 week the larvae moult from L3 to L4 and, after a migration of 2–3 months in the subcutaneous tissues, moult to immature adults (L5). The L5 larvae penetrate a systemic vein and migrate to the right side of the heart and pulmonary arteries within a few days, where they mature and mate after approximately 3–6 months, releasing microfilariae into the circulation and perpetuating their life cycle (**Figure 5.3**).

The life expectancy of *D. immitis* is approximately 5–6 years in dogs and 2–3 years in cats. In experimental infections, the adult worms in cats do not reach the same size as in dogs and their development is slower; therefore, the average prepatent period is longer in cats (8 months) than in dogs (5–6 months). Furthermore, the worm burden in cats is typically lower than in dogs and microfilaraemia is uncommon (<20% of infected cats) and, when present, it is inconstant and transient. Thus, cats are poor reservoirs of infection, as *D. immitis* is less likely to mature in this species and adults are short-lived when present. The frequency of infection caused by *D. immitis* in cats is related to that in dogs living in the same area, but the prevalence is usually lower. Given that cats, when compared with dogs, are 2–4 times less prone to attract mosquitoes, and considering that 25% of cats are naturally resistant to infection with *D. immitis*, the prevalence in cats is approximately 10% of that found in dogs.

Dirofilariasis is present in several countries, with a variable prevalence that depends on the canine population, the presence of mosquito vectors and the climate. The climate must be sufficiently warm to allow the presence of mosquitoes and the development of larval stages in the insects. For this reason, the prevalence of dirofilariasis varies with both geographical area and season. This is an important concept to consider when screening for the disease or planning a chemoprophylactic schedule.

The disease has been diagnosed throughout North America, in most European countries and in Africa, Asia and Australia. In non-endemic countries, such as the UK, dirofilariasis may be diagnosed in dogs that have travelled from or through countries where infection is prevalent. However, climate change can potentially increase the risk of the disease even in current non-endemic areas.

Table 5.2 Potential vectors of *Dirofilaria immitis*.

SPECIES	GEOGRAPHICAL AREA WHERE LARVAL DEVELOPMENT IN THE MOSQUITO HAS BEEN REPORTED	SPECIES	GEOGRAPHICAL AREA WHERE LARVAL DEVELOPMENT IN THE MOSQUITO HAS BEEN REPORTED
Aedes aegypti	Brazil, Nigeria, USA, Japan	*Anopheles francisoi*	Philippines
Aedes albopictus	Taiwan, Brazil, Italy, Japan	*Anopheles maculopennis*	Europe
Aedes atropalpus	USA	*Anopheles minimus flavirostris*	Philippines
Aedes canadensis	USA	*Anopheles plumbeus*	Europe
Aedes caspius	Italy, Spain**	*Anopheles punctipennis*	USA
Aedes cinereus	USA	*Anopheles quadrimaculatus*	USA
Aedes excrucians	USA	*Anopheles sinensis*	China
Aedes fijensis	Fiji	*Anopheles tesellatus*	Philippines
Aedes fitchii	USA	*Anopheles walkeri*	USA
Aedes geniculatus	Europe	*Armigeres subalbatus*	Taiwan
Aedes guamensis	Guam	*Coquillettida perturbans*	USA
Aedes infirmatus	USA	*Culex anulorostris*	Guam, Fiji, Oceana
Aedes koreicus	China	*Culex bitaeniorhyncus*	Philippines
Aedes notoscriptus	Australia	*Culex declarator*	Brazil*
Aedes pandani	Guam	*Culex erraticus*	USA
Aedes pempaensis	Africa	*Culex gelidus*	Philippines
Aedes poecilus	Philippines,	*Culex pipiens*	USA, Switzerland, Italy
Aedes polynesiensis	French Polynesia, Fiji, Samoa	*Culex pipiens quinquefasciatus*	Australia, Philippines, USA, Fiji, Japan, Taiwan, Brazil, Guam, Oceana, Africa, Singapore
Aedes pseudoscutellaris	Fiji		
Aedes punctor	Europe		
Aedes samoanus	Samoa	*Culex pipiens molestus*	England
Aedes scapularis	Brazil	*Culex pipiens pallens*	Japan, China
Aedes sierrensis	USA	*Culex restuans*	USA
Aedes sollicitans	USA	*Culex saltanensis*	Brazil*
Aedes sticticus	USA	*Culex sitiens*	Guam
Aedes stimulans	USA	*Culex tarsalis*	USA
Aedes taeniorhyncus	USA, Brazil, Guyana	Culex territans	USA
Aedes togoi	Japan, Taiwan	*Culex tritaeniorhynchus*	Japan, China, Malaysia
Aedes togoi	Japan, Thailand	*Culex tritaeniorhynchus summorosus*	Philippines
Aedes triseriatus	USA		
Aedes trivittatus	USA	*Mansonia annulata*	Malaysia
Aedes vexans	USA, Switzerland	*Mansonia bonneae*	Malaysia
Aedes vigilax	Australia	*Mansonia dives*	Malaysia
Aedes zoosophus	USA	*Mansonia Indiana*	Malaysia
Anopheles bradleyi	USA	*Mansonia titillans*	Argentina
Anopheles crucians	USA	*Mansonia uniformis*	Singapore, Philippines
Anopheles earlei	USA	*Wyeomyia bourrouli*	Brazil*

Modified and updated from Ludlam *et al.*, 1970; *larvae isolated at non-infective stage; **suspected vector, but larvae not isolated from mosquito.

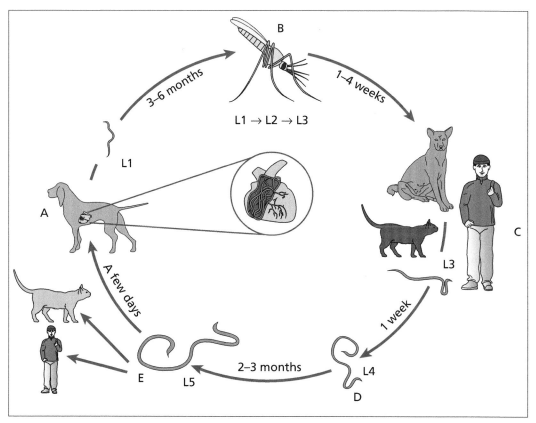

Fig. 5.3 Life cycle of *Dirofilaria immitis*. **(A)** Adult worms in the pulmonary arteries and right ventricle of the definitive host release immature larvae (L1 or microfilariae) into the circulation. Microfilaraemia is uncommon in cats and humans. **(B)** Microfilariae are ingested by a mosquito during a blood meal and they mature from L1 to L3 in the insect. **(C)** L3 larvae penetrate the local connective tissues of the host during a later blood meal. **(D)** The larvae moult from L3 to L4. **(E)** L4 mature in the subcutaneous tissues until they reach the pre-adult stage (L5). L5 larvae migrate to the right heart and pulmonary arteries where they mature and mate, releasing microfilariae into the circulation and perpetuating the life cycle.

Pathogenesis

Dirofilariasis is primarily a cardiopulmonary disease. The presence of adult nematodes in the pulmonary arteries causes proliferation of the intima with consequent narrowing and occlusion of the vessels and subsequent pulmonary hypertension and pulmonary infarction (**Figures 5.4–5.6**). Direct blockage by the adult worms is relatively rare. The severity and extent of lesions depend on the number and location of adult worms. The caudal lobar arteries are usually the most heavily parasitized. Severe pulmonary arterial disease may cause an increased permeability of lung vessels, with periarterial oedema and interstitial and alveolar cellular infiltration, which can result in irreversible pulmonary fibrosis. Pulmonary thromboembolism (PTE) is another potential sequela of dirofilariasis. It is initiated as a consequence of platelet aggregation following exposure of collagen secondary to endothelial damage induced by the parasite. Platelet aggregation may also be responsible for the release of platelet-derived growth factor (PDGF), which promotes proliferation of medial smooth muscle cells and fibroblasts. PTE

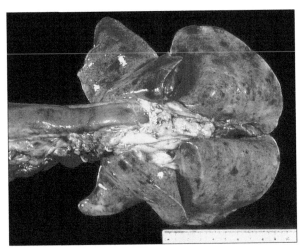

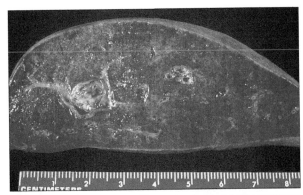

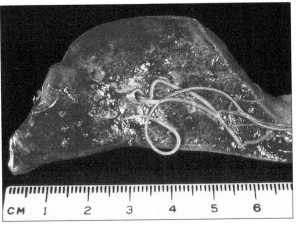

Figs. 5.4–5.6 Lungs of a dog with dirofilariasis. The presence of adult nematodes in the pulmonary arteries causes proliferation of the intima with consequent narrowing and occlusion of the vessels. Severe pulmonary arterial disease may cause increased permeability of lung vessels with periarterial oedema and interstitial and alveolar cellular infiltrate. (5.4, above) The entire lungs appear oedematous, with areas of haemorrhagic infarction. (5.5, above right) Section of a lung lobe showing inflammatory oedema and a large area of infarction. (5.6, right) Adult parasites in the lumen of a large pulmonary artery.

can also occur in response to adult worm death, either as a spontaneous event or induced by adulticidal treatment. Experimental intravenous administration of *D. immitis* extract induces shock in dogs and, even more often, in cats as a consequence of mast cell degranulation and histamine release. This phenomenon seems to be caused by an unknown substance contained in the parasite extract and may explain the circulatory collapse that is occasionally seen in dogs after the spontaneous death of parasites or adulticidal treatment.

In cases of severe infection, particularly where a large number of parasites mature concurrently, retrograde displacement from the pulmonary artery to the right ventricle, right atrium and venae cavae may occur (**Figures 5.7–5.9**). This induces incompetence of the tricuspid valve, which, in association with the concurrent pulmonary hypertension, is the cause of backward, right-sided heart failure (jugular distension, liver congestion and ascites; **Figure 5.10**). Additionally, in heavy burdens, erythrocyte membranes may be damaged as cells pass

through the mass of intravascular parasites, causing haemolysis and haemoglobinaemia. The presence of tricuspid incompetence, right-sided heart failure with hepatomegaly, poor cardiac output and intravascular haemolysis with resultant haemoglobinaemia and haemoglobinuria is referred to as 'caval syndrome'. Severe cases of caval syndrome can also be characterized by the presence of adult worms in the caudal vena cava and thromboembolic events accompanied by disseminated intravascular coagulation (DIC). The pathogenesis of caval syndrome is not fully understood, even though the retrograde displacement of adult nematodes from the pulmonary arteries to the right ventricle, right atrium and venae cavae, secondary to increased pulmonary pressure, seems the most plausible explanation.

Immune-complex glomerular disease is also reported commonly in dogs with dirofilariasis. It is characterized by protein-losing nephropathy (PLN), with hypoalbuminaemia and, eventually, reduced plasma antithrombin III (ATIII), which may exacerbate the development

Figs. 5.7–5.9 Necropsy specimens from a case of canine dirofilariasis. Right-side enlargement is primarily a consequence of the concomitant pulmonary hypertension. In cases of severe infestation, the migration of the parasites in the right ventricle and right atrium can contribute to the development of right heart enlargement. (5.7, right) Severe right ventricular enlargement (arrowheads). Hepatomegaly and liver congestion may also be appreciated. (5.8, below left) Magnification of the same heart. The right side appears significantly larger than the left. (5.9, below right) Section of the right ventricle showing numerous adult parasites.

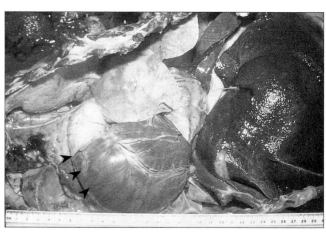

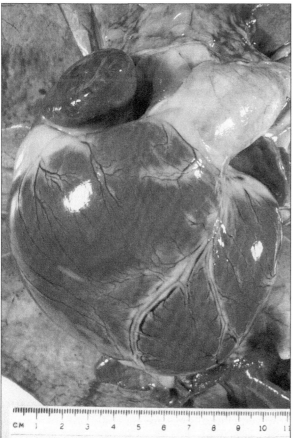

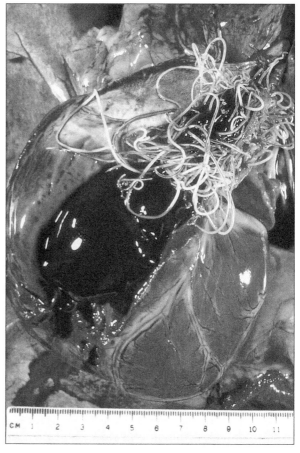

of PTE. The antigen that causes the immune-complex disease is unknown, but it could be a substance released by circulating microfilariae.

In cats, pulmonary hypertension, right-sided heart failure and caval syndrome are less common. In this species, the presence of parasites in the distal pulmonary arteries may induce a diffuse pulmonary infiltration and eosinophilic pneumonia. As in dogs, the subsequent death of adult parasites may cause acute pulmonary arterial infarction and the lung lobe involved can become haem-

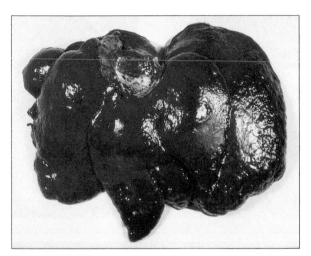

Fig. 5.10 Chronic hepatic congestion in a dog with caval syndrome. Hepatomegaly is present and the parenchyma appears dark as a consequence of blood stasis. Eventually, the liver parenchyma may become fibrotic with increased connective tissue and atrophy of the hepatocytes. These lesions are responsible for the portal hypertension and ascites.

orrhagic, with areas of oedema. If the cat survives the initial embolic lesion, recanalization around the obstruction occurs rapidly and pulmonary function can markedly improve within days, with remission of the clinical signs.

The pathogenesis of HWD in cats appears to follow different stages. The first phase begins after the arrival of juvenile larvae, 3 months after infection, into the caudal pulmonary arteries. Cats can develop severe pulmonary disease even in the absence of fully mature worms. During this phase, cats may experience acute episodes of coughing, dyspnoea or intermittent vomiting, known as feline heartworm-associated respiratory disease (HARD). Since most immature worms do not survive in cats after they reach the caudal pulmonary arteries, it is thought that this acute disease is related to the death and embolization of worms or worm fragments. This induces a strong inflammatory response in the vessels and pulmonary parenchyma, with subsequent infarction of the pulmonary parenchyma and circulatory collapse. Other signs of HARD may include neurological signs (e.g. ataxia, head tilt, blindness, circling or seizures) and sudden death.

If juvenile parasites develop into adult stages, suppression of the immune system and resolution of

clinical signs may occur. Once the adult parasites die (spontaneously or following medical treatment) the downregulation of the immune system terminates and the most severe form of the disease may appear. Indeed, the decomposing worms trigger a dramatic inflammatory and thromboembolic response, leading to sudden or acute death in approximately 20% of cats. In cats surviving the worm death, hyperplastic type II alveolar cells replace the normal type I cells, which may cause permanent respiratory dysfunction and chronic respiratory disease, representing a final stage of the disease. Ultimately, 80% of cats naturally infected by *D. immitis* self-cure.

Occasionally, adult worms can migrate to sites other than the heart and the pulmonary arteries and cause ectopic infection. Localization of *D. immitis* has been reported in the eye, central nervous system (cerebral arteries and lateral ventricles), systemic arteries and subcutaneous tissue. Ectopic infections are more commonly seen in cats than in dogs, suggesting that the parasite is not well adapted to feline hosts.

Much of the recent focus on heartworm immunology and pathophysiology has been on the role of *Wolbachia*. *Wolbachia* is an intracellular gram-negative bacterium belonging to the order Rickettsiales and is an endosymbiont of some pathogenic filarid nematodes. Antibodies against *Wolbachia* surface protein (WSP) have been detected in naturally infected dogs and cats. In experimentally infected cats, anti-WSP antibodies remain high even after the disappearance of antibodies to *D. immitis*. *Wolbachia* certainly plays a role in the pathogenesis of canine and feline heartworm infection, although the precise role remains unclear.

Clinical signs in dogs

Dirofilariasis may be completely asymptomatic; however, clinical signs are generally present in cases with a high worm burden and/or when there is a significant allergic response of the host to the parasite. Infected patients may present with an acute onset of clinical signs but, more often, the disease develops slowly and gradually. Furthermore, clinical signs of dirofilariasis are triggered or exacerbated by exertion, and patients that perform little exercise may never show overt signs of HWD. In dogs, coughing is the most common clinical sign, followed by tachypnoea and dyspnoea, exercise intolerance, chronic weight loss and syncope. In severe cases, haemoptisis can be present as a possible consequence of pulmonary arterial rupture. Jugular distension, hepatomegaly, ascites and marked exercise intolerance are typical signs of right-sided heart failure. In these cases, a systolic heart murmur or split second heart sound can be heard on thoracic auscultation, with a point of maximum intensity over the right apex. Hindlimb lameness and paresis have been described in dogs with aberrant arterial localization of the parasites.

Caval syndrome, a severe complication of HWD, is characterized by anorexia and weight loss, respiratory distress, haemoglobinuria secondary to intravascular haemolysis, signs of right-sided heart failure and possibly DIC. Its onset is due to a sudden increase in pulmonary arterial pressure (thromboembolism) with displacement of the majority of worms into the right cardiac chambers.

Diagnosis in dogs

Diagnostic investigations are justified only if there is a previous history of exposure to mosquitoes in an area where *D.immitis* infection is likely to be present.

Laboratory diagnosis of heartworm infection in dogs can be achieved by detecting circulating microfilariae or adult worm antigens in the blood. However, further diagnostic procedures are usually required to determine the severity of disease and identify the most suitable treatment.

Tests to identify microfilariae

Direct microscopic examination can be performed by examining a drop of fresh blood under the microscope. If present, the microfilariae can be easily identified because they can vigorously move the surrounding red blood cells. Although this method offers an easy and inexpensive diagnosis, it is not sufficiently sensitive, especially when there is a low concentration of microfilariae in the blood stream. Filtration methods (Difiltest®; Vetoquinol Inc.) and the modified 'Knott's test' (haemolysis, centrifugation and staining with methylene blue) are more sensitive and allow morphological examination of the microfilariae. Identification of microfilariae as *D.immitis* on the basis of morphology can be considered to be definitive proof of infection (specificity 100%) (**Figures 5.11a, b, Table 5.3**).

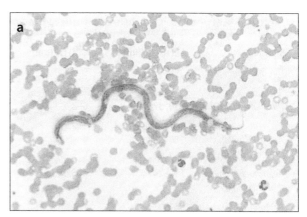

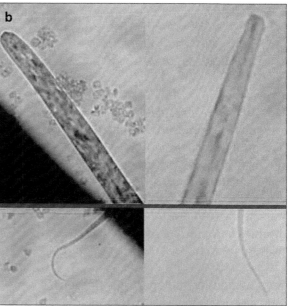

Figs. 5.11a, b (a) L1 larva (microfilaria) identified by the Knott's test. The larva is surrounded by red blood cells and its dark colour is due to the methylene blue staining (×100 magnification). (b) Microfilariae of *D. repens* (left) and *D. immitis* (right). *D. immitis* microfilaria are shorter (295–322 μm × 6–7.0 μm) and have a tapered head and a straight tail compared with the longer *D. repens* microfilariae (350–370 μm × 8–9.0 μm), which have a blunt head and a curved (umbrella handle-like) tail. The cephalic space of *D. repens* is further characterized by being short and commonly terminating with a distinct pair of nuclei that are separate from the remaining somatic nuclei of the microfilaria. The cephalic space of the smaller microfilariae of *D. immitis* is longer and does not have the distinct nuclei separated from the somatic column nuclei near the anterior end.

Table 5.3 **Morphological features of microfilariae from filarial worms of dogs and cats.**

SPECIES	LENGTH (µm)	WIDTH (µm)	FEATURES
Dirofilaria immitis[1]	295–322	5–7	No sheath, cephalic end tapered, tail straight with the end pointed
Dirofilaria repens[1]	350–370	6–8	No sheath, cephalic end obtuse, tail sharp and filiform ending as an umbrella handle
Acanthocheilonema reconditum[1]	260–283	4	No sheath, cephalic end obtuse with a prominent cephalic hook, tail button hooked and curved
Acanthocheilonema dracunculoides[2]	190–247	4–6.5	Sheath, cephalic end obtuse, caudla end sharp and extended
Cercopithifilaria grassi[1]	567	12–25	Sheath, caudal end slightly curved

[1] measurements obtained on Knott's test.

[2] measurements obtained from uterus of adult parasites.

However, up to 30% of dogs do not have circulating microfilariae even when they harbour adult worms. The presence of worms of the same sex, the immune reactivity of the host to microfilariae and administration of microfilaricidal drugs reduce dramatically the diagnostic yield obtained with these tests. Therefore, the sensitivity of test for microfilariae is considered insufficient to rule out the infection in case of negative test.

Tests to identify adult parasite antigens

Tests designed to detect *D. immitis* adult antigens based on ELISA or colloidal gold staining techniques are currently available as either 'in-house' tests or laboratory tests and their sensitivity and specificity approach 100%. These tests allow detection of specific circulating proteins released by the reproductive tract of mature female worms and can also provide information about worm burden. Cross-reactivity with other filarial parasites (i.e. *D. repens* and *Dipetalonema* species) does not occur. However, false-positive results can occur following cross-reactions of sera from dogs infected experimentally with *Angiostrongylus vasorum*. Because of this potential cross-reaction with *A. vasorum* with commercially available tests, simultaneous use of highly specific diagnostic methods for the differentiation of these two canine heartworms may be recommended in endemic regions. Sensitivity is also very high, although small worm burdens, presence of immature females or male only infections are common causes of low antigen titres and false-negative responses. Furthermore, antigens have occasionally been reported to be trapped by immune complexes, preventing detection by the antigen test (antigen masking phenomenon).

Haematology and biochemistry

Routine laboratory work-up is usually insufficient to provide a definitive diagnosis. Haematological examination often reveals eosinophilia and basophilia in the early stage of infection. Microfilariae can occasionally be seen on examination of the blood smear.

Serum biochemistry may show changes related to secondary organ involvement (e.g. increased hepatic enzymes or increased blood urea and creatinine in cases of hepatic or renal damage respectively). C-reactive protein (CRP), a blood marker of inflammation and a hallmark of the acute-phase response, has been shown to increase in dogs with HWD. This increase seems to be mostly related to vascular disease leading to pulmonary hypertension rather than the worm burden. The CRP level appears to be associated with the severity of the pulmonary vascular disease, which can persist even after adulticide therapy, suggesting a possible permanent pulmonary vascular damage.

Antibody testing for dirofilariasis

Antibody testing provides information about previous exposure, but not necessarily about current infection.

Consequently, antibody tests are more useful to rule out rather than confirm infection. These tests are no longer used in dogs, given their low specificity and the widespread availability of highly reliable antigen tests.

Polymerase chain reaction testing

Polymerase chain reaction (PCR)-based tests may represent a very sensitive and specific diagnostic tool for routine identification of mature and immature adult worms, especially in unconventional hosts. Direct PCR is capable of directly detecting first larval stages in the blood, third larval stages in the mosquito vector and fragments of mature stages of *Dirofilaria* species.

Thoracic radiography

Survey radiographs of the thorax may show, in advanced stages, a bulge at the level of the main pulmonary artery, enlarged and tortuous pulmonary arteries and an interstitial and/or alveolar pattern. An enlarged right side of the heart and caudal vena cava, hepatomegaly and ascites can be observed in cases of severe infection with caval syndrome. Although thoracic radiographs are useful to assess the severity of pulmonary lesions, they cannot provide information on worm burden. Indeed, some severe lung lesions can be associated with a low worm burden, while some sedentary dogs with large worm burdens may reveal trivial radiographic lesions (**Figures 5.12a, b**). Depending on the severity of the lesions, some radiographic findings can persist even after successful adulticide treatment.

Electrocardiography

Some electrocardiographic abnormalities can be observed in the last stage of the disease and they are mainly characterized by changes associated with right atrial and right ventricular remodelling, such as right bundle branch block, atrial fibrillation, supraventricular and ventricular ectopic beats.

Echocardiography

Echocardiography allows direct visualization of adult parasites in the main pulmonary artery and proximal tract of both caudal pulmonary arteries as double-lined

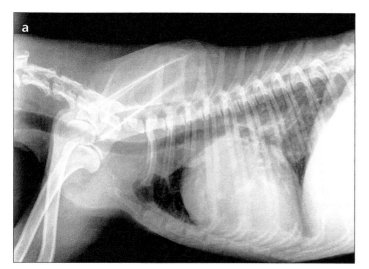
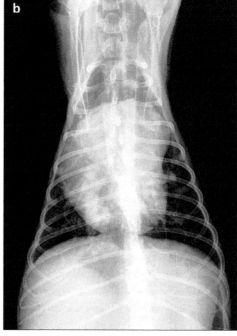

Figs. 5.12a, b Thoracic radiograph of an 8-year-old dog affected by heartworm disease. (a) Right lateral view. Observable lesions include clear enlargement of the cranial and main pulmonary arteries caused by pulmonary hypertension and a rounded cranial border of the cardiac silhouette suggesting right ventricular dilation. (b) Ventrodorsal view. The main pulmonary artery is enlarged, appearing as a distinct bulge at 2 o'clock of the cardiac silhouette. The reversed 'D shape' of the cardiac silhouette suggests right ventricle enlargement. Dilation of both caudal pulmonary arteries is also visible.

hyperechoic structures (**Figures 5.13a, b**) resulting from the echogenicity of the body wall of the parasite. Parasites can also occasionally be seen in the right ventricle, right atrium and caudal vena cava. In severe cases, echocardiography may also reveal signs of pulmonary hypertension (right ventricular hypertrophy, right atrial dilation and high-velocity tricuspid regurgitation)

(**Figures 5.13c, d**). Cardiac ultrasound can increase the accuracy in staging the disease and estimating the worm burden, both of which may affect treatment planning and the prognosis. Finally, ultrasonography can be particularly useful for detection of hepatomegaly, liver congestion and ascites and identification of parasites in ectopic lesions.

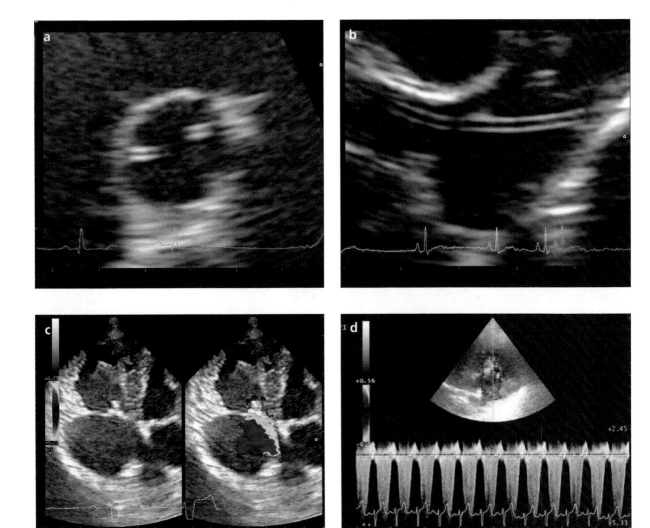

Figs. 5.13a–d Echocardiographic images of a dog affected by heartworm disease. (a) Right parasternal short-axis view; two adult worm echoes are visible in the transverse section of the right pulmonary artery. (b) Right parasternal short-axis view; an adult parasite is seen as double, short parallel lines floating across the right and main pulmonary artery. (c) Left parasternal apical four-chamber view. Right atrium and right ventricle appear dilated, while the colour flow Doppler examination shows systolic tricuspid regurgitation. (d) Continuous wave spectral Doppler interrogation of the tricuspid valve shows systolic valvular regurgitation. The peak velocity of the regurgitant flow allows estimation of systolic pulmonary pressure (approximately 5 m/s in this case, which equates to 100 mmHg of pulmonary pressure).

Therapy in dogs

Several strategies for HWD therapy should be considered, including conservative options. Prior to therapy, each patient should be thoroughly assessed and rated for risk of adverse reactions. Important factors to consider include the expected worm burden based on ELISA testing and echocardiographic examination, size and age of the dog, concurrent diseases, severity of pulmonary lesions and the possibility for stringently restricting exercise during and after adulticide therapy. According to these considerations, patients can be classified as having 'high' or 'low' risk of thromboembolic complications (**Table 5.4**).

Supportive therapy

Anti-inflammatory doses of glucocorticoids (e.g. prednisolone 0.5 mg/kg PO q24h or q12h for 5 days) can control pulmonary inflammation and possibly reduce the risk of thromboembolism. Thoracocentesis and abdominocentesis associated with diuretics (e.g. furosemide 1 mg/kg q12h) are often necessary to control signs of right-sided congestive heart failure. Digoxin (0.03–0.05 mg/kg PO q12h) and diltiazem sustained release (2–5 mg/kg PO q12h) should be administered, alone or in combination, to control atrial fibrillation with rapid ventricular response rate. The use of antiplatelet aggregation prophylaxis, such as aspirin (1–2 mg/kg PO q24h), is highly controversial and convincing evidence of its clinical benefit is lacking. Exercise restriction and, in selected cases, cage rest seem to be the most important measures to improve cardiopulmonary circulation and reduce signs associated with pulmonary hypertension.

Adulticide therapy

The severity of the heartworm infection should be carefully evaluated to determine the optimum treatment protocol and provide a more accurate prognosis. Adulticidal treatment consists of the administration of melarsomine dihydroclhloride, an arsenical compound of relatively new generation. Melarsomine is injected intramuscularly into the lumbar muscles at a recommended dose of 2.5 mg/kg, repeated after 24 hours. In order to reduce the risk of PTE, a more gradual two-step approach is recommended by injecting a single dose followed by administration of the standard pair of injections at least 50 days later. It appears that one administration of melarsomine can kill approximately 90% of male worms and 10% of female worms, therefore resulting in an approximately 50% reduction of the worm burden and reducing the risk of parasitic embolism and shock. For this reason, the three-injection alternative protocol represents the treatment of choice of the American Heartworm Society and of several academic teaching hospitals, regardless of disease stage.

PTE is an inevitable risk of a successful adulticide therapy. If several worms die simultaneously, widespread pulmonary thrombosis frequently develops. Mild thromboembolism may be clinically unobserved, but in severe cases, life-threatening respiratory distress can occur. These complications can be reduced by exercise restriction or, in selected cases, complete cage

Table 5.4 **Clinical classification of patients classified as having 'high' or 'low' risk of thromboembolic complications following adulticide treatment.**

LOW RISK OF THROMBOEMBOLIC COMPLICATIONS	HIGH RISK OF THROMBOEMBOLIC COMPLICATIONS
(dogs included in this group must satisfy all of these conditions)	(dogs that do not satisfy one or more of these conditions)
No clinical signs	Clinical signs related to the disease (e.g. coughing, syncope, ascites)
Normal thoracic radiographs	Abnormal thoracic radiographs
Low level of circulating antigens or a negative antigen test with circulating microfilariae	High level of circulating antigens
No worms visualized by echocardiography	Worms visualized by echocardiography
No concurrent diseases	Concurrent diseases
Possibility of exercise restriction	No possibility of exercise restriction

rest, for 30–40 days following treatment. Concomitant administration of calcium heparin and anti-inflammatory doses of glucocorticoids may also be indicated.

Certain macrolides have adulticidal properties and experimental studies have shown partial adulticidal properties of ivermectin when used continuously for 16 months at preventive doses (6–12 µg/kg PO monthly) and 100% adulticidal efficacy if administered continuously for over 30 months. While there may be a role for this therapeutic strategy in the very few and selected cases in which patient age, financial constraints or concurrent medical problems prohibit melarsomine therapy, ivermectin is not a substitute for the primary adulticidal approach, and this kind of therapeutic approach should be used cautiously. In fact, the adulticide effect of ivermectin is slow in action and it takes some time before heartworms are completely eliminated. Furthermore, older worms are slower to die when exposed to ivermectin and, in the meantime, the infection may persist and continue to cause organ damage and clinical signs.

There is also some evidence that treatment of *Wolbachia* organisms with doxycycline can improve clinical outcomes in dogs. Therefore, the American Heartworm Society currently recommends doxycycline (10 mg/kg PO q12h for 4 weeks) as part of a heartworm treatment protocol, and it should be given prior to melarsomine administration so that the organisms and their metabolites are reduced when worms die and fragment. A combination of ivermectin and doxycycline may be used instead of adulticide therapy if melarsomine administration is contraindicated or the patient's condition makes melarsomine treatment difficult.

Surgical removal

Surgical removal of heartworms has been well documented both in dogs and cats. This approach is always recommended when several worms appear to be located in the right cardiac chambers associated with signs of right-sided cardiac failure (caval syndrome). Surgical removal can be accomplished under general anaesthesia with flexible alligator forceps (e.g. Ishihara forceps) introduced via the jugular vein. Flexible alligator forceps inserted under fluoroscopic guidance can access the right cardiac chambers as well as the pulmonary arteries (**Figure 5.14**). Overall survival and recovery rate improves dramatically in dogs with high risk of PTE after successful surgical removal.

However, this procedure requires dedicated instrumentation and expertise, and the anaesthetic risk, possible damage to cardiac structures and the potential hazard of postoperative ventricular arrhythmias should be carefully evaluated. Transoesophageal echocardiography may represent a useful complementary tool to fluoroscopic guidance.

Clinical signs in cats

Although susceptible to infection, cats are somewhat resistant to *D. immitis*. Increased host resistance is reflected by the relatively low adult worm burden in natural infections (1–6 worms with 2–4 worms being the average burden). Furthermore, the prolonged prepatent period (8 months), the absent or transient microfilaraemia and the short life span of adult worms (2–3 years) are other facts suggesting that cats are not ideal hosts for *D. immitis*. Although changes in the pulmonary arteries and lungs following *Dirofilaria* infection seem similar to those observed in dogs, right cardiac chamber enlargement and right-sided heart failure are unusual finding in cats.

Most cats seem to tolerate *Dirofilaria* infection better than dogs and for a longer period of time. The most common clinical signs observed in cats are cough and dyspnoea, sometimes associated with vomiting. Diar-

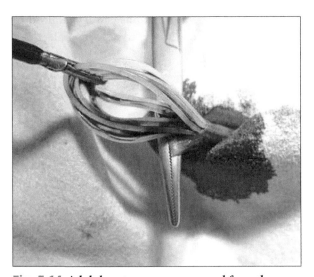

Fig. 5.14 Adult heartworms are removed from the pulmonary arteries via jugular vein access using flexible alligator forceps ('Ishihara' technique).

rhoea and weight loss can be occasionally observed. Sudden death in apparently healthy cats may also represent a possible outcome.

Diagnosis in cats
Tests to identify microfilariae
Since microfilaraemia in cats is unlikely, sensitivity of tests for detection of circulating microfilariae is very low, despite their high specificity.

Tests to identify adult parasite antigens
Tests detecting adult heartworm antigens can provide definitive proof of infections in cats because of their very high specificity. Unfortunately, false-negative results in cats are relatively common due to the typical low worm burden in this species or to infections caused by male adults or immature worms. Furthermore, negative results secondary to antigen masking are more common in cats than in dogs.

Antibody testing for dirofilariasis
Because of the low sensitivity of the above tests, detection of antibodies to adult heartworms can be particularly useful in cats. Antibody tests are currently available for routine screening of feline heartworm infection, either as 'in-house' tests or laboratory tests. Antibody testing provides information about previous expo-sure, but does not necessarily prove current infection. Consequently, antibody tests are more useful to rule out rather than confirm an infection. Cross-reactivity with other parasites or antibodies to abortive infections further reduces the test specificity.

Polymerase chain reaction testing for dirofilariasis
Although little information is available about the use of PCR to detect the presence of heartworms in cats, initial results suggest that this technology can provide a useful diagnostic tool to detect the low level *D. immitis* infection in feline HWD.

Thoracic radiography
Thoracic radiographs are an important tool for the diagnosis of feline HWD. Although thoracic abnormalities in some cases are absent or transient, typical findings include enlarged peripheral branches of the pulmonary arteries accompanied by varying degrees of pulmonary parenchymal disease (**Figure 5.15**). Unlike dogs, right-sided cardiomegaly is not considered a common radiographic finding in cats.

Non-selective angiocardiography
Non-selective angiocardiography is useful in visualizing the gross morphology of the pulmonary arteries

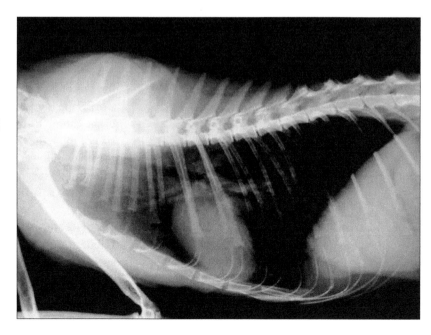

Fig. 5.15 Thoracic radiograph, right lateral view, of a 6-year-old female cat with sudden onset of severe dyspnoea caused by heartworm disease. Sudden truncation ('pruning') of the pulmonary arteries and peripheral undercirculation suggests the presence of pulmonary thromboembolism.

and sometimes heartworms can be seen as negative filling defects within opacified arteries.

Electrocardiography

Heartworm infections in cats rarely cause right-sided cardiac lesions and, consequently, electrocardiography is rarely abnormal in infected cats.

Echocardiography

Adult parasites are sometimes observed in the main pulmonary artery and proximal tract of both its peripheral branches (**Figure 5.16**). Specificity is virtually 100%, but sensitivity is affected by the ultrasonographical visualization of the pulmonary arteries, which is often reduced by acoustic impedance of the air-inflated lungs.

Transtracheal lavage

The presence of eosinophils in a tracheal wash, with or without eosinophilia, may be noted in cats 4–7 months after infection, although this finding is not specific and infection with other pulmonary parasites (e.g. *Paragonimus kellicotti*, *Aelurostrongylus abstrusus*), allergic pneumonitis and feline asthma should be ruled out.

The interpretation of heartworm diagnostic procedures and tests in cats is summarized in **Table 5.5**.

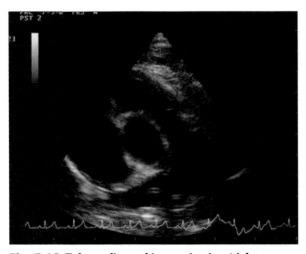

Fig. 5.16 Echocardiographic examination (right parasternal short-axis view) of an adult cat affected by heartworm disease. The pair of short parallel echoes indicates the presence of adult heartworms in the main pulmonary artery.

Therapy in cats
Supportive therapy

Cage rest, oxygen supplementation, fluid therapy, bronchodilators and injectable steroids (e.g. dexamethasone) can be used to stabilize those cats that become acutely ill. Prednisolone can be started at 0.5 mg/kg PO q24h or q12h for 4–5 days, tapering the dose to 0.25–0.5 mg/kg PO q48h. Higher doses may be indicated in case of acute respiratory distress secondary to parasitic embolization of dead worms.

Adulticide therapy

In cats, adulticidal treatment can be dangerous even in patients with low-grade infection, and the risk of PTE due to premature parasite death is high. Some cats undergo spontaneous clinical remission after the natural death of *D. immitis* adults and, therefore, adulticidal treatment may not be warranted. Thiacetarsamide is the only arsenical compound used in cats in the field. The use of this drug in cats is debatable since infected cats may develop acute respiratory distress or sudden death in the post-treatment period, most likely caused by parasite embolization following worm death.

The use of melarsomine in cats is not advised because of incomplete efficacy in killing worms with the same regimen used in dogs (2.5 mg/kg) and because of the high toxicity in this species.

Surgical removal

In cases of caval syndrome, or when a heavy worm burden is seen by echocardiography, surgical removal may be attempted. As described in dogs, adult worms can be extracted via the jugular vein using thin alligator forceps or basket catheters. The incidental rupture of worms during the procedure may result in the death of the cat (up to 30% of cases). Furthermore, the small size of the feline heart and pulmonary arteries makes the procedure very challenging. Because of these considerations, surgical removal of heartworms in cats is considered a particularly risky procedure.

Dirofilariasis in ferrets

Laboratory studies have shown that ferrets are highly susceptible to HWD, with infection and recovery rates similar to those observed in the dog. Microfilaraemia is minimal and transient, similar to that seen in heartworm-infected cats. A definitive diagnosis can be

Table 5.5 **Interpretation of heartworm diagnostic procedures and tests in cats.**

TEST	BRIEF DESCRIPTION	RESULT	INTERPRETATION	COMMENTS
Antibody test	Detects antibodies produced by the cat in response to presence of heartworm larvae. May detect infections as early as 8 weeks post transmission by mosquito	Negative	Lowers index of suspicion	Antibodies confirm infection with heartworm larvae, but do not confirm disease causality
		Positive	Increases index of suspicion; 50% or more of cats will have pulmonary arterial disease; confirms cat is at risk	
Antigen test	Detects antigen produced by the adult female heartworm	Negative	Lowers index of suspicion	Immature or male only worm infections are not detected. Heat treatment of samples prior to testing increases their sensitivity
		Positive	Diagnosis	
Thoracic radiography	Detects vascular enlargement (inflammation caused by young L5 and, later, hypertrophy), pulmonary parenchymal inflammation and oedema	Normal	No change to index of suspicion	Radiographic signs subjective and affected by clinical interpretation
		Signs consistent with feline heartworm disease	Enlarged arteries. Feline asthma like signs. Increases index of suspicion	
Echocardiography	Detects echogenic walls of the immature or mature heartworm residing in the lumen of the pulmonary arterial tree	No worms seen	No change to index of suspicion	Sonographer experience and equipment quality greatly influence accuracy rate
		Worms seen	Diagnosis	

Modified from the American Heartworm Society: Current Feline Guidelines for the Prevention, Diagnosis, and Management of Heartworm (*Dirofilaria immitis*) Infection in Cats (2014).

achieved using ELISA-based antigen tests and echocardiography. Prevention has been shown to be effective with currently used canine prophylactic pharmaceutical agents, but effective treatment of adult heartworms in ferrets has not yet been confirmed by controlled studies. Treatment with melarsomine has been reported in ferrets, but its efficacy is lower than in dogs and with a higher fatality rate secondary to thromboembolism. In one experimental study, a single injection of moxidectin (sustained release) was demonstrated to be an effective and safe therapeutic alternative.

Prophylaxis

Chemoprophylaxis is typically recommended for all pets living in endemic areas during the transmission period. Clinicians should be aware of the changing seasonality of mosquitoes in their geographical regions in order to prescribe chemoprophylaxis at the appropriate time of year. Taking into account that in urban areas the transmission may also occur in colder months, year-round chemoprophylaxis may represent a safer option. It is strategically important to rule out the presence of infection with adequate testing before starting any chemoprophylactic drugs.

Macrolides represent the most common and efficient prophylactic drugs. Ivermectin, milbemycin oxime and moxidectin, via the oral route, topical selamectin, moxidectin and eprinomectin, and sustained released injectable moxidectin are currently available on the market (with the exception of injectable moxidectin in USA). The prophylactic efficacy of macrolides is due to their ability to kill tissue-migrating L4 larvae of *D. immitis* up to the 5th–6th week of infection. Therefore, macrolides provide a high degree of protection when administered on a monthly basis or in sustained released formulation. Although some degree of adulticide effect has been documented for macrolides at a prophylactic dose, patients that have missed one or more months of prophylaxis should be tested for heartworm infection after 7–8 months.

A chemoprophylactic schedule should also be considered in non-endemic regions when pets have temporarily lived in, or travelled through, areas where HWD is endemic. If pets reside in an endemic area for <30 days, two administrations of a prophylactic agent immediately after their return to the country of origin would be sufficient to guarantee protection. Conversely, if pets are resident in an endemic area for >30 days, administration of a complete prophylactic regimen is recommended.

High doses of macrolides have been shown to be potentially toxic in about one-third of Collies, but side-effects are not observed when administered at the recommended doses that are considered therefore safe, even in ivermectin-sensitive Collies or related breeds.

Daily administration of diethylcarbamazine citrate (DEC) was used for decades as a protocol for HWD prevention. However, its use is now discouraged as macrolides provide a more practical, reliable and safer alternative. There is minimal residual action and discontinuation for only 2–3 days may eliminate protection. DEC does not have an immediate larvicidal effect and it should be administered daily during and for 2 months after exposure to infective mosquitoes.

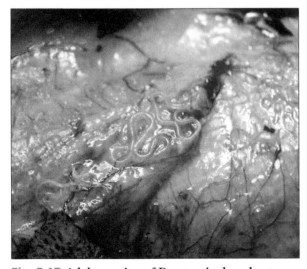

Fig. 5.17 **Adult parasites of *D. repens* in the subcutaneous tissues of an adult dog. This discovery was an incidental finding during surgery.**

SUBCUTANEOUS DIROFILARIASIS

Dirofilaria repens infection

Subcutaneous dirofilariasis is mainly caused by *D. repens* (**Figure 5.17**), which infects domestic dogs in Europe (especially Italy, Spain, Greece, ex-Yugoslavia and France), Africa and Asia, and bears in the USA and Canada. *D. repens* has also been reported in wild dogs, cats and foxes (**Table 5.1**). Subcutaneous dirofilariasis is transmitted by different species of mosquito (genera *Aedes*, *Anopheles* and *Culex*) to those involved in *D. immitis* transmission. However, the biological cycle of *D. repens* is very similar to that of *D. immitis* except that adult *D. repens* worms reside in subcutaneous tissues. The clinical significance of adult *D. repens* worms in dogs and cats has not been clearly defined. In most of these hosts, infection is completely asymptomatic, but nodular skin lesions have often been described in association with infection with typical cytological findings.

Treatment is achieved by surgical removal of nodules or minimally invasive removal of the parasites from skin lesions. Some macrolides are effective in preventing *D. repens* infections using the same prophylactic scheme described for *D. immitis*.

Dipetalonema reconditum (*Acanthocheilonema reconditum*) infection

This nematode is commonly found in dogs in the USA, Africa, Italy, Spain and Australia. Unlike *D. immitis*, *D. reconditum* infection is not limited to warm months because it is transmitted by fleas (*Ctenocephalides* species, *Pulex* species), ticks (*Rhipicephalus sanguineus*) and lice (*Linognathus* species) (**Table 5.1**). The biological cycle of *D. reconditum* is very similar to that of *D. repens* and the adults live within the dog's subcutaneous tissues. Development of L3 larvae in the intermediate host takes 7–19 days and the mechanism of entry into the definitive host is not definitely known. It is possible that the infected flea is ingested by the dog while grooming and L3 larvae are released and then penetrate the mucous membranes of the mouth. The prepatent period of *D. reconditum* is approximately 60–70 days.

The clinical significance of *D. reconditum* is limited, although it may induce eosinophilia. It may also interfere with the diagnosis of *D. immitis* infection if microscopic examination of a blood sample alone is used. The microfilariae of *D. reconditum* have a distinguishing cephalic hook and are smaller and narrower than *D. immitis* (**Table 5.1**).

Histochemical differentiation of *D. immitis, D. repens* and *D. reconditum* microfilariae

D. reconditum and *D. repens* can cause false positives in tests for circulating *D. immitis* microfilariae, but they can be differentiated with acid phosphatase staining. *D. immitis* microfilariae concentrate the dye in two regions, namely the excretory and anal pores, while *D. repens* shows an acid phosphatase reaction exclusively in the anal pore and *D. reconditum* stains evenly.

Cercopithifilaria infection

Filarids belonging to the genus *Cercopithifilaria* are transmitted by hard ticks (Ixodidae), and infect a range of host species, including dogs. Microfilariae are found in the dermis only and not in the bloodstream. Due to the fact that microfilariae cause limited clinical alterations and that skin samples necessary for the diagnosis are difficult to collect due to the invasive nature of a biopsy, *Cercopithifilaria* infection is probably underestimated. A few cases of canine polyarthritis associated with the infection have also been described.

HUMAN DIROFILARIASIS

Although humans are considered incidental hosts, *D. immitis* and *D. repens* infections are frequently reported in people and they represent an important zoonotic risk. The parasitic lesions are generally benign, but they may be misdiagnosed as more severe disease (i.e. tumours) and prompt unnecessary diagnostic and therapeutic procedures. Sometimes, sensitive organs such as the eyes are affected by the presence of the parasite.

D. immitis can cause pulmonary dirofilariasis in humans. This is normally caused by a single nematode that rarely reaches sexual maturation and, after having entered the right ventricle, dies and causes lung embolization and small lung infarctions, which subsequently appear as solitary nodules on thoracic radiography. Microfilaraemia and extrapulmonary dirofilariasis have also been described, but they represent rare events.

D. repens is commonly found in people in different body locations, including the conjunctiva, eyelid, scrotum, inguinal area, breast, arms and limbs. Diagnosis of human dirofilariasis depends mainly on micro-

scopic evaluation of the morphological characteristics of the nematode in histopathological specimens. A PCR-based assay has been validated to identify the different parasites in humans, animals and vectors.

CASE STUDY: HEARTWORM DISEASE (CAVAL SYNDROME)

History

Fog, an 8-year-old, neutered male, crossbred dog was referred with a history of having haemoglobinuria for the last 24 hours. The owner also reported that 2 months ago the dog had been coughing for a few weeks.

Clinical examination

The dog had hypothermia (body temperature 37.4°C); tachycardia and dyspnoea. On physical examination, the dog was depressed, dehydrated (5%) and had pale mucous membranes. Thoracic palpation revealed a thrill on the right side of the thorax and a loud (grade V/VI) systolic murmur was heard on the right side of the thorax (tricuspid valve).

Diagnostics
Haematology
Abnormal haematological findings (**Table 5.6**) included severe microangiopathic haemolytic anemia (**Figure 5.18**).

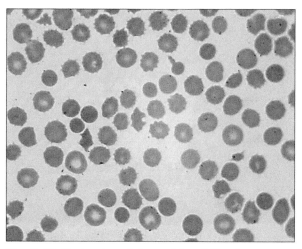

Fig. 5.18 **Evaluation of the peripheral blood smear (Romanowsky stain). There is severe thrombocytopenia and a few schistocytes and spherocytes can be observed. (Courtesy Dr W. Bertazzolo).**

PARAMETER	VALUE	REFERENCE RANGE
RBC	$2.75 \times 10^{12}/l$	5.5–8.5
Hb	65 g/l	100–180
Hct	0.174 l/l	0.35–0.55
MCV	63 fl	58–73 fl
MCH	23.8 pg	19–25 pg
MCHC	376 g/l	280–400
WBC	$22.3 \times 10^9/l$	6–17
Segmented neutrophils	$18.5 \times 10^9/l$	2.9–13.3
Band neutrophils	$1.3 \times 10^9/l$	0–0.3
Lymphocytes	$0.0 \times 10^9/l$	1–4.8
Monocytes	$0.2 \times 10^9/l$	0–1.3
Eosinophils	$1.1 \times 10^9/l$	0–1.2
Platelets	$37 \times 10^9/l$	120–600
Nucleated RBCs	6/100 WBCs	
Reticulocytes	5.8% (total $160 \times 10^9/l$)	

Table 5.6 Haematology findings.

Serum biochemistry

There was increased BUN (59.3 mmol/l; reference range 5.4–16.1), total bilirubin (25.7 μmol/l; reference range 0–10.3) and ALT (322 IU/l; reference range 0–110).

Urinalysis

There was severe haemoglobinuria.

Coagulation assays

Prothrombin time and partial thromboplastin time were both within the reference ranges.

Radiography

Thoracic radiographs (right lateral and dorsoventral views) revealed enlargement and tortuosity of the pulmonary arteries with mild right-sided cardiomegaly (**Figure 5.19**), bulging of the pulmonary trunk and dilation of the caudal pulmonary arteries with pruning of the right pulmonary artery (**Figure 5.20**, arrow).

Echocardiography

Cardiac ultrasound examination showed several adult heartworms (double-lined echoes) moving into the right cardiac chambers through the tricuspid valve (**Figures 5.21, 5.22**) and indirect signs of pulmonary hypertension (i.e. enlarged pulmonary arteries).

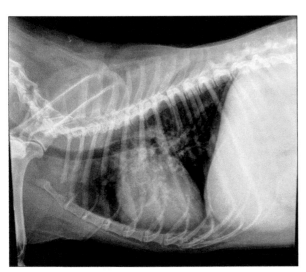

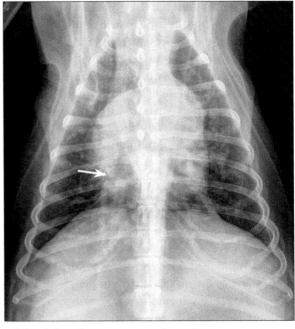

Figs. 5.19, 5.20 Right lateral (5.19, above) and dorsoventral (5.20, right) thoracic radiographs showing enlargement and tortuosity of pulmonary arteries with mild right-sided cardiomegaly, bulging of the pulmonary trunk, dilation of the caudal pulmonary arteries and pruning of the right pulmonary artery (arrow).

Antigen testing for *Dirofilaria immitis*
Positive to a high level (Snap Idexx HW®).

Knott's test
Positive for circulating microfilariae of *D. immitis* (L1).

Treatment
Fog underwent surgical heartworm removal via the jugular vein (by the Ishiahara technique). A total of 14 heartworms (eight female and six male) were removed from the right atrium and ventricle. No worms were found in the pulmonary arteries. After surgery, the dog

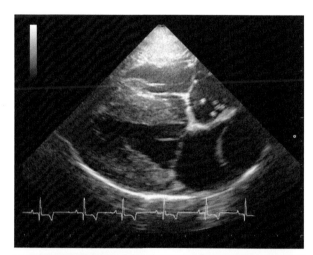

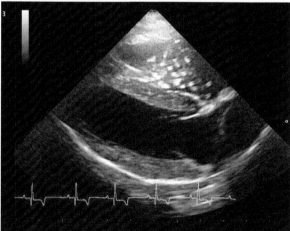

Figs. 5.21, 5.22 Ecochardiography (right parasternal long-axis view) showing several filarid worm echoes moving into the right cardiac chambers through the tricuspid valve. The right pulmonary artery (cross-section) appears dilated.

was hospitalized and received intravenous fluids and prednisolone (1 mg/kg SC q24h). There was a dramatic clinical improvement within 12 hours; the dog started eating and the haemoglobinuria disappeared (**Figure 5.23**). Two days later, Fog was discharged and the owners were instructed to keep him in a small cage and to visit the hospital for a recheck in 28 days.

Outcome
After 28 days, Fog had recovered completely. He was bright, alert and responsive during the return visit. Clinical examination, haematology and biochemistry parameters were all normal. Radiographic and echocardiographic signs of pulmonary hypertension were, however, still present. The owner was therefore instructed to limit his physical activity, to start chemprophylaxis for heartworm disease and to have the referring veterinarian perform an antigen test for *D. immitis* 3 months later. That examination was negative.

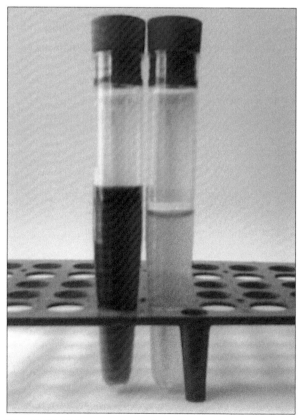

Fig. 5.23 Urine samples before (left) and a few hours after (right) heartworm removal.

FURTHER READING

Albanese F, Abramo F, Braglia C *et al*. (2013) Nodular lesions due to infestation by *Dirofilaria repens* in dogs from Italy. *Veterinary Dermatology* **24:**255–256.

Kramer L, Genchi C (2014) Where are we with *Wolbachia* and doxycycline: an in-depth review of the current state of our knowledge. *Veterinary Parasitology* **206:**1–4.

Lee AC, Atkins CE (2010) Understanding feline heartworm infection: disease, diagnosis, and treatment. *Top Companion Animal Medicine* **25:**224–230.

Liotta JL, Sandhu GK, Rishniw M *et al*. (2013) Differentiation of the microfilariae of *Dirofilaria immitis* and *Dirofilaria repens* in stained blood films. *Journal of Parasitology* **99:**421–425.

Mavropoulou A, Gnudi G, Grandi G *et al*. (2014) Clinical assessment of post-adulticide complications in *Dirofilaria immitis*-naturally infected dogs treated with doxycycline and ivermectin. *Veterinary Parasitology* **205:**211–215.

McCall JW, Genchi C, Kramer LH *et al*. (2008) Heartworm disease in animals and humans. *Advances in Parasitology* **66:**193–285.

Park H-J, Lee S-E, Lee W-J *et al*. (2014) Prevalence of *Dirofilaria immitis* infection in stray cats by nested PCR in Korea. *Korean Journal of Parasitology* **52:**691–694.

Schnyder M, Deplazes P (2012) Cross-reactions of sera from dogs infected with *Angiostrongylus vasorum* in commercially available *Dirofilaria immitis* test kits. *Parasites and Vectors* **13:**258.

Silbermayr K, Eigner B, Duscher GG *et al*. (2014) The detection of different *Dirofilaria* species using direct PCR technique. *Parasitology Research* **113:**513–516.

Small MT, Atkins CE, Gordon SG *et al*. (2008) Use of a nitinol gooseneck snare catheter for removal of adult *Dirofilaria immitis* in two cats. *Journal of the American Veterinary Medical Association* **233:**1441–1445.

Venco L, Bertazzolo W, Giordano G *et al*. (2014) Evaluation of C-reactive protein as a clinical biomarker in naturally heartworm-infected dogs: a field study. *Veterinary Parasitology* **206:**48–54.

Venco L, Genchi M, Genchi C *et al*. (2011) Can heartworm prevalence in dogs be used as provisional data for assessing the prevalence of the infection in cats? *Veterinary Parasitology* **176:**300–303.

Chapter 6

Babesiosis and Cytauxzoonosis

Peter Irwin

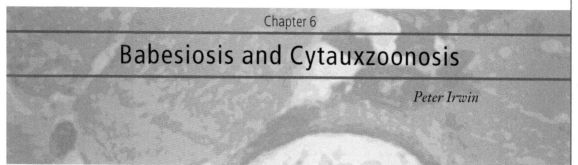

BABESIOSIS

BACKGROUND, AETIOLOGY AND EPIDEMIOLOGY

Babesiosis is caused by tick-borne intraerythrocytic protozoan parasites of the genus *Babesia* and is one of the most common infections of animals worldwide. Babesiosis (also referred to as piroplasmosis) occurs in domesticated dogs and cats, wild Canidae (wolves, foxes, jackals and dingoes) and wild Felidae (leopards, lions), and is an emerging zoonosis in humans. Babesiosis was originally viewed as a predominantly tropical and subtropical disease in dogs and cats, but in recent times it has been recognized with increasing frequency in temperate regions of the world.

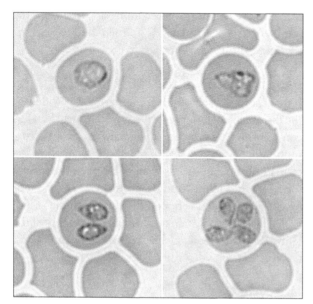

Fig. 6.1 Large piroplasms of the dog (*Babesia canis vogeli*, northern Australia) demonstrating a variety of morphological forms.

The taxonomic classification of *Babesia* species places them in the phylum Apicomplexa, the order Piroplasmida and the family Babesiidae. This classification was originally based on morphological characteristics of the intraerythrocytic parasites (merozoites and trophozoites) and other life cycle observations; however, the traditional methods of classification have been replaced by molecular genetic techniques, as phenotypic features alone are not sufficient for species differentiation. Molecular phylogenetic analysis has been useful not only for defining the relationships between individual *Babesia* species, but also for further elucidating the association between *Babesia* and closely related piroplasms such as *Theileria* species and *Cytauxzoon* species. The erythrocytic stages of all three genera are similar, yet they are differentiated phylogenetically and by the presence of distinct exoerythrocytic life cycle stages within the vertebrate host for *Theileria* and *Cytauxzoon* and by transovarial transmission, which is a feature of *Babesia* species.

Babesia species of the dog

Babesia parasites have been grouped informally into 'small' *Babesia* and 'large' *Babesia* when observed during microscopic examination of a blood film, and this remains a useful and practical starting point for identification in the clinical setting (**Figure 6.1**). Both types are recognized in dogs; the larger piroplasm that was originally referred to as simply *B. canis* is now understood to represent at least five different species (**Table 6.1**). The geographical region and species of enzootic tick provide the best guide for the clinician about the most probable identity of these piroplasms in any given locality, but ultimately molecular techniques are required to provide certainty. Returning home after travel, either when dogs accompany owners on holiday or for hunting purposes, has resulted in an alarming increase in reports of canine vector-borne pathogens in regions where these diseases were previously unknown.

Table 6.1 Piroplasms affecting domestic dogs and cats, their tick vectors and a guide to their virulence.

HOST	TYPE	SIZE (µm)	PIROPLASM SPECIES (FIRST DESCRIPTION)*	DISTRIBUTION (ESTABLISHED/ SPORADIC)	TICK VECTOR	VIRULENCE
Dog	Large	2 × 5	*Babesia canis canis* (1895)	Southern Europe, Central Europe	*Dermacentor reticulatus*	Moderate–severe
			Babesia canis vogeli (1937)	Africa, Asia, North and South America, Australia, Europe	*Rhipicephalus sanguineus*	Mild–moderate
	Small	0.8–1.2 × 3.2	*Babesia canis rossi* (1910)	Southern Africa	*Haemaphysalis leachi*	Severe
			Babesia gibsoni (1910)	Asia, North America, Australia, Europe	*Haemaphysalis longicornis, Haemaphysalis bispinosa, Rhipicephalus sanguineus?*	Moderate–severe
			Babesia conradae (1991)	California	Unknown	Moderate–severe
			Babesia microti-like (originally *Theileria annae*) (2000)	Northern Spain	*Ixodes hexagonus?*	Mild–moderate
Cat		1 × 2.25–2.5	*Babesia felis* (1929)	Africa	Unknown	Mild–moderate
		1 × 2	*Cytauxzoon felis* (1979)	Southern States USA, Zimbabwe	*Amblyomma americanum*	Moderate–severe

* Published isolates only

Until relatively recent times it was assumed that *Babesia gibsoni* was the only small piroplasm in dogs (**Figure 6.2**). It was originally described from India early in the last century and is considered to be widespread and endemic throughout Asia. The full geographical range of *B. gibsoni*, as with the other canine piroplasms, has yet to be elucidated in detail, but the organism has been found in dogs in the Middle East, parts of Africa, North America, Europe and most recently in Australia (**Table 6.1**). Reports of *B. gibsoni* from countries outside Asia are increasing, notably in dog breeds used for fighting activities, and it may become established in these areas if a competent vector is present.

With widespread use of molecular techniques, new canine piroplasms are discovered regularly, including those that are classified phylogenetically as *Theileria* species rather than strictly aligning with the Babesiidae (**Table 6.1**). Some are closely related to piroplasms found in wildlife, suggesting that dogs become inadvertently infected when they encroach into the sylvatic life cycles of these piroplasms and are bitten by ticks that normally feed on local wildlife hosts. A small *B. microti*-like organism (originally named *Theileria annae*) that causes serious illness in dogs was originally reported in northwestern Spain, but has now been found recently in red foxes and ticks in other parts of Europe (**Table 6.1**). With the advent of highly sensitive and specific molecular techniques, the range and diversity of piroplasm species is only now becoming apparent, and the number of species isolated from the blood of dogs (or their ticks) is likely to continue to grow.

Babesia species of the cat

Feline babesiosis has not been researched as widely as the disease in dogs, but regardless, it appears to be a less common clinical problem. *Babesia felis* in Africa is currently the best known cause of babesiosis in domestic cats (**Figure 6.3**). The association between the species found in wild felines and domesticated cats is under investigation and it is hoped that future studies using molecular tools will help to clarify the taxonomy of the feline *Babesia*. Another closely related feline piroplasm, *Cytauxzoon felis*, is described later in this chapter.

Life cycle

In general, *Babesia* parasites are transmitted to their vertebrate hosts by the 'hard' ticks (Ixodidae) (**Figure 6.4**). Infective sporozoites are injected into the vertebrate

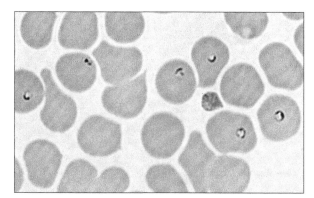

Fig. 6.2 Small piroplasms of the dog (*Babesia gibsoni*, Malaysia). Note the small, single piroplasms in each erythrocyte. (Courtesy Dr E.C. Yeoh)

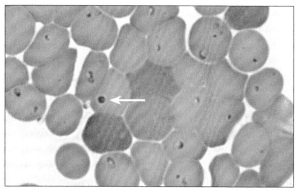

Fig. 6.3 *Babesia felis* piroplasms in a cat with acute babesiosis (South Africa). Note the high parasitaemia and wide variety of morphological forms. There is also evidence of erythrocyte regeneration and the presence of single Howell-Jolly body (arrow). (Courtesy Dr T Schoeman)

Fig. 6.4 Life cycle of *Babesia* in the dog and invertebrate host. (1) Sporozoites injected into bloodstream by feeding tick. (2) Trophozoite (ring form). (3) Merozoite. (4) Binary fission. (5) Paired trophozoites. (6) Infected erythrocytes ingested by feeding tick. (7) Lysis of erythrocyte in tick gut. (8) Gamont development and fusion. (9) Kinete formation. (10) Kinete migration from gut to other tissues within the tick, notably ovaries and salivary glands. (11) Development of sporokinetes in ovaries (ensuring transovarial transmission). (12) Development of sporokinetes to form a large, multinuclear sporont (containing many sporozoites). (13) Release of sporozoites from salivary gland during feeding. (Adapted from Melhom H, Walldorf V (1988) Life cycles. In: *Parasitology in Focus: Facts and Fiction* (ed. H Melhom) Springer-Verlag, Berlin.)

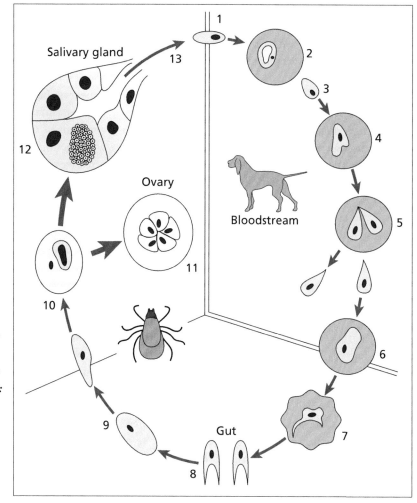

host within saliva during engorgement of the tick. These organisms then invade, feed and divide by binary fission within, and rupture erythrocytes during repeated phases of asexual reproduction, releasing merozoites that find and invade other erythrocytes (**Figure 6.5**). In chronic infections it is assumed that babesial parasites become sequestered within the capillary networks of the spleen, liver and other organs, from where they are released periodically into circulation. Transmission to the vector may occur at any time that a parasitaemia exists. After ingestion by the tick, the complex processes of migration and sexual reproduction (gamogony and sporogony) take place, resulting in sporozoite formation in the cells of the tick's salivary glands. While tick transmission is the major source of infection, babesiosis may also occur after transfusion of infected blood, in neonates after transplacental transfer, and from blood exchanged between individuals while fighting.

Epidemiology

In endemic regions the prevalence of antibodies directed against *Babesia* ranges from 3.8% to 80%, with the highest seroprevalence rates reported from animal refuges and greyhound kennels. A higher prevalence of babesiosis has been reported in male dogs and, generally, younger dogs (and cats) are more likely to develop clinical disease. The efficiency of tick control largely determines the risk of infection to individual household pets. A higher prevalence of *B. felis* infection has been observed in Siamese and Oriental cats in South Africa, and dog breeds used for fighting (e.g. Pit Bulltype) are overrepresented in reports of *B. gibsoni* infections outside Asia. As noted previously, wildlife may act as a reservoir of piroplasms for domestic pets in some regions, but further studies are required to better understand this epidemiology.

Babesiosis is considered to be an emerging disease in many parts of the world. Veterinarians should retain a high degree of clinical suspicion when investigating haemolytic anaemia and thrombocytopenia, and should include questions relating to the pet's travel history during consultation. An increasing number of cases of canine babesiosis are reported in regions where the disease was not previously known to exist (e.g. northern Europe). Possible reasons for this include changing ecological and environmental circumstances that favour the establishment of vector ticks in previ-

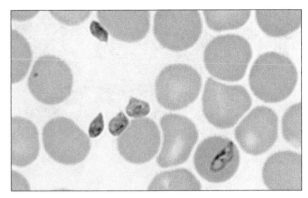

Fig. 6.5 **Free merozoites of Babesia canis.**

ously non-enzootic regions, and the increasing ease of international pet travel associated with the relaxation of national quarantine regulations. The brown dog tick *Rhipicephalus sanguineus* is particularly adaptable and may become established in homes with central heating well beyond its usual enzootic range.

Concurrent infection with other haemoparasites, notably *Ehrlichia* species, haemotropic *Mycoplasma* species, *Hepatozoon* species and other species of *Babesia*, appears to be a common occurrence in endemic regions and potentially complicates the diagnosis and management of individuals by the veterinarian. Multiple co-infections are difficult to diagnose without highly sensitive tests such as polymerase chain reaction (PCR).

PATHOGENESIS

The severity of babesiosis in dogs and cats ranges from the development of mild anaemia to widespread organ failure and death. The critical determinant of this variable pathogenesis is the species or strain of *Babesia* parasite, yet other factors such as the age and immune status of the host and the presence of concurrent infections or illness are also important. While haemolytic anaemia is the principal mechanism contributing to the pathogenesis of babesiosis, it has been recognized for many years that the level of parasitaemia does not correlate well with the degree of anaemia, suggesting that multiple factors contribute to erythrocyte destruction. Direct parasite-induced red cell damage, increased osmotic fragility of infected cells, oxidative injury and secondary immune-mediated attack of the erythrocyte membrane result in a combination of intravascular and extravascular haemolysis.

The wide spectrum of clinical signs associated with canine babesiosis has led to the classification of uncomplicated and complicated forms.

Uncomplicated babesiosis

Uncomplicated babesiosis is generally associated with thrombocytopenia, mild-to-moderate anaemia, lethargy, weakness and hepatosplenomegaly, and is typical of *B. canis vogeli* infections, for example. Pyrexia, when it occurs, is attributed to the release of endogenous pyrogens and inflammatory mediators from inflamed and hypoxic tissue.

Complicated babesiosis

Complicated babesiosis refers to manifestations that cannot be explained as a consequence of a haemolytic crisis alone (**Table 6.2**). This form of babesiosis has been extensively studied with respect to virulent babesial species in the USA, southern Africa and Europe, and is characterized by severe anaemia and dysfunction of one or more organs. Cerebral babesiosis causes severe neurological dysfunction (seizures, stupor and coma), which is often peracute and associated with congestion, haemorrhage and sequestration of parasitized erythrocytes in cerebral capillaries. Hypotension and systemic inflammation are associated with the activation of cytokines and potent humoral agents such as kallikrein, complement and the coagulation systems. Consumption of platelets and clotting factors may result in haemorrhagic diatheses. Renal dysfunction has been attributed to the development of haemoglobinuric nephrosis, but this probably requires additional processes such as hypoxia and reduced renal perfusion to become clinically evident (**Figures 6.6, 6.7**). A shift in haemoglobin–oxygen dissociation dynamics has been reported to occur in dogs with virulent babesiosis, leading to less efficient oxygen off-loading in capillaries, further compounding poor tissue oxygenation caused by the anaemia. Metabolic (lactic) acidosis in babesiosis has been attributed to anaemic hypoxia and capillary pooling. Recently, mixed respiratory and metabolic acid–base disturbances have been described in dogs with complicated babesiosis. With the buffering capacity of blood adversely compromised by low haemoglobin concentrations, arterial pH is reported to vary from severe acidaemia to alkalaemia. Mortality in complicated babesiosis often exceeds 80%.

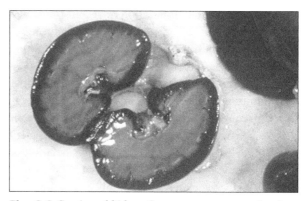

Fig. 6.6 Sectioned kidney from a necropsy examination of a puppy that died of acute babesiosis demonstrating the gross appearance of haemoglobinuric nephrosis in the renal cortex.

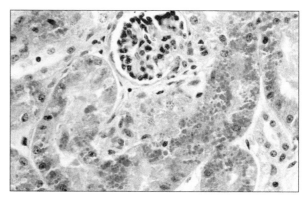

Fig. 6.7 Haemoglobinuric nephrosis. High-power view of the renal cortex of the specimen in Figure 6.6 demonstrating hyaline droplet formation in the proximal tubules, confirmed to be haemoglobin by subsequent naphthol black staining.

CLINICAL SIGNS

Canine babesiosis

Veterinarians should be mindful that the clinical picture of canine babesiosis might be complicated by concurrent infection with pathogens that share the same tick vector or result from sequential infections by different ticks. The most severe forms of the disease in adult dogs are generally associated with virulent infections (*B. canis rossi*, *B. canis canis*, *B. gibsoni*, the Californian piroplasm and *B. microti*-like species). Ticks may or may not be found on the animal at the time of presentation in endemic regions, but there is usually a history of known tick infestation or recent travel to a tick-enzootic region.

Peracute babesiosis is characterized by the rapid onset of collapse. Clinical findings are typical of hypotensive shock and include pale mucous membranes (sometimes with cyanosis), rapid heart rate and weak pulse, profound weakness and mental depression. Fever may be present, but hypothermia is a more consistent finding in this state. Severe intravascular haemolysis leads to haemoglobinuria ('red water'). This presentation is usually associated with complicated babesiosis, referred to in the previous section, and affected dogs develop signs that reflect widespread organ dysfunction associated with hypotension, hypoxaemia and extensive tissue damage such as anuria or oliguria, neurological dysfunction, coagulopathies and acute respiratory distress (**Table 6.2**). A rapid deterioration to coma and death is the usual outcome of peracute babesiosis.

Acute babesiosis is the clinical state that most veterinarians will encounter. Recurrent episodes may occur in some dogs infected with more virulent strains of the parasite (e.g. *B. canis canis*, *B. gibsoni*). Dogs with acute anaemia may have been unwell for a few days with non-specific signs such as anorexia, depression, vomiting and lethargy (**Figure 6.8**). The most consistent finding on physical examination is pallor of the mucous membranes, with a variable occurrence of fever, hepatosplenomegaly, icterus and dehydration (**Table 6.3**). Congested mucous membranes are also occasionally reported. Petechial and ecchymotic haemorrhages may be observed on the gums or ventral abdomen in some dogs, consistent with the presence of concurrent thrombocytopenia or thrombocytopathy. This may also suggest concomitant infection with another organism. Urine obtained from dogs with acute *B. canis* infection is typically brown or dark yellow–orange, reflecting a mixture of haemoglobinuria and bilirubinuria. The patient's serum is often overtly haemolysed or icteric. A variety of atypical manifestations of severe babesiosis (e.g. dermal necrosis, myositis and polyarthritis) have been reported, but the possibility of these being attributable to co-infection has not been examined in detail.

It is likely that most dogs that survive the initial infection become lifelong carriers of the parasite despite appropriate treatment and resolution of the original signs. Secondary immune-mediated complications such as anaemia, thrombocytopenia and glomerulone-

Table 6.2 **Features of complicated babesiosis.**
Anaemia (PCV <0.15 l/l)
Renal dysfunction
Hepatic dysfunction
Cerebral complications
Rhabdomyolysis
Pulmonary oedema
Consumptive coagulopathy (DIC)
Mixed acid–base disturbances

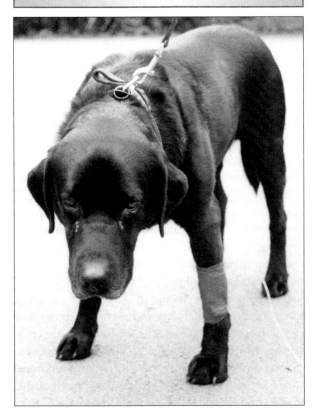

Fig. 6.8 Acute babesiosis (*B. canis canis*) causing severe weakness and haemolytic anaemia in a 6-year-old Labrador Retriever.

phritis may develop, but the long-term consequences of chronic infection are poorly understood. Many dogs remain subclinical, in a state referred to as premunity, despite intermittent, low parasitaemias. Recrudescence of intraerythrocytic parasites into the bloodstream may occur following stressful situations, immunosuppressive therapy or concurrent disease (e.g. cancer). In some individuals this leads to a further significant disease

Table 6.3 **Clinical features of babesiosis.**

UNCOMPLICATED		COMPLICATED
Mild-to-moderate anaemia (PCV 0.15–0.35 l/l)	Severe anaemia (PCV <0.15 l/l)	Severe anaemia (PCV <0.15 l/l)
May be asymptomatic	Lethargy	Dark red urine (haemoglobinuria)
Lethargy	Weakness	Oliguria or anuria
Fever	Fever	Shock-like state
Hepatosplenomegaly	Anorexia	Tachypnoea, dyspnoea, cough
Anorexia	Vomiting	Neurological signs (depression, collapse, seizures, vestibular signs, coma)
Pallor	Dehydration	Petechial and ecchymotic haemorrhage
Mild icterus	Dark red urine (haemoglobinuria)	Vomiting
	Icterus	
Low to moderate mortality	Low to moderate mortality	High mortality

episode, yet others may develop only a mild anaemia and intermittent pyrexia.

Chronic babesiosis has also been associated with non-specific signs such as anorexia, weight loss and lymphadenomegaly. Although recurrent infections in the same dog may occur, in practice it is rarely possible to distinguish between recrudescence and a novel infection in endemic regions.

Feline babesiosis

South Africa appears to be the only country where feline babesiosis is currently recognized as a clinical entity in domestic cats, where it manifests as an afebrile, chronic, low-grade disease. Presentation of cats to the veterinarian may be delayed when compared with dogs, due in part to the more introverted nature of cats and to the failure of the owners to recognize early signs of illness. Furthermore, cats are able to tolerate more severe anaemia than dogs without showing signs. Anorexia, depression and pallor were the clinical signs attributed to feline babesiosis most commonly in one study, with weight loss, icterus, constipation and pica recorded less frequently. Pyrexia is not a feature of feline babesiosis. The highest prevalence of disease occurs in young adult cats (<3 years old) during the spring and summer in enzootic regions. Complications of feline babesiosis are wide ranging and include hepatopathy, renal failure,

pulmonary oedema, cerebral signs and immune-mediated haemolytic anaemia. Concurrent infections with feline immunodeficiency virus, feline leukaemia virus and haemotropic *Mycoplasma* species may occur in older individuals. It is probable that young cats in enzootic areas contract the infection early in life and become subclinical carriers.

DIAGNOSIS

The definitive diagnosis of babesiosis currently requires visualization of the parasite during light microscopic examination of a blood smear. The DNA of the organism is amplified by PCR and the identity is then confirmed by sequencing the amplified DNA.

Identification of the *Babesia* species, or at least a distinction between 'small' and 'large' babesial organisms, is important with regard to the choice of therapeutic agent. The search for *Babesia*-infected erythrocytes in a blood smear may be tedious and time-consuming when the parasitaemia is low, yet is greatly facilitated by the preparation of good quality blood films (see **Table 4.1**). Blood smear examination should be done in the clinic and the result can be available within minutes. Most of the in-house rapid staining systems are sufficient to adequately stain intraerythrocytic piroplasms if performed correctly. The blood smear should be viewed through a cover slip, which is placed over the slide on a drop of microscope oil, or resin fixative (e.g. DPX) if a permanent mount is to be made. Large *Babesia* trophozoites can be seen using an objective lens magnification of ×40, but oil-immersion (×100 objective lens) is required for accurate identification of small babesial parasites. *Babesia* parasites should be differentiated from stain artefact and *Mycoplasma* species by a magenta staining nucleus and their blue and white cytoplasm (see **Figures 6.1, 6.2**). In cats, *Cytauxzoon felis* appears very similar to *Babesia* species and accurate differentiation may require molecular techniques. Parasitaemias in cats with *B. felis* infection are variable and range from very low in chronic disease to extremely high in acute cases (see **Figure 6.3**).

The physical properties of erythrocytes are altered after infection by *Babesia* parasites. Infected red cells become rigid, slowing down their passage through capillary networks. Large numbers of parasitized cells may be observed in capillary networks (**Figure 6.9**), a phenomenon that is possibly explained by the tendency of the parasite to proliferate locally in certain capillary beds or by the tendency of parasitized erythrocytes to autoagglutinate. This characteristic is useful for diagnosis, as higher parasitaemias may be demonstrated in blood samples collected from the ear tip (**Figure 6.10**) and claw. Erythrocytes parasitized by the larger *Babesia* species are less dense than normal red cells and they concentrate in a layer immediately below the buffy coat within a haematocrit tube (**Figures 6.11, 6.12**). Par-

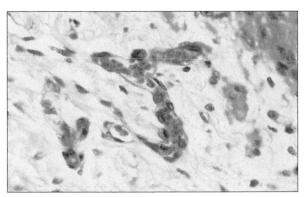

Fig. 6.9 High-power view showing the accumulation of large numbers of parasitized erythrocytes within a capillary.

asitized erythrocytes also tend to be found in greater numbers around the periphery of the blood film and in the 'feather edge' at the end of the smear.

Haematological analysis typically reveals thrombocytopenia, haemolytic anaemia, characterized by a regenerative anaemia, and leucocytosis. In peracute cases the anaemia is normochromic and normocytic, with erythron regeneration only evident after 2–3 days. Large 'reactive' lymphocytes (**Figure 6.13**) may be observed in chronic babesiosis, indicating antigenic stimulation, but they are also associated with other infectious disease states. Thrombocytopenia is very common in babesiosis, although its clinical significance is unclear. Platelet counts are rarely critical (<10 × 10⁹/l), typically within the range 20–90 × 10⁹/l,

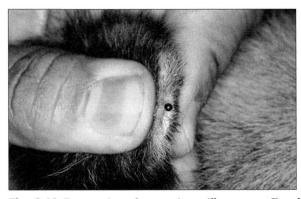
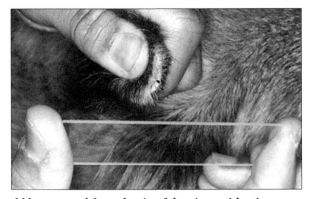

Fig. 6.10 Preparation of an ear tip capillary smear. Fur should be removed from the tip of the pinna with scissors or electric clippers and the skin cleaned with a dry swab to remove skin squames and dirt. The ear tip should be gently pricked with a fine (25-gauge) needle and pressure applied to squeeze out a droplet of blood (left). A clean microscope slide is touched onto the drop of blood and a smear is made in the usual way (right).

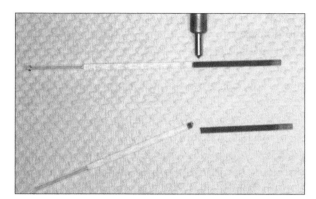

Fig. 6.11 Erythrocytes containing large *Babesia* piroplasms accumulate just beneath the white cell layer (buffy coat) in a microhaematocrit tube. The tube should be cracked at this point with a diamond pencil to obtain a sample for a blood smear.

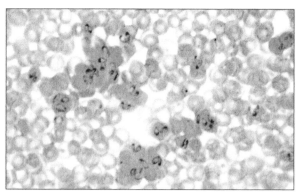

Fig. 6.12 High-power view of concentrated parasitized erythrocytes obtained from beneath the buffy coat (see Figure 6.11).

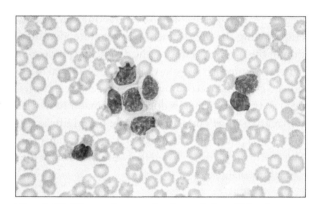

Fig. 6.13 Photomicrograph of a peripheral blood smear demonstrating 'reactive' lymphocytes, which are a common feature of chronic babesiosis.

Table 6.4 **Differential diagnosis of haemolytic anaemia in dogs.**	
AGE OF DOG	**DISORDER**
Neonates and young dogs	Neonatal isoerythrolysis
	Babesiosis
	Inherited erythrocyte defects (rare)
	Transfusion reactions
Older dogs	Immune-mediated haemolytic anaemia
	Babesiosis
	Heinz body anaemia (onion poisoning and various drug toxicities)
	Anticoagulant toxicity
	Dirofilariasis (caval syndrome)
	Transfusion reactions
	Acute zinc and copper toxicosis
	Neoplasia (microangiopathic haemolysis)

and overt signs of a bleeding diathesis (i.e. petechial and ecchymotic haemorrhages) are relatively unusual. Concurrent infections (e.g. ehrlichiosis) might further exacerbate the potential for bleeding by causing platelet dysfunction. Autoagglutination has been reported in babesiosis and up to 80% of dogs give a positive result in direct antiglobulin (Coombs) tests, making a search for parasites imperative in order to make the correct diagnosis. Immune-mediated haemolytic anaemia is the main differential diagnosis for babesiosis but other causes of haemolysis should be considered (**Table 6.4**).

Serum biochemistry results are non-specific in babesiosis. Extravascular red cell lysis results in elevated serum bilirubin in both dogs and cats. Acute hepatocellular injury leads to markedly elevated levels of alanine aminotransferase (ALT) and alkaline phosphatase (ALP) in dogs, while ALP and gamma glutamyl transferase are generally normal in cats with babesiosis. Azotaemia was recorded in 36% of dogs with Spanish piroplasm (*T. annae*) infection in northwest Spain and was associated with a high risk of mortality. Hyperkalaemia and hypoglycaemia have been reported in pups with acute intravascular haemolysis.

Serum proteins are usually normal, but hyperglobulinaemia with hypoalbuminaemia has been recorded in some chronic cases of babesiosis.

Because of the difficulty associated with microscopic detection of babesial organisms, a variety of serological tests have been developed. These facilitate the identification of animals that have been exposed to *Babesia* parasites, but provide little information about the individual's current infection status. The IFAT seems to be the most reliable assay for clinical purposes and is offered by commercial diagnostic laboratories in the USA and Europe. Specific methodologies vary between laboratories and the clinician should seek advice from the laboratory regarding accepted cut-off values. Unfortunately, cross-reactivity between the canine babesial species often necessitates positive identification of the organism by microscopy. Antibodies to *Babesia* may also cross-react with other apicomplexan parasites, giving further potential for false-positive serology.

Amplification of *Babesia* DNA using PCR is a highly sensitive technique that is becoming widely available. It is very useful for the detection of subclinical carriers in specific situations (e.g. before importation into *Babesia*-free regions) and for screening potential blood donors, and for confirming the species identity of the infection.

It is worth reiterating that the discovery of *Babesia* parasites in a blood film should always be viewed in the light of the clinical findings and other laboratory test results. It is not uncommon to find an occasional infected red cell in the blood of a clinically normal dog living in an endemic region.

TREATMENT

Issues to be considered when treating pets with babesiosis should include the clinical status of the patient, the degree of anaemia, the identity of the organism and its level of parasitaemia, and the potential for drug toxicity (especially if there is a history of previous anti-babesial therapy). In all but mild, uncomplicated cases, hospitalization and a combination of specific anti-babesial therapy and supportive care are necessary. Complicated babesiosis provides a challenge for even the most experienced intensive care clinicians.

Specific therapy

Randomized controlled trials to test the efficacy of anti-babesial treatments in dogs and cats have not been reported. With the exception of the recent introduction of atovaquone and azithromycin for the treatment of small *Babesia* infections, little has changed in the last 10 years with regard to the therapeutic options for babesiosis. A wide variety of therapeutic regimens have been tried, including quinoline and acridine derivatives, diamidine derivatives, azo-naphthalene dyes, various anti-malarial formulations and assorted antibiotics, yet few have gained acceptance for being consistently reliable and safe. Rarely, if ever, do any of these drugs sterilize the babesial infection and it may be preferable to induce a subclinical state of premunity in endemic regions where ongoing challenge is to be expected.

The choice of anti-babesial drug is determined largely by the species of *Babesia* infecting the patient, emphasizing the importance of an accurate identification of the piroplasm during the diagnostic process. In general, imidocarb is preferred for large babesial infections, a combination of atovaquone and azithromycin is used to treat *B. gibsoni* in dogs and primaquine is used for treating *B. felis* infections (**Table 6.5**). Differences in national pharmaceutical registration laws may mean that many of the drugs listed in **Table 6.5** are not universally available.

Imidocarb dipropionate

Imidocarb is an aromatic diamidine of the carbanilide series. In common with other diamidine derivatives, it interferes with parasite DNA metabolism and aerobic glycolysis, is rapidly effective and is slowly metabolized from the host. While it is generally safe for use in very young dogs with babesiosis, side-effects of imidocarb include pain at the site of injection and signs attributed to cholinergic properties of the drug, such as vomiting, diarrhoea, salivation, muscle tremor and restlessness (**Table 6.5**).

Atovaquone

Atovaquone belongs to the class of naphthoquinone anti-protozoal drugs used to treat pneumocystis pneumonia, toxoplasmosis, malaria and babesiosis in humans, alone or with other drugs. In dogs, atovaquone has been used in combination with azithromycin (a macrolide antibiotic) or proguanil (an anti-malarial) for the treatment of *B. gibsoni* and *B. conradae* infections (**Table 6.5**). Limited observational and controlled studies suggest that while atovaquone drug combinations are both safe and efficacious in many dogs, resulting in a rapid clinical improvement and clearance of piroplasm DNA from the bloodstream, there are also reports of it failing to clear these parasites, even with repeated doses, as a result of drug resistance conferred by mutation of the organism's cytochrome b gene. Proguanil may cause gastrointestinal side-effects in some dogs.

Diminazene

Diminazene is a diamidine derivative used for the treatment of trypanosome and piroplasm infections. A single intramuscular dose is recommended for

Table 6.5 **Anti-babesial drug therapy.**

HOST	BABESIA TYPE	DRUG NAME (AND SALT)	TRADE NAME(S)	RECOMMENDED DOSE	FREQUENCY	NOTES/ COMMENTS
Dog	Large	Imidocarb (dipropionate and dihydrochloride)	Imizol, Carbesia, Forray 65	5 mg/kg SC or IM	Repeat after 14 days	Pain at site of injection and nodule may develop at site of injection. Anticholinergic signs controlled with atropine (0.05mg/kg SC)
		Trypan blue	Trypan blue SS, Trypan blue Kyron	10 mg/kg IV		Tissue irritant, use as 1% solution. Reversible staining of body tissues occurs
	Large and small	Phenamidine (isethionate)	Oxopirvédine, Phenamidine, Lomadine	15 mg/kg SC	Once or repeat after 24 hours	Nausea, vomiting and CNS signs are common side-effects
		Pentamidine (isethionate)	Pentam 300	16.5 mg/kg IM	Repeat after 24 hours	
		Diminazine (aceturate and diaceturate)	Berenil, Ganaseg Veriben, Babezine, Dimisol	3.5 mg/kg IM	Once	Unpredictable toxicity, CNS signs may be severe. Berenil and Ganaseg contain antipyrone
	Small	Parvaquone	Clexon	20 mg/kg SC	Once	
		Atovaquone, atovaquone and azithromycin, or proguanil	Wellvone, Zithromax, Mepron	13.3 mg/kg PO q8h (atovaquone); 10 mg/kg PO q24h together for 10 days (atovaquone and azithromycin); 7-10 mg/kg PO (proguanil)	10 days / 10 days	Vomiting is common
		Clindamycin, metronidazole and doxycycline combination		25 mg/kg q12h PO (clindamycin); 15 mg/kg PO q12h (metronidazole); 5 mg/kg PO q12h (doxycycline)		
Cat	B. felis	Primaquine (phosphate)	Primaquine	0.5 mg/kg PO	Once	

the treatment of canine babesiosis (**Table 6.5**). The main disadvantage of diminazene is its low therapeutic index and, although the development of toxicity is dose-related in most dogs, there appears to be variable susceptibility between individuals and idiosyncratic reactions occur. Signs of toxicity can develop as soon as 1 hour after injection in some cases, or they may be delayed for up to 48 hours. Affected dogs show signs of central vestibular disease, including ataxia, rolling, vertical nystagmus and conscious proprioceptive deficits that may progress to opisthotonos, paralysis and death. Mild cases usually recover spontaneously, but the worst affected dogs develop irreversible neurological deterioration. There is no antidote for diamidine poisoning so treatment should consist of supportive care. The toxicity of diminazene is cumulative and repeat injections should be avoided for at least 14 days. There have been additional concerns about the use of diminazene in severe, complicated babesiosis due to its hypotensive and anticholinergic effects. For such cases it is advisable to start intensive supportive therapy prior to administering the anti-babesial drug. Furthermore, some clinicians prefer to use another anti-babesial drug (e.g. trypan blue) initially in these cases. Diminazene is also safe for use in very young dogs with babesiosis, but strict attention must be paid to the individual's body weight to avoid overdosing.

Other anti-babesial drugs

Trypan blue was one of the earliest drugs to be used for canine babesiosis, but experience with this drug appears to be limited to South Africa. It is relatively safe and is thought to suppress parasite numbers by preventing their invasion of erythrocytes. Primaquine is an anti-malarial that is considered to be the most effective drug against *B. felis* infection (**Table 6.5**). Although it reduces the parasitaemia (which can be extremely high in cats), primaquine does not sterilize the infection. Accurate dosage calculations are required in cats in order to avoid toxicity; however, vomiting is a common side-effect at the recommended dose rate. Parvaquone, an anti-theilerial drug used in cattle, has been used to treat small canine piroplasms with some success (**Table 6.5**), and there is anecdotal information that doxycycline is effective against both large and small canine piroplasms, but convincing evidence for this claim is currently unavailable.

Supportive care for babesiosis

Proactive supportive care is an integral component of the treatment of a dog or cat with babesiosis (**Table 6.6**). Regular patient monitoring should include assessment of mucous membrane colour, hydration status, respiratory rate and pattern and urine production, and laboratory evaluation of packed cell volume (PCV), serum total protein (TP), electrolytes and acid–base status. In dogs with severe anaemia, normalizing circulatory status is best accomplished by blood transfusion. Both the rapidity of onset and the degree of anaemia should be considered when assessing the need to provide additional red cells. Blood transfusion is generally determined by the clinical status of the patient, but is advisable in dogs with a PCV of <0.20 l/l and cats with a PCV of <0.15 l/l. While in dogs it is preferable to confirm compatibility of the donor blood prior to transfusion by cross-matching, in cats this is mandatory owing to the high prevalence of alloantibodies in this species. The development of 'in-house' blood-typing cards has greatly facilitated the assessment of donor-recipient blood compatibility in recent years (**Figure 6.14**). Fresh whole blood transfusions are preferred for complicated babesiosis cases, but packed red cells are adequate in other cases (**Table 6.7**).

Crystalline fluid therapy should be given with caution in anaemic patients so as to avoid causing further haemodilution or exacerbating respiratory distress. Oxygen therapy does not alleviate the hypoxia in anaemic states, but is indicated for the therapy of pulmonary oedema in complicated babesiosis. Bicarbonate therapy continues to attract controversy and its use is best restricted to institutions where acid–base status can be regularly assessed and interpreted. Organ dysfunction associated with complicated babesiosis should be managed according to the general guidelines provided in current critical care manuals. A detailed review pertaining to the supportive treatment of canine babesiosis has been published (see Further Reading). Glucocorticoids, including dexamethasone and prednisolone (or prednisone), have been recommended by some authors, but their benefits in babesiosis are currently unproven.

PREVENTION AND CONTROL

As with any tick-transmitted disease, removing all possibility of exposure to the vector is the best way to prevent

Table 6.6 **Drugs used for supportive care of canine babesiosis.**

	UNCOMPLICATED	COMPLICATED
MILD	MODERATE–SEVERE	
Anti-babesial drug	Anti-babesial drug	Anti-babesial drug (combination therapy?)
	Blood transfusion (packed RBCs or whole blood)	Blood transfusion (whole blood)
	Crystalloid infusion if dehydrated	Crystalloid and colloid infusion as dictated by patient's status
	Dexamethasone? (0.2mg/kg IV once)	Dexamethasone? (0.2 mg/kg IV once)
	Outpatient medication	**Pulmonary oedema**
	Prednisolone?	Frusemide (2–4 mg/kg IV or SC q6–8h)
		Oxygen therapy
		Acute kidney injury
		Frusemide (2–4 mg/kg IV q6–8h)
		Mannitol 10% (1–2 g/kg IV once) or
		Dopamine (1–5 μg/kg/min IV)
		Disseminated intravascular coagulation
		Plasma transfusion with heparin (75 units/kg added to plasma bag)
		Heparin (75 mg/kg SC q8h)
		Outpatient medication
		Prednisolone?

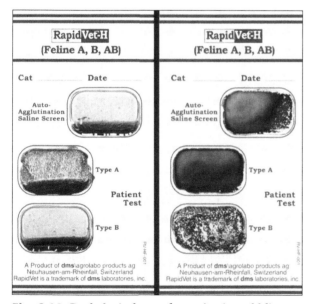

Fig. 6.14 Cards for in-house determination of feline blood types. The presence of agglutination indicates the blood type. The sample on the left is type A and the sample on the right is type B.

Table 6.7 **Formulae for blood transfusion.**

Whole blood transfusion:

Blood volume to be transfused =

$$k \times \text{body weight (kg)} \times \frac{(\text{required PCV} - \text{recipient PCV})}{\text{PCV of donated blood}}$$

Constant 'k' = 90 in dogs, 60 in cats

Packed red blood cell (pRBC) transfusion:

Infusion of 10 ml/kg pRBC will increase the recipient's PCV by approximately 10% (0.1 l/l) babesiosis. However, this is rarely achievable in endemic areas despite attentive ectoparasite control. Regular spraying, dipping or bathing with topical acaricidal preparations in accordance with the manufacturers' instructions should be practised in regions where tick challenge is continual (see **Table 1.2**). For dogs that are visiting tick-enzootic regions for a short time, and in cats that may have increased susceptibility to the toxicity of many acaricidal preparations, fipronil spray or 'spot-on' is a suitable choice, with a reasonable prophylactic effect. Owners should be encouraged to search their pets daily for ticks and, once found, to physically remove and dispose of them. Tick 'removers' are available and the use of these devices (and the wearing of gloves) may help to reduce the chance of inadvertent exposure of the owner to other potentially infectious agents within the tick (e.g. *Borrelia* species).

Several drugs have been investigated for their prophylactic potential against babesiosis, yet none have been consistently reliable in this regard. Experimental studies have suggested that a single dose of imidocarb dipropionate (6 mg/kg) protects dogs from *Babesia* challenge for up to 8 weeks, and that doxycycline at 5 mg/kg/day ameliorates the severity of disease when challenged with virulent *B. canis*. Higher doses of both drugs may protect more effectively for longer periods, but the potential toxicity of imidocarb and the overuse of doxycycline would be of concern. Reliance on such strategies cannot be recommended.

Vaccines made from cell culture-attenuated antigens have been developed for immunization against *B. canis canis* and are available commercially. While these vaccines do not prevent infection, they limit the parasitaemia and ameliorate the clinical signs and laboratory changes that occur after acute infection. The use of vaccines containing *B. canis canis* antigen only is restricted to Europe, as cross-protection against other *Babesia* parasites of dogs (e.g. *B. canis rossi* and *B. gibsoni*) does not develop. However, when mixed *B. canis canis* and *B. canis rossi* antigens are incorporated into a vaccine, heterologous protection is induced.

ZOONOTIC POTENTIAL/PUBLIC HEALTH SIGNIFICANCE

Babesiosis is an emerging zoonosis in many parts of the world, yet the common babesial parasites of companion animals described in this chapter are not implicated in zoonotic transmission. Babesiosis in people is associated with a spectrum of clinical signs, ranging from asymptomatic infections to severe illness and death. The majority of human cases of babesiosis around the world are thought to be caused by piroplasms of wildlife, and molecular analysis has provided significant insight to the identity of these zoonotic infections in recent years (see **Table 6.1**). *Babesia microti*, a parasite of rodents, is the main cause of human babesiosis in north America, and a complex of closely related parasites (*Babesia microti*-like) have been also reported in Europe, Asia, and Africa. Although uncommon, human babesiosis in Europe is associated with greater morbidity (and mortality) and is usually caused by the bovine pathogen *B. divergens*, although a second organism, *B. venatorum* (EU-1), is increasingly reported in people.

CYTAUXZOONOSIS

BACKGROUND, AETIOLOGY AND EPIDEMIOLOGY

Cytauxzoonosis is a tick-transmitted protozoal disease of growing clinical importance for domestic cats in the southern USA. The causative agent is *Cytauxzoon felis*, which is recognized to have both pre-erythrocytic and erythrocytic phases of its life cycle in the vertebrate host. Members of the genus *Cytauxzoon*, which occur in wild felines in most continents, are differentiated from *Theileria* species based on the fact that schizogony in *Cytauxzoon* occurs in macrophages, while schizogony in *Theileria* occurs in lymphocytes. However, it is clear that *C. felis* not only shares morphological characteristics with organisms of the genera *Theileria* and *Babesia*, but it is also closely related on a molecular basis to the smaller piroplasms *B. rodhaini* and *T. equi*.

The natural host is the bobcat (*Lynx rufus*) and recent research indicates that domestic cats that survive infection may become chronically infected and likely act as reservoirs of infection for naïve felines. Natural *C. felis* infection may result from transmission by an attached tick, ingestion of infected ticks or by inoculation of infected blood or tissue during fights, notably with bobcats. The highest incidence of disease occurs during early summer through to autumn, corresponding to the time when ticks are most active. More than one individual in a multicat household may be affected and it is wise to check the other cats when the disease is first diagnosed.

The life cycle of *C. felis* is poorly understood. It is suspected that *Dermacentor variabilis* is the principal vector for natural transmission and is responsible for injecting infective sporozoites from its salivary glands into the mammalian host. Schizonts develop primarily within tissue histiocytes in many organs and go on to release merozoites, which invade monocytes and erythrocytes. In cats that survive initial infection, low-level erythrocytic parasitaemias can persist for many years.

PATHOGENESIS

Infection of domestic cats with the schizogenous stage typically results in a rapidly progressive systemic disease with a high mortality rate. In natural infections with *C. felis* there is an apparent variation in pathogenicity that may be associated with geographical location. Some cats survive and develop chronic parasitaemia. The pathogenesis of cytauxzoonosis is attributed to the schizogenous phase, which causes mechanical obstruction to blood flow through various organs, notably the lungs, and results in a shock-like state. Vascular occlusion and damage are further associated with the release of inflammatory mediators and development of disseminated intravascular coagulation (DIC). Intravascular and extravascular haemolysis occur as a result of erythrocyte invasion by merozoites.

CLINICAL SIGNS

The tissue schizont phase of infection with *C. felis* is responsible for the clinical signs. Soon after infection, affected cats develop non-specific signs such as anorexia, lymphadenomegaly, fever and lethargy, but the course of the disease is usually rapid, with the onset of a severe clinical syndrome characterized by dehydration, pallor, dyspnoea, icterus, recumbency and death. Thoracic radiographs may reveal enlarged and tortuous pulmonary vessels as a result of vascular occlusion by the tissue stages (**Figures 6.15, 6.16**). Usually, by the time the cat is presented, it is severely ill. Most cats die within 9–15 days following infection by virulent strains, regardless of treatment.

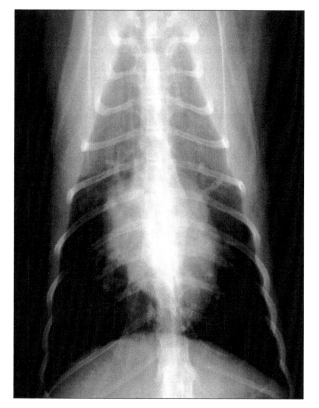

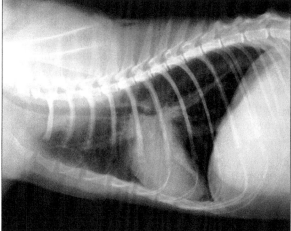

Figs. 6.15, 6.16 Ventrodorsal (6.15, left) and lateral (6.16, above) radiographs of the thorax of a cat with cytauxzoonosis. The pulmonary vessels are enlarged and appear increased in number. The margins are slightly hazy due to a moderate diffuse increase in interstitial opacity, with a mild bronchial component. Faint pleural fissure lines indicate a small volume of pleural effusion. (Courtesy Dr N Lester)

DIAGNOSIS

Diagnosis of cytauxzoonosis is made by identification of intraerythrocytic piroplasms in blood smears stained with Wright's stain or Giemsa (**Figure 6.17**). There is no serological assay available commercially at the current time. Parasitaemias are typically low (1–4%), although in some acute infections as many as 25% of the red cells may be infected. *C. felis* is a small piroplasm (see **Table 6.1**) that must be differentiated from *Babesia felis*, which is very similar in size and appearance, by light microscopy; however, *B. felis* is confined geographically to southern Africa. *C. felis* appears in a number of morphological varieties including the signet-ring form, bipolar oval forms, tetrads and dark-staining 'dots', the latter of which may be mistaken for a more common and widespread parasite of cats, haemotropic *Mycoplasma* species, the cause of feline infectious anaemia (see Chapter 7). A unique, yet uncommon, finding in cytauxzoonosis is the appearance of tissue phase schizonts in blood smears and buffy coat preparations. However, these forms are best demonstrated in impression smears from bone marrow, spleen or lymph nodes, where they are typically numerous (**Figure 6.18**).

Haematology and serum biochemistry abnormalities are typical of haemolytic anaemia. Initially, the anaemia is normochromic and normocytic, but it progresses to a strong regenerative response, characterized by the presence of nucleated red cells by the time of death. Moderate to severe leucopenia is typical and thrombocytopenia, sometimes profound, is commonly reported with or without DIC. Prolongation of clotting times (prothrombin time and activated partial thromboplastin time) has been recorded and been used to support a diagnosis of DIC, but concentrations of fibrin degradation products are variable. The plasma appears icteric on the last day or two of life and is associated with a high serum concentration of bilirubin. Other clinicopathological changes that have been recorded in cases of cytauxzoonosis include hyperglycaemia, hypokalaemia, hypocholesterolaemia and elevations in serum ALT and ALP; however, these changes may be minimal in acutely affected individuals, which typically die before such abnormalities are recorded.

Necropsy findings in cats that have died of cytauxzoonosis include pallor and icterus of the tissues, petechial and ecchymotic haemorrhages on the serosal surfaces of organs, oedematous lymph nodes and lungs, and hepatosplenomegaly. Diagnosis may be confirmed by histological examination of the tissues. Large numbers of mononuclear phagocytes containing schizonts are visible in the veins of most organs, including the liver, lung, spleen, lymph nodes, kidneys and central nervous system.

TREATMENT AND CONTROL

A diagnosis of cytauxzoonosis carries a grave prognosis, with high mortality rates despite treatment. Of the specific therapies that appear to help ameliorate the acute disease, imidocarb dipropionate and the combination

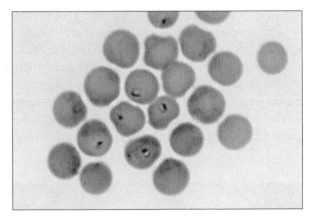

Fig. 6.17 *Cytauxzoon felis* piroplasms in a domestic cat with terminal cytauxzoonosis (Oklahoma, USA). (Courtesy Dr J. Meinkoth)

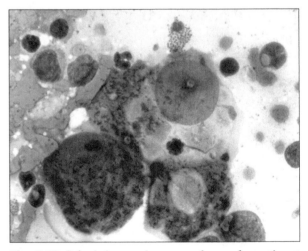

Fig. 6.18 Splenic impression smear from a domestic cat that died from cytauxzoonosis. Note the large schizont-laden macrophages. (Courtesy Dr J. Meinkoth)

of atovaquone and azithromycin have shown most promise (**Table 6.8**). Early administration of subcutaneous heparin, together with fluid therapy and blood transfusions, may also be beneficial in the management of DIC, but controlled studies are lacking.

ZOONOTIC POTENTIAL/PUBLIC HEALTH SIGNIFICANCE

There is currently no recognized zoonotic potential of *C. felis* infection.

Table 6.8 **Treatment of cats with cytauxzoonosis.**

TYPE OF THERAPY	DRUG/MEDICATION	TRADE NAME(S)	RECOMMENDED DOSE	FREQUENCY	NOTES/COMMENTS
Specific	Diminazine aceturate	Ganaseg, Berenil	2 mg/kg IM	Once	Haemolysis and icterus may worsen transiently after injection
	Imidocarb dipropionate	Imizol	2 mg/kg IM	Repeat after 3–7 days	Anticholinergic signs (vomiting, diarrhoea, miosis, 3rd eyelid prolapse and muscle fasciculations) controlled by atropine (at 0.05 mg/kg SC)
Supportive	Crystalloid fluid therapy	-	To correct dehydration and provide maintenance	Ongoing	Care to avoid excess haemodilution
	Blood transfusion	-	Refer to Table 6.7	As required	Blood typing or cross-match is necessary to ascertain compatibility of donor blood
	Heparin	-	100–150 units/kg SC	q8h	Reduce dose gradually to avoid rebound hypercoagulability

CASE STUDY: MIXED VECTOR-BORNE INFECTIONS IN A DOG

History

Misty, a 6-year-old neutered female Terrier, presented because she had been lethargic (preferring to lie in her basket and reluctant to go for walks) for the previous 2 days and was refusing to eat. Misty had been a stray and was obtained from an animal shelter 9 months earlier, but she had been well for the time she had been with the new owners except for an incident about 6 weeks earlier in which she was involved in a fight with a Pit Bull Terrier, during which she received lacerations to her neck and left forelimb. The wounds were treated surgically at the clinic, a 10-day course of cephalexin was prescribed and she had appeared to recover well, although the owners report that she had become fearful in the presence of other dogs.

Physical examination

Clinical examination revealed a quiet patient, body condition score 4/9, temperature 38.7°C, respiratory rate 25/minute and heart rate 100/minute. The wounds on the neck and leg had healed well, but the veterinarian noted that Misty had pale mucous membranes, capillary refill time (CRT) <1 second and mild dehydration.

Assessment

Lethargy, anorexia, pallor and dehydration were noted as the medical problems in this dog. The pallor was considered to be significant, indicative of anaemia or poor peripheral perfusion; however, the normal CRT and mild dehydration suggested that anaemia was the more likely cause.

In-house laboratory testing

In-house testing included microhaematocrit (PCV 0.20 l/l, TS 78 g/l), a peripheral blood film examination and testing for infectious diseases using a bench top immunochromatographic kit (Snap 4Dx Plus™, Idexx Laboratories). Anaemia was confirmed and an in-house examination of the blood film indicated a regenerative process (anisocytosis, polychromasia and occasional spherocytes). Very few platelets were observed. In addition, Mitsy was positive for the presence of antibodies to *Ehrlichia* species and heartworm antigen (**Figure 6.19**). A tentative diagnosis of immune-mediated haemolytic anaemia (IMHA), ehrlichiosis and heartworm infection was made and treatment was started with prednisolone (1 mg/kg PO q12h), doxycycline (10 mg/kg PO q24h) and IV fluid therapy. Blood samples (in EDTA and lithium heparin) and a urine sample (free catch) were sent to a commercial laboratory for testing.

External laboratory testing

Laboratory test results, available the next day, confirmed anaemia (red cell count 3.89×10^{12}/l [reference range: 5.70–8.80]; haemoglobin 112 g/l [reference range: 129–184]) and thrombocytopenia (platelet count 23×10^{9}/l [reference range: 200–500]), but in addition the pathologist reported observation of intraerythrocytic inclusions consistent with a small piroplasm infection (**Figure 6.20**). *Babesia gibsoni* was suspected and confirmed by subsequent PCR testing, as was *E. canis* infection. Additional laboratory abnormalities included hypoalbuminaemia (18 g/l [reference range: 25–38]), hyperglobulinaemia (50 g/l [reference range: 25–45]) and a mild (1+) proteinuria.

Diagnosis

Babesiosis associated with *B. gibsoni* infection, canine monocytic ehrlichiosis and heartworm infection.

Treatment

The combination treatment for *B. gibsoni* of azithromycin (10 mg/kg q24h PO) and atovaquone (13.3 mg/kg q8h PO) was started immediately and continued for 10 days; the doxycycline treatment started previously was continued (for 28 days), but the prednisolone therapy was stopped over a period of 2 days. Further treatment of the heartworm infection was considered (http://heartwormsociety.org/images/pdf/2014-AHS-Canine-Guidelines.pdf), but was postponed pending the outcome of treatment for the other two infections.

Outcome

Misty responded favourably to fluid therapy and the combined drug treatments and started to eat within 24 hours. She was discharged from hospital after 3 days, at which time her PCV was 0.28 l/l. Follow-up laboratory testing 1 week later revealed normalization of the red blood cell count, haemoglobin concentration and serum albumin concentration, although mild hyperproteinaemia and thrombocytopenia persisted. The *Babesia* PCR was repeated after 1 month and was negative; *E. canis* was not re-tested.

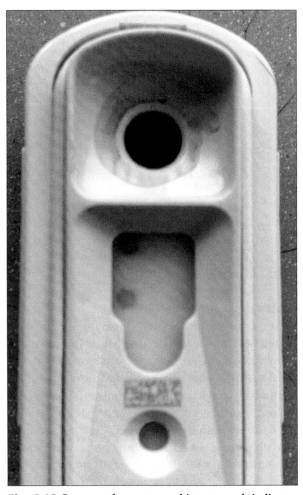

Fig. 6.19 Immunochromatographic test result indicating a positive result for *Ehrlichia* species (bottom left) and heartworm (bottom right) and a positive sample control (top left).

Comments

An initial diagnosis of IMHA was made on the basis of in-house testing. The cause was unknown at the time, but the clinician thought that secondary IMHA as a drug reaction to the previously prescribed cephalexin was a possibility. *B. gibsoni* parasites are often difficult to see on blood film examination, so a careful evaluation using oil-immersion and a high-power objective (×100) is advised. The earlier history of a dog fight is very important in this case, especially as the fight was with a Pit Bull Terrier. This breed is known to be over-represented for babesiosis and in this case *B. gibsoni* infection is presumed to have occurred during blood exchanged during fighting. Occasional cases of babesiosis, such as this one, have been reported in non-Pit Bull Terriers following fights with this breed. Thrombocytopenia is a common laboratory abnormality with both babesiosis and ehrlichiosis. In this case it was not known when the dog had become infected with *E. canis* or *Dirofilaria immitis*; the dog had been a stray and had not been tested previously for vector-borne disease, although she had been receiving combined ectoparasite and heartworm prophylaxis since being obtained from the animal shelter. Antibodies to *E. canis* may remain for many months to years following infection.

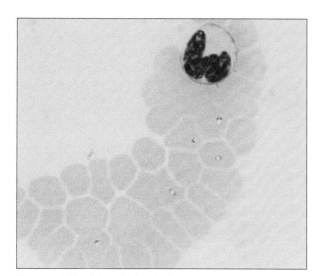

Fig. 6.20 Peripheral blood film showing five small intraerythrocytic inclusions: *Babesia gibsoni* infection.

FURTHER READING

Babesiosis

Holm LP, Kerr MG, Trees AJ *et al.* (2006) Fatal babesiosis in an untravelled British dog. *Veterinary Record* **159:**179–180.

Irwin PJ (2009) Canine babesiosis: from molecular taxonomy to control. *Parasites & Vectors* **2(S1):**1–9.

Jefferies R, Ryan UM, Jardine J *et al.* (2007) Blood, bull terriers and babesiosis: further evidence for direct transmission of *Babesia gibsoni* in dogs. *Australian Veterinary Journal* **85:**459–463.

Kjemtrup AM, Wainwright K, Miller M *et al.* (2006) *Babesia conradae*, sp. nov., a small canine *Babesia* identified in California. *Veterinary Parasitology* **138:**103–111.

Matijatko V, Kiš I, Torti M *et al.* (2009) Septic shock in canine babesiosis. *Veterinary Parasitology* **162:**263–270.

Sakuma M, Setoguchi A, Endo Y (2009) Possible emergence of drug-resistant variants of *Babesia gibsoni* in clinical cases treated with atovaquone and azithromycin. *Journal of Veterinary Internal Medicine* **23:**493–498.

Yeagley TJ, Reichard MV, Hempstead JE *et al.* (2009) Detection of *Babesia gibsoni* and the canine small *Babesia* 'Spanish isolate' in blood samples obtained from dogs confiscated from dog fighting operations. *Journal of the American Veterinary Medical Association* **235:**535–539.

Cytauxzoonosis

Cohn LA, Birkenheuer AJ, Brunker JD *et al.* (2011) Efficacy of atovaquone and azithromycin or imidocarb dipropionate in cats with acute cytauxzoonosis. *Journal of Veterinary Internal Medicine* **25:**55–60.

Lewis KM, Cohn LA, Marr HS *et al.* (2014) Failure of efficacy and adverse events associated with dose-intense diminazene diaceturate treatment of chronic *Cytauxzoon felis* infection in five cats. *Journal of Feline Medicine and Surgery* **16:**157–163.

Chapter 7

Haemoplasmosis

Emi Barker
Séverine Tasker

BACKGROUND, AETIOLOGY AND EPIDEMIOLOGY

The haemotropic mycoplasmas (haemoplasmas) are a group of uncultivatable bacteria within the genus *Mycoplasma*. They have worldwide distribution and can infect a wide variety of mammals, including domesticated dogs and cats, wild felidae (e.g. Iberian lynx, Eurasian lynx, European wildcat, Iriomote cat, lion, puma, jaguar, oncilla, Geoffroy's cat, margay and ocelot) and wild canidae (e.g. European wolves, coyotes, bush dog and raccoon dog). They parasitize the surface of erythrocytes and can induce variable degrees of haemolytic anaemia (haemoplasmosis) (**Figure 7.1**).

Haemoplasmas were previously classified as rickettsial organisms within the genera *Eperythrozoon* and *Haemobartonella* due to their obligate parasitism, small size, erythrocyte tropism and suspected arthropod transmission. However, following molecular phylogenetic analysis they were subsequently reclassified as mycoplasmas within the family Mycoplasmataceae. Certain phenotypic characteristics of the haemoplasmas, including their small size (~0.3–0.8 μm), small genome (0.51–1.16 Mbp), fastidious growth requirements (they are currently uncultivatable *in vitro*) and lack of a cell wall, supported their reclassification. Their uncultivatable status limits full characterization, therefore the '*Candidatus*' prefix is applied to newly described haemoplasmas.

Feline haemoplasmas

At least three haemoplasma species have been shown to infect cats: *Mycoplasma haemofelis* (previously the Ohio strain, or large form of *Haemobartonella felis*), '*Candidatus* Mycoplasma haemominutum' (previously the California strain, or small form of *Haemobartonella felis*) and '*Candidatus* Mycoplasma turicensis'. Epidemiological studies have identified DNA from a further two hae-

moplasmas in domestic cats: '*Candidatus* Mycoplasma haematoparvum'-like haemoplasma and '*Candidatus* Mycoplasma haemominutum'-like haemoplasma.

Feline haemoplasma species vary in pathogenicity. *Mycoplasma haemofelis* is the most pathogenic, and can cause moderate to severe, Coombs-positive, haemolytic anaemia (feline infectious anaemia) in immunocompetent cats. '*Ca*. M. haemominutum' and '*Ca*. M. turicensis' are less pathogenic, but can result in a decreased haematocrit, which may or may not be clinically significant. Co-infections with all three feline haemoplasma species have been described frequently. The whole genome sequences of *M. haemofelis* and '*Ca*. M. haemominutum' have been determined.

Canine haemoplasmas

At least two haemoplasma species have been shown to infect dogs: *Mycoplasma haemocanis* and '*Candidatus* M. haematoparvum'. Epidemiological studies have identified DNA from a further four haemoplasmas in domes-

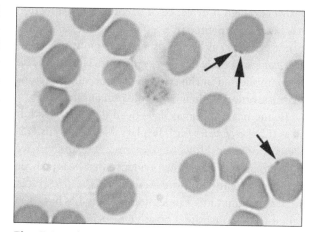

Fig. 7.1 A thin blood smear revealing *Mycoplasma haemofelis* (arrows) on the surface of feline erythrocytes during acute infection.

tic dogs: '*Ca*. M. haemominutum'-like haemoplasma, '*Ca*. M. turicensis'-like haemoplasma, '*Candidatus* Mycoplasma haemobos'-like haemoplasma and *Mycoplasma ovis*-like haemoplasma.

Fewer data are available regarding the pathogenesis of canine haemoplasmas. Co-infections with both canine haemoplasma species are common. Case reports have described both *M. haemocanis* and '*Ca*. M. haematoparvum' in association with anaemia, most commonly in splenectomized dogs, those receiving chemotherapeutic agents and those infected with other haemoparasites. The whole genome sequence of *M. haemocanis* has been determined.

Transmission

Early studies demonstrated transmission of *M. haemocanis* between splenectomized dogs by the brown dog tick, *Rhipicephalus sanguineus*, including transstadial and transovarian transfer within the tick. However, these studies were based on cytological diagnosis of infection and have not been repeated using molecular methods to determine infecting species and to confirm absence of haemoplasma infection prior to tick exposure. Epidemiological studies support an arthropod-borne mechanism of transmission. A lower prevalence of both *M. haemocanis* and '*Ca*. M. haematoparvum' is seen in cooler climates and higher prevalence seen in warmer climates that support *R. sanguineus*. In regions where climate does not support survival of *R. sanguineus*, haemoplasma-positive dogs frequently had a history of travel to regions where *Rhipicephalus* ticks are endemic. However, high prevalence of haemoplasma infection has been documented in a region where *R. sanguineus* is not endemic, although other arthropods (fleas and *Haemaphysalis leachi* ticks) were present. Ticks have also been implicated in the transmission of feline haemoplasmas; however, their exact role remains unclear.

Feline haemoplasmas have been detected in adult fleas (*Ctenocephalides felis*), flea larvae and flea dirt collected from cats. However, experimental studies have failed to provide conclusive evidence that fleas provide a common route of transmission of *M. haemofelis* or '*Ca*. M. haemominutum'. Epidemiological studies have also failed to demonstrate a positive association between haemoplasma infection and presence of flea infestation.

Both feline and canine haemoplasmas may be transmitted via parenteral administration of infected blood products, either experimentally or iatrogenically. Successful transmission may also occur following experimental ingestion of infected blood products, although this route is less consistent. The oral route is suspected to be a natural mechanism of transmission in Japanese fighting dogs and in cats with increased likelihood of aggressive interaction with other cats (e.g. male, outdoor access, cat bite abscesses). Haemoplasma DNA has been detected in the saliva of acutely infected cats, which could provide another route of transmission; however, this has not been supported experimentally. Vertical transfer of haemoplasma infection is suspected to occur, in cats at least, with the cytological diagnosis of haemoplasma infection in very young kittens and queens reported. However the exact route of transmission (i.e. transplacental or transmammary) has not been investigated.

Epidemiology

Reported haemoplasma prevalence from polymerase chain reaction (PCR)-based epidemiological studies vary significantly, likely reflecting factors such as the varying nature of the cats and dogs being sampled in the different studies (e.g. healthy versus sick/hospitalized/anaemic populations; pet versus feral), detection methods (conventional PCR with sequencing versus species-specific qPCR) and/or geographical variation. **Tables 7.1** and **7.2** describe haemoplasma prevalence in at-risk cats and dogs, respectively (predominantly anaemic or sick populations), and risk factors identified.

The three main feline haemoplasma species have been detected worldwide, with both dual and triple haemoplasma infections occurring naturally. '*Ca*. M. haemominutum' is typically the most prevalent of the feline haemoplasmas (up to 46.7%), with similar prevalence between healthy and sick or anaemic cats within the same geographical region and no association between '*Ca*. M. haemominutum' status and presence of anaemia in most studies. Feline haemoplasmas *M. haemofelis* and '*Ca*. M. turicensis' are less prevalent. Within sick cat populations, *M. haemofelis* is identified in up to 21.3% of samples, although a prevalence of ~5% is more typical. The two main canine haemoplasma species have also been detected worldwide, with *M. haemocanis* typically more prevalent than '*Ca*. M. haematoparvum'.

Data regarding risk factors for feline haemoplasma infections are limited by small numbers of infected cats,

Table 7.1 **Selected feline haemoplasma PCR-based prevalence studies and risk factors.**

REFERENCE	COUNTRY	NUMBER ENROLLED	HEALTH STATUS	% POSITIVE SAMPLES				RISK FACTORS FOR INFECTION
				HP	Mhf	CMhm	CMt	
Ghazisaeedi *et al.* 2014	Iran	100	100% sick	22.0	14.0	12.0	4.0	Older; male; lower HCT/RBC/Hb (all HP)
Lobetti *et al.* 2012	South Africa	102	100% sick	25.5	3.9	21.6	0	Lower HCT; lower WBC; lower platelets (Mhf)
Roura *et al.* 2010	Spain	191	60% sick	12.3	3.7	9.9	0.5	FIV status; outdoor access; male (all HP). (Not associated: age; breed; health status; FeLV status)
Gentilini *et al.* 2009	Italy	307	Mostly sick	18.9	5.9	17.3	1.3	FIV status; summer season (all HP). Low HCT/RBC/Hb/ MCHC; higher WBC (Mhf). (Not associated: age; breed; gender; FeLV status; anaemia [all HP]]
Sykes *et al.* 2007	USA	263	99% sick; 51% anaemic	18.0	0.4	15.6	0.4	(Not associated: FeLV status [CMhm])
Sykes *et al.* 2008	USA	310	Anaemic or HP suspected	27.4	4.8	23.2	6.5	Male (all HP). FIV/FeLV status; reticulocytosis (Mhf). Increased MCV (Mhf/CMhm). (Not associated: FIV/FeLV status [CMhm/CMt])
Willi *et al.* 2006a	Switzerland	713	89% sick (14% HP suspected)	11.6	1.5	10	1.3	Older; male; outdoor; geographical region; CMt status; CKD (CMhm). Male; geographical region (Mhf). (Not associated: FIV/FeLV status [CMhm]; anaemia [CMhm/Mhf])
Tasker *et al.* 2003; Willi *et al.* 2006b	UK	426	72% sick	19.2	1.6	17.1	2.3	Older; male (CMhm)
Tasker *et al.* 2004; Willi *et al.* 2006b	Australia	147	95% sick	32	4.8	23.8	10.2	Older; male; lower HCT; non-pedigree (CMhm). Copy number negatively correlated with HCT (Mhf)

HP, haemoplasma; Mhf, *M. haemofelis*; CMhm, '*Ca*. M. haemominutum'; CMt, '*Ca*. M. turicensis'; HCT, haematocrit; RBC, red blood cell count; Hb, haemoglobin concentration; MCHC, mean corpuscular haemoglobin concentration; WBC, white blood cell count; FIV, feline immunodeficiency virus; FeLV, feline leukaemia virus; CKD, chronic kidney disease.

limited data regarding samples and conflicting results. Some studies found male gender, older age and positive retroviral status to be associated with haemoplasma infection, particularly with '*Ca*. M. haemominutum', while others have not found this link. Outdoor access and presence of cat bite abscesses were also found by some to be associated with haemoplasma infection. The higher prevalence of '*Ca*. M. haemominutum' in older cats could represent a cumulative risk and increased likelihood of carrier status as compared with other feline haemoplasmas. Increased incidence in

outdoor, male cats could represent increased roaming, resulting in increased exposure to infected individuals or unknown vectors and increased likelihood of aggressive contact with infected cats.

Both feline immunodeficiency virus (FIV) and feline leukaemia virus (FeLV) infection have been found associated with haemoplasma infection in some studies, although FIV infection is more consistently identified as a risk factor. It is unclear whether a positive retrovirus status renders individuals more susceptible to haemoplasma infection or vice versa, or whether transmis-

Table 7.2 Selected canine haemoplasma PCR-based prevalence studies and risk factors.

REFERENCE	COUNTRY	NUMBER ENROLLED	HEALTH STATUS	% POSITIVE SAMPLES			RISK FACTORS FOR INFECTION
				HP	Mhc	CMhp	
Compton *et al.* 2012	USA	383	Sick	1.3	0.3	1.0	n/a
Roura *et al.* 2010	Spain	182	Sick	14.3	14.3	0.6	Other vector-borne infections (all HP). (Not associated: age; sex; anaemia; health-status [all HP])
Barker *et al.* 2010b	Trinidad	184	Sick	8.7	6.0	6.0	(Not associated: age; sex; haematological parameters [all HP])
Novacco *et al.* 2010	Italy	600	Sick	9.5	4.5	5.8	Cross-breed; kennelled cf. private home; mange (all HP). (Not associated: sex; HCT; health-status [all HP])
	Spain	200		2.5	0.5	2.0	
	Portugal	50		40	40	0	
Wengi *et al.* 2008	Switzerland	882	Sick	1.2	0.9	0.3	(Not associated: age; sex; anaemia [all HP])
Kenny *et al.* 2004	France	460	Sick	15.4	5.9	12.2	n/a

Mhf, *M. haemocanis*; CMhp, '*Ca.* M. haematoparvum'; HP, haemoplasma; sick, samples collected for clinical diagnostic purposes.

sion of haemoplasma shares risk factors with retrovirus transmission. Co-infection with FeLV has been associated with a more significant anaemia following '*Ca.* M. haemominutum' infection. Experimentally, FIV infection does not appear to enhance the pathogenicity of haemoplasmas; however, chronic FIV infection has been shown to modify the acute phase response to haemoplasma infection.

Fewer data are available regarding risk factors for canine haemoplasma infection. Male dogs appear to be at increased risk of *M. haemocanis* infection, particularly those specifically used for dog fighting. Group kennelling, as compared with residence in private homes, was also found to be a risk factor in one study. Concurrent infection with other haemoparasites was also found to be a risk factor for *M. haemocanis* infection and could represent a common vector or immunocompromise from one infection or the other increasing susceptibility.

PATHOGENESIS

Erythrocytes infected with *M. haemofelis* have a significantly reduced half-life, attributed to a combination of destruction (intravascular and/or extravascular haemolysis) and temporary removal from the circula-

tion during sequestration by the reticuloendothelial system, in particular the spleen. Direct mechanical effects of the haemoplasma, such as erythrocyte membrane damage (surface erosions) and altered lipid concentrations increase erythrocyte fragility and increase the risk of membrane shearing, particularly during passage through narrow blood vessels. Destruction can also occur as a result of 'bystander' effects of a direct immune response following attachment of antibody to the cell membrane, with subsequent complement activation leading to intravascular haemolysis, or as a result of targeted phagocytosis by the reticuloendothelial system, to extravascular haemolysis.

CLINICAL SIGNS

Many of the clinical signs reported with haemoplasmosis result from anaemia and activation of the reticuloendothelial system. The severity of the anaemia can range from mild and unapparent to life-threatening. Factors believed to influence clinical presentation include host factors (e.g. age, presence or absence of spleen [in dogs], concurrent disease and immunosuppressive therapy) and haemoplasma factors (e.g. infecting species, strain).

Cats with acute *M. haemofelis* infection may present with lethargy, depression, inappetence, pica, weight loss and weakness. Clinical examination findings may include pyrexia, pallor, icterus, cardiac (haemic) murmurs, lymphadenomegaly, tachypnoea, tachycardia and weak or hyperdynamic femoral pulses (**Figure 7.2**). In severe cases, cats may become dehydrated, hypothermic, collapsed and exhibit neurological signs (i.e. vocalization, coma). Hepatosplenomegaly may also be apparent, due to a combination of increased macrophage activity within the spleen, splenic sequestration of erythrocytes and extramedullary haematopoiesis. In experimental studies, clinical signs were not reported in cats infected with '*Ca*. M. haemominutum', although significant decreases in red cell parameters (i.e. number, haemoglobin concentration and haematocrit) did occur during acute infection. However, retrospective studies of cats have identified anaemia in some cats naturally infected with '*Ca*. M. haemominutum' in the absence of other recognized causes. '*Ca*. M. turicensis' has been inconsistently associated with clinical haemolytic anaemia.

Dogs with acute haemoplasmosis have presented with clinical signs ranging from progressive weakness and lethargy, to acute collapse, months to years following splenectomy. Clinical examination findings were consistent with anaemia (i.e. weakness, pale mucous membranes, tachycardia and hyperdynamic pulses).

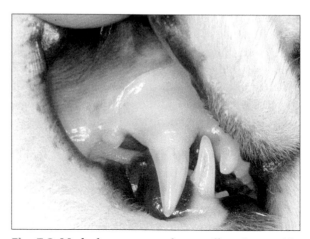

Fig. 7.2 Marked mucous membrane pallor of a cat with acute haemoplasmosis.

DIAGNOSIS

Routine laboratory findings

Laboratory abnormalities in cats and dogs with clinical haemoplasmosis are similar. Haematology typically reveals a moderate to severe regenerative anaemia, with macrocytosis, anisocytosis, polychromasia, Howell–Jolly bodies, reticulocytosis and (in severely affected cats) normoblastaemia. Persistent erythrocyte autoagglutination or Coombs test positivity may be present. Reticulocyte evaluation using new methylene blue staining should be interpreted cautiously as haemoplasma-infected erythrocytes may have a similar punctate appearance. Infrequently, the anaemia may appear non-regenerative where insufficient time has lapsed for an appropriate bone marrow response (i.e. pre-regenerative) or where concurrent bone marrow disease (e.g. FeLV infection) is present. No specific leucogram findings are pathognomonic: the neutrophil count may be increased, normal or decreased; the monocyte count may be increased or normal; and a lymphopenia may or may not be present. Platelet numbers are typically normal, but may be reduced.

Serum biochemistry may reveal increased hepatocellular enzyme activity, most likely secondary to hypoxic damage. Tissue hypoxia and poor peripheral perfusion may also result in metabolic acidosis. A mild to moderate hyperbilirubinaemia may be present secondary to the haemolytic anaemia or systemic inflammation. Prerenal azotaemia may be present in collapsed or dehydrated cases.

Specific diagnosis

Cytological evaluation of thin blood smears using light microscopy for the diagnosis of haemoplasmosis has poor sensitivity and specificity. False-positive results can occur with stain precipitation, basophilic stippling and Howell–Jolly bodies. False-negative results can occur due to low copy number within samples or dissociation of organisms from the erythrocyte surface (post-collection artefact). During experimental infection with *M. haemofelis*, copy numbers frequently cycle, with organisms visible <50% of the time during acute infection and at an even lower frequency during the chronic/carrier state. The diminutive size of '*Ca*. M. haemominutum' limits its visualization on blood smears and it is typically not visible in chronically infected cats. To date, even during acute infection, '*Ca*. M. turicensis' has not been visualized using light microscopy due to low copy number. In contrast, as the canine haemoplasma *M. haemocanis* can form chains (**Figure 7.3**) it may be more easily differentiated from stain artefact on light microscopy if the copy number is sufficiently high.

Currently, PCR assays are the diagnostic test of choice for haemoplasma infection in cats and dogs. Conventional and quantitative real-time PCR diagnostic assays typically target the 16S rRNA gene and may be genus- or species-specific. These assays are highly specific and are far more sensitive than cytological examination of blood smears; however, when animals only have very low haemoplasma copy numbers in the blood (e.g. healthy carrier animals or following antibiotic administration) below the lower limit of PCR detection, they may yield PCR-negative results despite being haemoplasma infected.

Serological diagnosis of haemoplasmosis is not currently available commercially. Recently, enzyme-linked immunosorbent assays (ELISAs) based on recombinant *M. haemofelis* DnaK, an immunodominant protein of haemoplasmas, have been developed for research purposes to detect a humoral response to haemoplasma infection in cats. However, these ELISAs are not species-specific and more work is required to determine their specificity for use in the clinical setting.

TREATMENT

Both supportive and specific treatment is indicated for cats and dogs with clinical signs and laboratory abnormalities consistent with haemoplasmosis. However, as no treatment regimen has yet been identified that com-

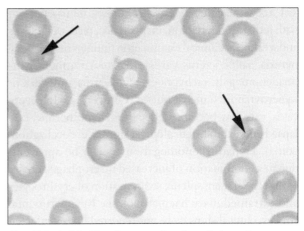

Fig. 7.3 A thin blood smear showing chains of *Mycoplasma haemocanis* (arrows) on the surface of canine erythrocytes during acute infection.

pletely eliminates the organism, antibiotic administration to clinically healthy animals that are PCR positive is not currently recommended.

Specific therapy for haemoplasmosis

Antibiotics belonging to the tetracycline (e.g. oxytetracycline, doxycycline) and fluoroquinolone (e.g. enrofloxacin, marbofloxacin, pradofloxacin) groups have been shown to have efficacy in treating the clinical signs of haemoplasmosis (**Table 7.3**). However, neither tetracycline nor fluoroquinolone protocols studied to date have demonstrated consistent efficacy at eliminating infection. There also appears to be a variable response to antibiotics both between infect-

Table 7.3 **Drugs used for therapy of haemoplasmosis.**

DRUG NAME	RECOMMENDED DOSE	NOTES/COMMENTS
Doxycycline	5 mg/kg PO q12h or 10 mg/kg PO q24h	Associated with gastrointestinal adverse effects, particularly oesophagitis
Oxytetracycline	25 mg/kg PO q8h	Best administered on an empty stomach. Not recommended due to availability of more efficacious drugs
Enrofloxacin	5 mg/kg PO q24h	Not recommended in cats due to association, albeit rarely, with irreversible retinal toxicity as an idiosyncratic reaction
Marbofloxacin	2 mg/kg PO q24h	
Pradofloxacin	5–10 mg/kg PO q24h	May be more effective at clearing *M. haemofelis* than doxycycline

ing haemoplasma species and isolates. Marbofloxacin administration resulted in a significant decrease in *M. haemofelis* copy number, which persisted following termination of treatment. In contrast, marbofloxacin administration resulted in a more conservative decrease in '*Ca*. M. haemominutum' copy number, which was not sustained following termination of treatment. Response of *M. haemocanis* to doxycycline in splenectomized dogs is variable, with apparent clearance of the organism in one case to recurrence of clinical signs following termination of treatment in another.

Doxycycline is currently preferred as the first-line therapy for suspected or confirmed haemoplasmosis, due to fewer adverse effects than other tetracyclines and concurrent activity against other infectious agents capable of inducing anaemia (e.g. *Anaplasma phagocytophilum*, *Bartonella* species, *Ehrlichia canis*-like organism and *Francisella tularensis*). However, oesophageal strictures subsequent to doxycycline administration have been reported with some formulations, therefore administration should be accompanied either by a water or food swallow. Marbofloxacin or pradofloxacin are suitable second-line alternatives to doxycycline. The majority of cats exhibit a clinical response within 14 days of starting treatment, and this duration of administration has been used effectively in a number of experimental studies. However, many feline practitioners treat cats with naturally acquired infection for 3–6 weeks if possible.

Supportive care for haemoplasmosis

Supportive care is an integral component in the treatment of canine and feline haemoplasmosis. This should include correction of dehydration with fluid therapy and, if the anaemia is severe, blood transfusion or treatment with a haemoglobin-based oxygen-carrying solution. A packed cell volume (PCV) of 20% is often used as a 'transfusion trigger' in dogs with acute anaemia; however, anaemic dogs and cats with signs consistent with decompensated anaemia (tachycardia, weakness, tachypnoea and metabolic acidaemia) are best treated with a whole blood or packed red blood cell transfusion regardless of PCV. Packed red blood cell transfusions, where available, are preferable when volume overload is a concern. Oxygen therapy should be provided pending stabilization of the patient's oxygen-carrying capacity.

Haemoglobin-based oxygen-carrying solutions can provide both short-term oxygen-carrying support and increase the circulatory volume due to their potent colloidal properties. However, they should be used with caution in normovolaemic patients (particularly cats, where anaemia has been associated with a circulatory volume overload), where excessive fluid administration may result in volume overload.

Administration of glucocorticoids to cats and dogs with suspected haemoplasmosis is controversial. Their efficacy is unproven, they are not required for a clinical response and immunosuppressive doses of glucocorticoids have been used experimentally to enhance bacteraemia and induce reactivation of latent infection. However, they may have a role in severe cases with documented immune-mediated destruction and/or in cases refractory to antibiosis.

PREVENTION AND CONTROL

In case arthropod vectors are involved in transmission, regular ectoparasite control would appear prudent. Similarly, avoidance of other risk factors could minimize the possibility of infection (i.e. restricting outdoor access, preventing violent interactions between individuals, and screening of blood donors). As the carrier status cannot be eliminated, infected individuals should not be considered for blood donors.

ZOONOTIC POTENTIAL/PUBLIC HEALTH SIGNIFICANCE

Individual case reports have described the detection of haemoplasma DNA within the blood of human patients in Brazil, China, the USA and the UK. Limited PCR-based human epidemiological studies have failed to detect significant infections and although human haemoplasma infections have been reported in China, these descriptions have not described clinical disease, PCR methodology or infecting species, making interpretation difficult. Only one report has documented severe haemolytic anaemia in association with the detection of haemoplasma DNA; in that report the haemoplasma species described was novel, with an as yet unknown definitive host. Of the companion animal haemoplasmas, DNA matching *M. haemofelis* was detected in a Brazilian man with concurrent *Bartonella henselae* and human immunodeficiency virus infection, *M. haemofelis*-like or *M. haemocanis*-like DNA was detected in the blood of a splenectomized patient with systemic lupus erythematosus, and DNA matching '*Ca.* M. haematoparvum' was detected in a female veterinarian with concurrent *B. henselae* and *Anaplasma platys* infection. The Brazilian man owned two *M. haemofelis*-infected cats and was described as having multiple cat scratches and bites. The female veterinarian was described as having received frequent animal bites and scratches from a wide variety of animal species (including cats, dogs and wide variety of arthropods).

As the route of zoonotic transmission of animal haemoplasmas remains unproven, advising on preventive care is difficult. Avoidance of skin trauma (bites, scratches) in people in contact with animals, and regular ectoparasite control of the animals in case arthropod vectors are involved in transmission, would appear prudent. The available case reports suggest that haemoplasma-associated disease is more likely in immunocompromised humans, therefore an increased level of care should be recommended in such cases.

CASE STUDY

Signalment

An 8-month-old, neutered female, domestic shorthair cat.

History

Indoor/outdoor access. No history of travel outside the UK. Fully vaccinated. Up to date with both ectoparasiticide and endoparasiticide medication. Two-week history of lethargy and weight loss. Twenty-four hour history of anorexia, weakness and tachypnoea.

Clinical examination findings

Quiet, but alert and responsive. Lean body condition (condition score 4/9). Mild pyrexia (39.5°C). Tachypnoea (60 breaths/min), tachycardia (204 beats/min), pale mucous membranes, prominent spleen on abdominal palpation and a grade 2/6 left basilar systolic heart murmur.

Investigation

Complete blood count revealed a strongly regenerative, severe anaemia with agglutination visible on the smear (**Tabe 7.4**). A direct Coombs test was weakly positive

Table 7.4 Haematology findings.

PARAMETER	DAY 1	DAY 6	DAY 29	REFERENCE RANGE
Reticulocytes	350			$<60.0 \times 10^9$/l
Hb	**3.44**	**6.32**	8.18	8.00–15.00 g/dl
Hct	**11.3**	**21.1**	26.5	25.0–45.0 %
RBC	**1.79**	**3.08**	5.55	5.50–10.00 $\times 10^{12}$/l
MCV	**63.2**	**68.6**	47.7	40.0–55.0 fl
MCH	**19.3**	**20.5**	14.8	12.5–17.0 pg
MCHC	30.5	**29.9**	30.9	30.0–35.0 g/dl
Platelets	42*	34*	144*	200–700 $\times 10^9$/l
Nucleated RBCs	**15.9**	**1.4**	-	$\times 10^9$/l
WBCs (corrected for NRBCs)	14.50	**19.40**	11.20	4.90–19.00 $\times 10^9$/l
Neutrophils	**12.95**	**15.94**	9.30	2.40–12.50 $\times 10^9$/l
Lymphocytes	1.46	2.14	1.46	1.40–6.00 $\times 10^9$/l
Monocytes	0.15	**0.78**	0.34	0.10–0.70 $\times 10^9$/l
Eosinophils	0.00	0.39	0.11	$<1.60 \times 10^9$/l
Basophils	0.00	**0.19**	0.00	$<0.10 \times 10^9$/l

Day 1 blood film examination: polychromasia++, macrocytic red blood cells+, anisocytosis+++. Agglutination present on film. Macrothrombocytes seen on film. *Platelets appear clumped, platelets plentiful.

Day 6 blood film examination: polychromasia++, anisocytosis++. Macrothrombocytes seen on film. *Platelets appear clumped, platelets plentiful.

Day 29 blood film examination: anisocytosis+. Macrothrombocytes seen on film. *Platelets appear clumped, platelets plentiful.

Abnormalities are highlighted in bold.

for polyvalent feline Coombs reagent and IgG at 37°C and negative for IgM. At 4°C there was agglutination in all test wells. Serum biochemistry (**Table 7.5**) revealed a severe hyperbilirubinaemia and a moderate increase in ALT activity. Urinalysis revealed only bilirubinuria. The cat was blood type B.

Thoracic radiography revealed a rounded globular appearance to the heart, with prominent pulmonary vessels (**Figure 7.4**). These changes were considered consistent with anaemia. Abdominal ultrasound

Table 7.5 **Serum biochemistry findings.**

PARAMETER	DAY 1	DAY 6	DAY 29	REFERENCE RANGE
Urea	7.2			6.5–10.5 mmol/l
Creatinine	**40**			133–175 µmol/l
Total protein	**73.5**	**71.0**	75.3	77.0–91.0 g/l
Albumin	29.1	28.3	27.0	24.0–35.0 g/l
Globulin	44.4	42.7	48.3	21.0–51.0 g/l
Albumin/ globulin ratio	0.66	0.66	0.56	0.4–1.30
ALT	**212**	**126**	34	15–45 IU/l
ALP	15	13	14	15–60 IU/l
Total bilirubin	**31.4**	**14.8**	3.2	<10.0 µmol/l
Sodium	145.5	142.3		149.0–157.0 mmol/l
Potassium	3.99	3.69		4.00–5.00 mmol/l
Chloride	110	112		115–130 mmol/l
Calcium	2.47	2.35		2.30–2.50 mmol/l
Phosphate	1.41	0.97		0.95–1.55 mmol/l
Glucose	7.3	5.7		3.5–6 .0 mmol/l

Abnormalities are highlighted in bold.

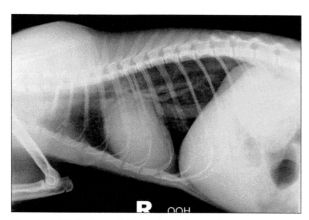

Fig. 7.4 **Right lateral thoracic radiograph demonstrating a rounded cardiac silhouette and prominent pulmonary vessels.**

revealed prominent abdominal lymph nodes, but these were of normal size and echotexture. The liver, gall-bladder, biliary tree and pancreas were unremarkable. There was no evidence of obstruction to the common bile duct. An echocardiogram showed no evidence of structural heart disease.

ELISAs for FeLV antigen and FIV antibodies were negative. PCR for *M. haemofelis* was positive with a cycle threshold of 22.4 (corresponding to an esti-mated organism number of 4×10^7/ml blood). PCRs for '*Ca.* M. haemominutum' and '*Ca.* M. turicensis' were negative.

Treatment

The clinicopathological changes were most consistent with an immune-mediated haemolytic anaemia, with increases in ALT activity secondary to tissue hypoxia. The cat received supportive care including an oxy-globin transfusion (0.25–0.5 ml/kg/hour; total volume of 5–10 ml/kg) and doxycycline (5mg/kg PO q12h). A whole blood transfusion was considered; however, her uncommon blood type (type B) and lack of available donor cat precluded this. The cat made a rapid clinical improvement with resolution of agglutination, increase in haematocrit and decrease in hyperbilirubinaemia. The doxycycline was continued for a total of 4 weeks, at which time the cat was clinically normal.

Discussion

Anaemia is a common clinical problem in feline prac-tice and is broadly categorized into pre-regenerative, regenerative (i.e. haemolytic or blood loss) or non-regenerative (i.e. bone marrow disorders or reduced erythropoietin production/activity). Haemolytic anaemia may be primary (autoimmune) or secondary, caused by various infectious diseases (e.g. haemoplas-mas, FeLV, FIV, feline infectious peritonitis [FIP], *Babesia felis*, *Cytauxzoon felis*), hereditary disease (e.g. pyruvate kinase deficiency), exposure to chemicals (e.g. antibiotics, methimazole, *Allium* species plants), severe hypophosphataemia, neoplasia (e.g. lymphoprolifera-tive or myeloproliferative disorders) or the presence of alloantibodies (e.g. neonatal isoerythrolysis, transfusion reaction). In this case, a lack of travel history excluded *B. felis* and *Cytauxzoon felis* infection and there was no history of recent drug administration or toxin access. There was no evidence on blood analysis or imaging to suggest a neoplastic process or FIP. A positive *M. hae-mofelis* PCR and rapid response to doxycycline and sup-portive care, supported a diagnosis of haemoplasmosis.

FURTHER READING

Barker EN, Helps CR, Heesom KJ *et al.* (2010a) Detection of humoral response using a recombinant heat shock protein 70 (dnaK) of *Mycoplasma haemofelis* in experimentally and naturally hemoplasma infected cats. *Clinical and Vaccine Immunology* **17:**1926–1932.

Barker EN, Tasker S, Day MJ *et al.* (2010b) Development and use of real-time PCR to detect and quantify *Mycoplasma haemocanis* and 'Candidatus *Mycoplasma haematoparvum*' in dogs. *Veterinary Microbiology* **140:**167–170.

Compton SM, Maggi RG, Breitschwerdt EB (2012) Candidatus *Mycoplasma haematoparvum* and *Mycoplasma haemocanis* infections in dogs from the United States. *Comparative Immunology, Microbiology and Infectious Diseases* **35:**557–562.

Gentilini F, Novacco M, Turba ME *et al.* (2009) Use of combined conventional and real-time PCR to determine the epidemiology of feline haemoplasma infections in northern Italy. *Journal of Feline Medicine and Surgery* **11:**277–285.

Ghazisaeedi F, Atyabi N, Zahrai Salehi T *et al.* (2014) A molecular study of hemotropic mycoplasmas (haemoplasmas) in cats in Iran. *Veterinary Clinical Pathology* **43:**381–386.

Kenny MJ, Shaw SE, Beugnet F *et al.* (2004) Demonstration of two distinct hemotropic mycoplasmas in French dogs. *Journal of Clinical Microbiology* **42:**5397–5399.

Korman R, Ceron J-J, Knowles TG *et al.* (2012) Acute phase response to *Mycoplasma haemofelis* and 'Candidatus Mycoplasma haemominutum' infection in FIV-infected and non FIV-infected cats. *Veterinary Journal* **193:**433–438.

Lappin MR (2014) Feline haemoplasmas are not transmitted by *Ctenocephalides felis*. *Symposium of the CVBD World Forum*, Barcelona.

Lobetti R, Lappin MR (2012) Prevalence of *Toxoplasma gondii*, *Bartonella* species, and haemoplasma infection in cats in South Africa. *Journal of Feline Medicine and Surgery* **14:**857–862.

Maggi RG, Compton SM, Trull CL *et al.* (2013) Infection with hemotropic *Mycoplasma* species in patients with or without extensive arthropod or animal contact. *Journal of Clinical Microbiology* **51:**32–37.

Marie JL, Shaw SE, Langton DA *et al.* (2009) Sub-clinical infection of dogs from the Ivory Coast and Gabon with *Ehrlichia*, *Anaplasma*, *Mycoplasma* and *Rickettsia* species. *Clinical Microbiology and Infection* **15:**284–285.

Novacco M, Meli ML, Gentilini F *et al.* (2010) Prevalence and geographical distribution of canine hemotropic mycoplasma infections in Mediterranean countries and analysis of risk factors for infection. *Veterinary Microbiology* **142:**276–284.

Roura X, Peters IR, Altet L *et al.* (2010) Real-time PCR detection of hemotropic mycoplasmas in healthy and unhealthy cats and dogs from the Barcelona area of Spain. *Journal of Veterinary Diagnostic Investigation* **22:**270–274.

Steer J, Tasker S, Barker EN *et al.* (2011) A novel hemotropic *Mycoplasma* (hemoplasma) in a patient with hemolytic anemia and pyrexia. *Clinical Infectious Diseases* **53:**e147–e151.

Sykes JE, Drazenovich NL, Ball LM *et al.* (2007) Use of conventional and real-time polymerase chain reaction to determine the epidemiology of hemoplasma infections in anemic and nonanemic cats. *Journal of Veterinary Internal Medicine* **21:**685–693.

Sykes JE, Terry JC, Lindsay LL et al. (2008) Prevalences of various hemoplasma species among cats in the United States with possible hemoplasmosis. *Journal of the the American Veterinary Medical Association* **232:**372–379.

Tasker S, Binns SH, Day MJ *et al.* (2003) Use of a PCR assay to assess the prevalence and risk factors for *Mycoplasma haemofelis* and 'Candidatus *Mycoplasma haemominutum*' in cats in the United Kingdom. *Veterinary Record* **152:**193–198.

Tasker S, Braddock JA, Baral R *et al.* (2004) Diagnosis of feline haemoplasma infection in Australian cats using a real-time PCR assay. *Journal of Feline Medicine and Surgery* **6:**345–354.

Weingart C, Tasker S, Kohn B Infection with haemoplasma species in 22 cats with anaemia. *Journal of Feline Medicine and Surgery*, in press.

Wengi N, Willi B, Boretti FS *et al.* (2008) Real-time PCR-based prevalence study, infection follow-up and molecular characterization of canine hemotropic mycoplasmas. *Veterinary Microbiology* **126:**132–141.

Willi B, Boretti FS, Baumgartner C et al. (2006a) Prevalence, risk factor analysis and follow-up of infections caused by three feline hemoplasma species in cats in Switzerland. *Journal of Clinical Microbiology* **44**:961–969.

Willi B, Tasker S, Boretti FS et al. (2006b) Phylogenetic analysis of 'Candidatus *Mycoplasma turicensis*' isolates from pet cats in the United Kingdom, Australia, and South Africa, with analysis of risk factors for infection. *Journal of Clinical Microbiology* **44**:4430–4435.

Woods JE, Brewer MM, Hawley JR et al. (2005) Evaluation of experimental transmission of '*Candidatus* Mycoplasma haemominutum' and *Mycoplasma haemofelis* by *Ctenocephalides felis* to cats. *American Journal of Veterinary Research* **66**:1008–1012.

Woods JE, Wisnewski N, Lappin MR (2006) Attempted transmission of '*Candidatus* Mycoplasma haemominutum' and *Mycoplasma haemofelis* by feeding cats infected *Ctenocephalides felis*. *American Journal of Veterinary Research* **67**:494–497.

Chapter 8

Hepatozoonosis

Gad Baneth
Nancy Vincent-Johnson

CANINE HEPATOZOONOSIS

Background, aetiology and epidemiology

Canine hepatozoonosis is a tick-borne disease caused by apicomplexan protozoa from the family Hepatozoidae. Two distinct species of *Hepatozoon* are known to infect dogs: *Hepatozoon canis* and *Hepatozoon americanum*.

H. canis infection (HCI) was first reported from India in 1905 and has since been described in southern Europe, the Middle East, Africa, southeast Asia and North and South America (**Figure 8.1**). *H. canis* infects the haemolymphatic tissues and causes anaemia and lethargy. *H. americanum* infection (HAI) is an emerging disease in the USA that has expanded north and east from Texas, where it was originally detected in 1978, to several southeastern states, with occasional cases reported in diverse locations across the USA including Washington, California, Nebraska, Vermont and Virginia. This organism infects primarily muscular tissues and induces severe myositis and lameness. *H. americanum* was initially considered to be a strain of *H. canis*, until it was described as a separate species in 1997. The species distinction was based on differences in the clinical disease manifestations, tissue tropism, pathological characteristics, parasite morphology and tick vectors. Subsequent genetic and antigenic comparative studies have supported the separate species classification (**Table 8.1**). Although *H. americanum* is diagnosed more frequently than *H. canis* in the USA, *H. canis* has been identified in dogs from several southern states, and co-infections with *H. americanum* and *H. canis* have been reported. Recently, the first case of *H. canis* in a red fox from the USA was reported in West Virginia. The main vector of *H. canis* is the brown dog tick, *Rhipicephalus sanguineus*, which is found in warm and temperate regions all over the world. It is also transmitted by the tick *Amblyomma ovale* in South America. The

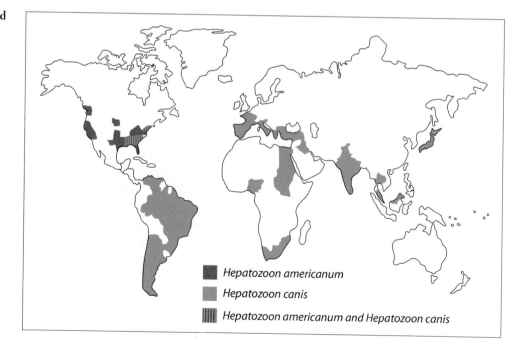

Fig. 8.1 **Reported geographical distributions of *H. canis* and *H. americanum* in domestic dogs.**

Hepatozoon americanum

Hepatozoon canis

Hepatozoon americanum and Hepatozoon canis

Table 8.1 **Comparison of *Hepatozoon americanum* and *Hepatozoon canis* infections.**

	H. americanum	*H. canis*
Main clinical signs	Lameness, muscular hyperaesthesia, fluctuating fever, lethargy, mucopurulent ocular discharge	Fever, lethargy, emaciation
Severity of signs	Severe; signs may wax and wane	Often mild. A severe disease is seen in dogs with a high parasitaemia
Haematological findings		
Extreme leucocytosis	Common, may be as high as $200 \times 10^9/l$	Rare, found in dogs with a high parasitaemia
Peripheral blood gamonts	Rare	Common
Parasitaemia	Usually <0.1% of leucocytes	1–100% of neutrophils
Anaemia	Common	Common
Radiographic abnormalities	Periosteal proliferation of long bones	Non-specific
Main diagnostic method	Demonstration of cysts and pyogranulomas in muscle biopsy, PCR	Detection of gamonts in blood smears, PCR
Primary target tissues	Skeletal muscle, cardiac muscle	Spleen, bone marrow, lymph nodes
Histopathological abnormalities	Pyogranulomatous myositis	Splenitis, hepatitis, pneumonia
Distinct tissue parasitic forms	'Onion skin' cyst	'Wheel spoke' meront
Vector tick	*Amblyomma maculatum*	*Rhipicephalus sanguineus*, *Amblyomma ovale*
Therapy	Combination of trimethoprim/sulphonamide and pyrimethamine and clindamycin or single agent ponazuril followed by long-term decoquinate	Imidocarb dipropionate

Gulf Coast tick *Amblyomma maculatum* is the vector of *H. americanum*. *A. maculatum* exists in the southern part of North America, throughout Central America and in the northern part of South America. In the USA, *A. maculatum* was once confined to the warm, humid regions along the Gulf and South Atlantic coasts, but its geographical range has expanded to reach as far inland as Kansas, Arizona, Arkansas, Missouri, Indiana, Kentucky and Tennessee, and as far north along the Atlantic coast as Virginia, West Virginia, Maryland and Delaware. Both of the *Hepatozoon* species that infect dogs are transmitted transstadially from the nymph to the adult stage in their tick vectors. Larval *A. maculatum* ticks can also become infected and transmit *H. americanum* as newly moulted nymphs or adults, and larval *R. sanguineus* can transmit *H. canis* transstadially to the nymph stage.

While *H. canis* appears to be a parasite of canines that is well adapted to dogs and causes only mild clinical signs in the majority of infections, it appears that *H. americanum* is less adapted to parasitic co-existence in the dog, causing a severe disease in most cases. It is likely a parasite of some other animal in North America and is transmitted to dogs either through ingestion of ticks that feed as nymphs or larvae on the natural host or through predation of wild animals and subsequent ingestion of paratenic host tissues. Gamonts and meronts of a *Hepatozoon* species have been reported in coyotes, bobcats and ocelots in the USA. The majority of these animals were in good physical condition at the time of capture. *H. americanum* has been transmitted successfully to coyote puppies from *A. maculatum* ticks that had previously fed on infected dogs. In contrast to the infected adult animals, puppies developed clinical signs of myasthenia, pain, ocular discharge, leucocytosis and inappetence. They also developed bone lesions typically seen in dogs with HAI and one pup was infective to nymphal *A. maculatum* ticks. Surveys of free ranging coyotes in Oklahoma showed that 40–50% were infected naturally with *H. americanum*.

Life cycle and transmission

The life cycles of *H. canis* (**Figure 8.2**) and *H. americanum* (**Figure 8.3**) include two hosts: the tick as a definitive host in which the sexual part of the cycle takes place, and a dog or other mammal as an intermediate host in which asexual reproduction of the parasite occurs. Nymphal or larval ticks engorge with gamont-infected leucocytes while feeding on blood from an infected intermediate host. Gamonts are freed from the leucocytes, associate in pairs in syzygy and transform into male and female gametes. Fertilization occurs and results in the formation of zygotes that develop to

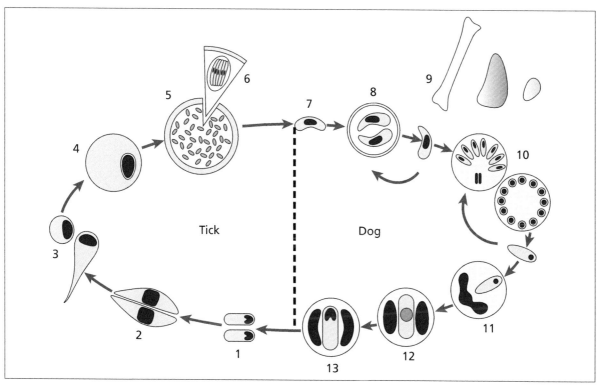

Fig. 8.2 Stages in the life cycles of *H. canis*. (1) Gamonts ingested by a tick during a blood meal from a parasitaemic dog are released from neutrophils. (2) Gamonts associate in syzgy during gametogony. (3) Male and female gametes transform prior to fertilization. (4) A zygote develops into an early oocyst. (5) During sporogony, numerous sporocysts are formed within the oocysts. (6) Each sporocyst contains several elongated sporozoites. (7) After ingestion of an infected tick, sporozoites are released from the oocysts and penetrate the dog's intestinal tract. The sporozoites disseminate to target tissues mainly to haemolymphatic organs. (8) Meronts containing macromeronts are formed during merogony in the haemolymphatic tissues. (9) Merozoites release from ruptured mature meronts and repeat the cycle of merogony. (10) Elongated micromerozoites are formed within a 'wheel spoke'-type meront. (11) Micromerozoites free from mature meronts and invade neutrophils. (12) Gamonts develop within neutrophils in the haemolymphatic organs. (13) Neutrophils containing mature gamonts enter the blood circulation and are ingested by a tick upon taking in a blood meal

oocysts. Each mature oocyst (**Figures 8.4–8.6**) contains numerous sporocysts (>200 for *H. americanum*) and 10–26 sporozoites develop within each sporocyst (**Figure 8.7**). After the tick moults, oocysts are found within the tick's haemocoele and each tick may carry thousands of infective sporozoites. *Hepatozoon* parasites have not been shown to migrate to tick salivary glands or mouthparts. Thus, transmission occurs by ingestion of an infected tick and not by a tick bite.

Once ingested by a dog or other susceptible mammal, the sporozoites of either species are released from the oocysts, penetrate the intestinal wall and are transported (possibly within a phagocytic cell) to target tissues and organs. *H. canis* disseminates via the blood or lymph and primarily infects the spleen, lymph nodes and bone marrow, where merogony takes place. Two forms of *H. canis* meronts are found in infected tissues: one type containing 2–4 macromerozoites (**Figure 8.8**) and a second type containing more than 20 elongated micromerozoites (**Figure 8.9**). When the meront matures and ruptures, merozoites are released and penetrate neutrophils, in which they develop into gamonts that circulate in peripheral blood. *H. americanum* has an affinity for skeletal

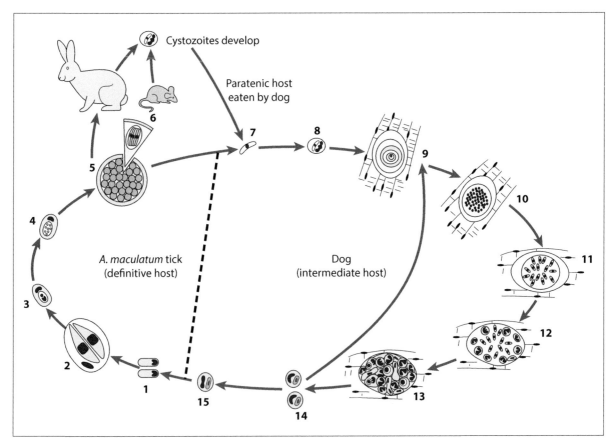

Fig. 8.3 Stages in the life cycles of *H. americanum*. (1) Gamonts ingested by a tick during a blood meal from a parasitaemic dog are released from leucocytes. (2) Gamonts associate and undergo gametogony, after which association (syzygy) and fertilization takes place within a tick gut cell. (3) Zygote development within a tick host cell. (4) Sporogony and formation of early sporocysts within the developing oocyst. (5) The mature oocyst contains over 200 sporocysts. (6) Each sporocyst contains 10–26 elongated sporozoites. The infected tick may also be ingested by a paratenic host (e.g. rabbit or rodent) and cystozoites may develop within that host. If the paratenic host is eaten by a dog, sporozoites may be released in the dog's intestine, thereby continuing the life cycle. (7) After ingestion of an infected tick, sporozoites are released from the oocysts and penetrate the dog's intestinal tract. (8) Sporozoites enter host cells and disseminate to target organs, mainly to skeletal and cardiac muscle. (9) Layers of mucopolysaccharides are laid down around the parasite and host cell forming an 'onion skin'-shaped cyst. (10) The parasite undergoes merogony within the cyst. (11) Mature merozoites are formed in the cyst. (12) Rupture of the cyst is followed by release of merozoites and induction of a local inflammatory response. (13) A pyogranuloma with intense vascularization is created where the cyst existed. Leucocytes are invaded by merozoites. (14) Some of the merozoites develop into gamonts, while others may disseminate to other muscular tissues and repeat merogony. (15) Mature gamonts in leucocytes enter the blood circulation and are ingested by a tick upon taking in a blood meal.

and cardiac muscle tissue, where it develops between myocytes within host cells that have been determined to be of monocytic origin. Mucopolysaccharide layers encyst the host cell in the muscle (**Figure 8.10**), where the parasite subsequently undergoes merogony. At maturation the cyst ruptures, releasing merozoites into adjacent tissue. Inflammatory cells are recruited to the area and become infected, each with a single zoite. A pyogranuloma forms where the cyst once existed (**Figure 8.11**). Two stages of *H. americanum*

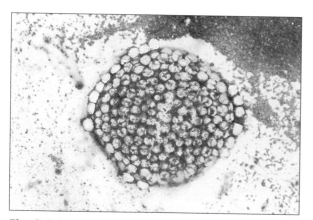

Fig. 8.4 An *H. americanum* oocyst containing numerous sporocysts.

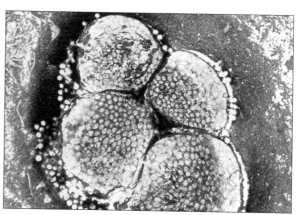

Fig. 8.5 Four attached *H. americanum* oocysts in a hemocoele smear.

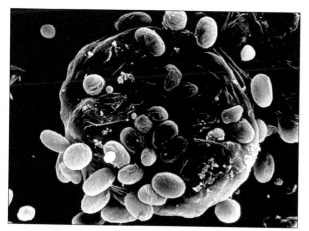

Fig. 8.6 Scanning electron microscope image of an *H. canis* oocyst. The oocyst is enveloped by a membrane and surrounded by free sporocysts.

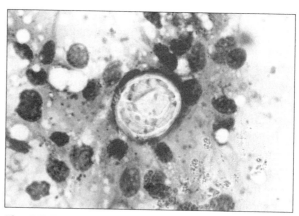

Fig. 8.7 *H. americanum* sporocyst containing sporozoites.

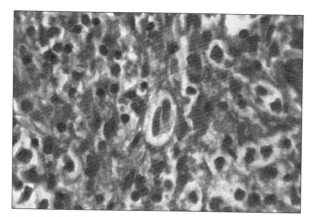

Fig. 8.8 Two *H. canis* macromerozoites in a section of spleen from an experimentally infected dog.

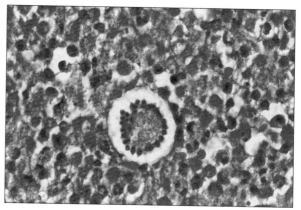

Fig. 8.9 *H. canis* meront containing micromerozoites shaped in a 'wheel spoke' form in a section of spleen from a naturally infected dog.

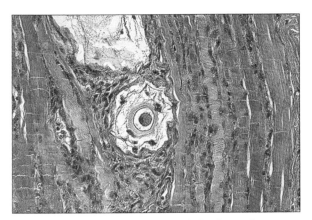

Fig. 8.10 *H. americanum* cyst in skeletal muscle. Infrequently, the cyst is found with a developing or mature meront with merozoites.

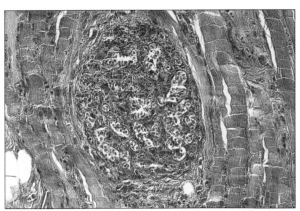

Fig. 8.11 A pyogranuloma in muscle tissue from a dog with *H. americanum* infection.

have been observed within macrophages of pyogranulomas: merozoites and, presumably, developing gamonts. Intense angiogenesis within the pyogranuloma results in a highly vascular structure through which the infected macrophages are able to enter the circulation to either become circulating gamonts or distribute merozoites to distant sites to repeat the asexual reproduction cycle. The life cycle of both *Hepatozoon* species is completed when ticks ingest blood infected with gamonts.

Experimental infections have shown that *H. canis* completes its development in the dog with the appearance of peripheral blood gamonts within 28 days post infection. The time from attachment of nymphs on an infected dog to development of mature oocysts infective to dogs in the adult tick, which moulted from the nymph, was 53 days. *H. americanum* completes its life cycle in the dog within 32 days. The development of *H. americanum* in nymphal *A. maculatum* ticks from feeding to the observation of mature oocysts in the haemocoele of a newly moulted adult tick requires 42 days.

Other modes of transmission exist. As with *Toxoplasma gondii*, some species of *Hepatozoon* can be transmitted through predation and ingestion of cysts present in tissues of paratenic hosts. Experimentally, laboratory raised rodents and rabbits fed *H. americanum* oocysts developed cystozoites but not meronts or gamonts. *Hepatozoon*-free dogs fed cystozoite-laden tissue from these animals became infected with *H. americanum* and developed classical clinical signs. Surveys of various wildlife species have shown that numerous vertebrates

harbour *Hepatozoon* species; DNA sequences obtained from rabbits were most closely related to those obtained from carnivores, although none were identified as *H. americanum*. The potential importance of this alternate mode of transmission is illustrated by an investigation of a natural outbreak in a pack of Beagles. Four to 6 weeks after a group of hunting Beagles was allowed to consume the carcass of a wild rabbit, all dogs in the group developed clinical signs of *H. americanum* infection, while dogs that consistently hunted with this group of dogs, but did not consume the carcass, did not become infected. Vertical transmission of *H. canis* has also been reported in puppies born to an infected dam and raised in a tick-free environment. The importance of this mode of transmission in the epidemiology of the disease has not yet been determined.

Pathogenesis

Most dogs infected with *H. canis* appear to undergo a mild infection associated with a limited degree of inflammatory reaction. However, HCI may vary from being apparently asymptomatic in dogs with a low parasitaemia to life threatening in animals that present with a high parasitaemia. HCI can be influenced by immune suppression due to co-existing infectious agents, an immature immune system in young animals or the presence of a primary immunodeficiency. Immune suppression influences the pathogenesis of new *H. canis* infections or the reactivation of pre-existing ones. Treatment with an immunosuppressive dose of prednisolone is followed by the appearance of *H. canis* parasitaemia in dogs with experimental HCI.

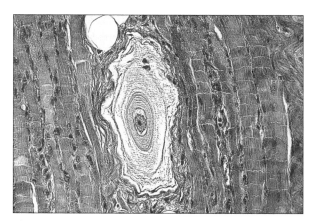

Fig. 8.12 *H. americanum* cyst. The round-to-oval 'onion skin' cysts are 250–500 μm in diameter. The outer portion of the cyst is made up of concentric layers of fine, pale blue-staining laminar membranes. A developing parasite may sometimes be observed at the centre of the cyst.

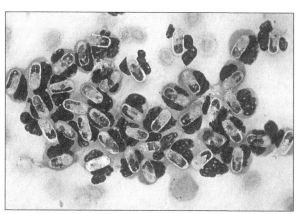

Fig. 8.13 *H. canis* gamonts on the edge of a blood smear from a naturally infected dog with extreme leucocytosis and a high parasitaemia approaching 100% of the neutrophils.

Concurrent HCI and infection with other canine pathogens are common; reported co-infections include parvovirus, *Ehrlichia canis*, *Anaplasma platys*, *Toxoplasma gondii*, *Neospora caninum* and *Leishmania infantum*.

In contrast, immunosuppression or concurrent illness is not necessary to induce clinical disease in dogs infected with *H. americanum*. The earliest lesions in skeletal muscle are noted 3 weeks post exposure, when the parasite may be seen within the host cell. Over time, the host cell produces the mucopolysaccharide lamellar membranes around itself to form the 'onion skin' cyst unique to *H. americanum* infection (**Figure 8.12**). Some cysts undergo merogony very rapidly while others appear to enter dormancy. Clinical signs start 4–6 weeks after infection and result from the pyogranulomatous inflammatory response that occurs after the encysted mature meront ruptures, releasing merozoites into the surrounding tissue.

With *H. americanum*, a single infecting episode can cause persistent infection due to repeated cycles of merogony. In a naturally infected dog that was followed over a 5.5 year period, characteristic lesions of *H. americanum* were seen repeatedly on muscle biopsy and the dog remained infective to nymphal *A. maculatum* ticks throughout that time period. Latent cysts may be found years after the initial diagnosis in clinically recovered dogs. These cysts have the potential to reactivate, producing continued cycles of asexual reproduction,

resulting in the waxing and waning pattern of clinical signs and relapse following treatment.

Clinical signs

Hepatozoon canis

Infection with *H. canis* may be subclinical in some animals but produce severe and fatal disease in others. It is difficult to characterize the clinical signs of HCI because: (1) dogs with low parasitaemia may be apparently asymptomatic; (2) the non-specific nature of changes such as pale mucous membranes due to anaemia and lethargy; and (3) the involvement of concurrent diseases in some of the cases. Mild disease is common and is usually associated with low-level *H. canis* parasitaemia (1–5%), frequently in association with a concurrent disease. A more severe disease, characterized by lethargy, fever and severe weight loss, is found in dogs with high parasitaemia, often approaching 100% of circulating neutrophils (**Figure 8.13**). Dogs presenting with both leucocytosis and high parasitaemia may have a massive number of circulating gamonts (>50,000 gamonts/mm^3). This extensive parasitism takes its toll on the canine host by demanding nutrients and energy, by direct injury to the affected tissues and by activating the different branches of the immune system. This massive parasitic load may lead to extreme loss of weight and cachexia in dogs with a high parasitaemia, although the dogs sometimes maintain a good appetite.

Hepatozoon americanum

Dogs infected with *H. americanum* are often presented with gait abnormalities ranging from stiffness to complete recumbency, generalized pain and deterioration of body condition. On physical examination the most common findings include fever, pain or hyperaesthesia, muscle atrophy, weakness, depression, reluctance to rise and mucopurulent ocular discharge (**Figure 8.14**). Body temperature tends to correlate directly with waxing and waning of clinical signs and may range from normal to 41°C.

Hyperaesthesia and/or generalized pain result from both pyogranulomatous inflammation in skeletal muscle and the periosteal reaction that causes bony proliferation. Pain can manifest as cervical, back, joint or generalized pain and clinical signs may resemble those of meningitis or discospondylitis. Affected dogs may display a 'His Master's Voice' stance as a result of guarding the cervical region (**Figure 8.15**). Muscle atrophy becomes apparent with chronic disease and can result in secondary weakness. Most dogs maintain a relatively normal appetite throughout the course of the disease. Despite this, weight loss is common due to muscle atrophy and chronic cachexia. Mucopurulent ocular discharge is common and is sometimes associated with decreased tear production. It may coincide with fever spikes and owners often report that the ocular discharge is the first noticeable sign of clinical relapse. Transient diarrhoea, often bloody, has been reported. Less frequently reported clinical signs include polyuria and polydipsia, abnormal lung sounds or cough, pale mucous membranes and lymphadenomegaly.

Laboratory findings

Most dogs with HCI have white blood cell counts within the reference range. However, dogs with a high parasitaemia frequently have extreme neutrophilia (up to 150×10^9/l), although it is less common than in dogs with HAI. Normocytic, normochromic non-regenerative anaemia is the most common haematological abnormality reported in HCI. Less frequently, a regenerative anaemia, sometimes severe, may be seen. In a case-controlled study of dogs with *H. canis* parasitaemia admitted to a veterinary teaching hospital in Israel, dogs with hepatozoonosis were significantly more anaemic than the control hospital population admitted with other diseases, and dogs with high parasitaemia were more anaemic and had higher leucocyte counts than both the controls and the dogs with low parasitaemia. Thrombocytopenia and proteinuria have also been reported in HCI.

In dogs with HAI, the most outstanding haematological abnormality is marked leucocytosis, characterized by neutrophilia. The white blood cell count typically ranges from $20–200 \times 10^9$/l, with reported means of 76.8 and 85.7×10^9/l. A mild to moderate normocytic, normochromic, non-regenerative anaemia

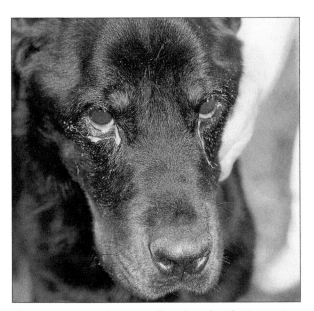

Fig. 8.14 Rottweiler naturally infected with *H. americanum*, with typical mucopurulent ocular discharge and facial muscle atrophy.

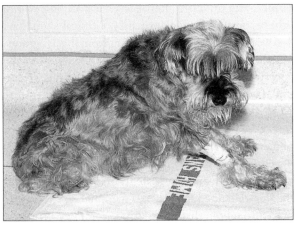

Fig. 8.15 Miniature Schnauzer naturally infected with *H. americanum* exhibiting a 'His Master's Voice' stance due to severe musculoskeletal pain and excessive stiffness.

is typical. Thrombocytosis, with platelet counts of 422–916 × 10⁹/l, occurs in a considerable number of dogs. Thrombocytopenia is rare unless there is concurrent infection with *Ehrlichia canis*, *Anaplasma platys*, *Rickettsia rickettsii* or other tick-borne organisms.

Abnormalities in serum biochemistry in highly parasitaemic dogs with HCI include hyperproteinaemia with hyperglobulinaemia and hypoalbuminaemia, and increased creatine kinase (CK) and alkaline phosphatase (ALP) activities. In dogs with HAI the most common biochemical changes are a mild elevation in ALP and decreased albumin. Artefactual hypoglycaemia (in the range of 2.22–3.33 mmol/l and occasionally as low as 0.28 mmol/l) due to increased *in-vitro* metabolism by the elevated number of white blood cells may be seen if sodium fluoride is not used for sample collection. The low albumin has been attributed to decreased protein intake, chronic inflammation or renal loss. Blood urea nitrogen (BUN) is also frequently decreased below the reference range. Surprisingly, CK activity is typically normal despite the myositis caused by *H. americanum*. Although the decreases in albumin and BUN are suggestive of hepatic failure, both fasting and postprandial bile acids are usually within the reference range or only slightly elevated.

Radiographic findings

Dogs with HAI commonly develop osteoproliferative lesions. Periosteal new bone formation is typically disseminated and symmetrical and is usually most frequent and severe on the diaphysis of the long bones. The radiographical appearance of the bony lesions ranges from subtle bone irregularity to a dramatic smooth laminar thickening (**Figure 8.16**). A study of the formation of the bone lesions after experimental infection with *H. americanum* revealed that the stages of morphological development of the lesions very closely resemble those of hypertrophic osteopathy.

Diagnosis

HCI is usually diagnosed by microscopical detection of *H. canis* gamonts in the cytoplasm of neutrophils, and rarely monocytes, on Giemsa- or Wright's-stained blood smears. They have an ellipsoidal shape, are about 11 × 4 μm and are enveloped in a thick membrane (**Figure 8.17**). Between 0.5% and 5% of the neutrophils are commonly infected, although this may reach as high as

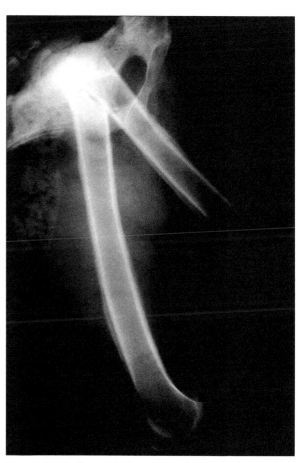

Fig. 8.16 Radiograph showing periosteal proliferation of the femurs and pelvic bones in *H. americanum* infection. Bone lesions range from rough irregularity to smooth laminar thickening such as in this case.

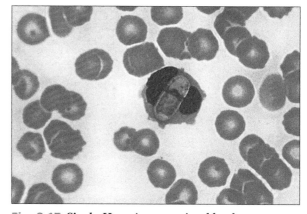

Fig. 8.17 Single *H. canis* gamont in a blood smear from a naturally infected dog. Note the ellipsoidal shape of the gamont compressing the lobulated neutrophil nucleus toward the cell membrane.

100% in heavy infections. A case-controlled study of dogs with *H. canis* parasitaemia admitted to a veterinary hospital in Israel indicated that 15% had a high number of circulating parasites (>800 gamonts/mm^3).

In contrast to *H. canis*, gamonts are found infrequently on blood smears from dogs infected with *H. americanum*. When they are identified, it is usually in very low numbers, rarely exceeding 0.1% of the leucocytes examined (**Figure 8.18**). Gamonts may exit the leucocytes rapidly after blood is drawn, leaving behind an empty capsule that is difficult to identify. Consequently, blood smears should be made rapidly after sampling to enhance identification. Buffy coat smears will also increase the chance of gamont detection. Bone marrow aspirates usually show granulocytic hyperplasia with an increased myeloid:erythroid ratio, and lymph node aspirates often reveal lymphoid hyperplasia. However, neither procedure is useful in making a definitive diagnosis, as organisms are rarely seen in these samples.

Radiography of the limbs or pelvis can be used for screening a suspected animal because many dogs with HAI will show periosteal proliferation. However, muscle biopsy is a more consistent method of diagnosis of HAI, as it typically reveals the unique cyst and pyogranuloma formation associated with *H. americanum* (see **Figures 8.10–8.12**). Myositis with muscle atrophy, necrosis and infiltration of inflammatory cells between muscle fibres is a frequent finding. The parasites are distributed widely in the muscle tissue, but multiple biopsies are recommended to increase the chances of detecting the organism, especially in early or low-level infections. The biceps femoris, semitendinosus and epaxial muscles are recommended sites for biopsy sampling.

An indirect immunofluorescent antibody test (IFAT) and western blot for the detection of anti-*H. canis* antibodies were developed using gamont antigens (**Figure 8.19**). The IFAT has been used for epidemiological studies in Israel and Japan. A survey of dogs from Israel showed that 33% had been exposed to the parasite, as indicated by the presence of anti-*H. canis* antibodies. Only 3% of the seropositive dogs had detectable blood gamonts and only 1% had severe clinical signs associated with the infection. This indicates that although there is a wide exposure to *H. canis*, most infections are probably subclinical. IgM and IgG class antibodies to *H. canis* were detected by an IFAT in experimentally infected dogs as early as 16 and 22 days post infection, respectively, well in advance of gamont detection by microscopy at 28 days post infection. Antibodies detected by an IFAT may be formed against conserved antigens found in earlier life cycle stages of *H. canis*.

Sera from dogs infected with *H. americanum* showed only a low degree of cross-reactivity to *H. canis* antigens by an IFAT. However, an ELISA for *H. americanum*, using sporozoites as antigen, was reported to have a sensitivity of 93% and a specificity of 96% when compared with muscle biopsy.

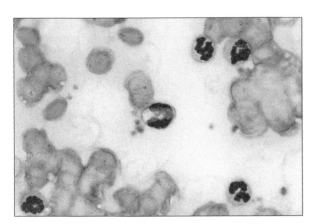

Fig. 8.18 Blood smear showing a gamont of *H. americanum* in a leucocyte. Although similar in appearance, the gamonts of *H. americanum* are slightly smaller in size than those of *H. canis* (8.8 × 3.9 µm as compared with 11 × 4 µm).

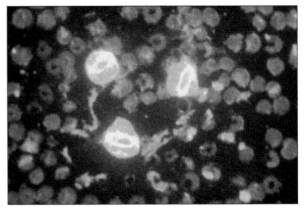

Fig. 8.19 Indirect immunofluorescent antibody test for the detection of antibodies against *H. canis*. Note the specific fluorescence of the gamont membranes in the positive reaction shown.

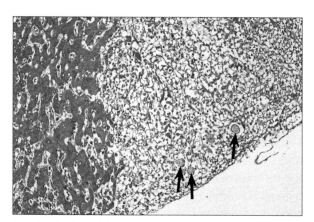

Fig. 8.20 Hepatitis associated with *H. canis* meronts in a section of liver from a dog with a high parasitaemia. Arrows indicate the location of *H. canis* meronts.

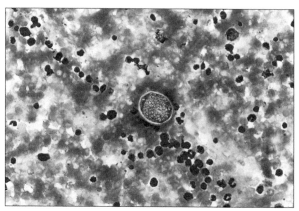

Fig. 8.21 Developing *H. canis* meront in a cytological preparation from a bone marrow aspirate.

Highly sensitive and specific quantitative real-time polymerase chain reaction (PCR) tests, which detect the 18S rRNA gene and can distinguish between *H. americanum* and *H. canis*, have been developed. They can detect as few as seven genomic copies per ml of blood. However, false negatives are possible when there are extremely low numbers of circulating gamonts, which may occur in very acute or very chronic cases; a muscle biopsy should be performed in suspect cases when PCR is negative. Because the tests are quantitative, they are useful in monitoring the effectiveness of treatment over time

Postmortem findings

HCI may be found as an incidental finding in histopathological specimens from dogs from endemic areas. In dogs with a low parasitaemia, few tissue lesions may be identified. However, necropsy examinations of dogs with a high parasitaemia reveal hepatitis (**Figure 8.20**), pneumonia and glomerulonephritis associated with numerous *H. canis* meronts. Meronts and developing gamonts are also found in the lymph nodes, spleen and bone marrow (**Figure 8.21**). *H. canis* meronts are usually round to oval, about 30 μm in diameter and include elongated micromerozoites with defined nuclei. A cross-section of the meront through the midshaft of the micromerozoites reveals a form with a central core mass surrounded by a circle of micromerozoite nuclei, which is often referred to as a 'wheel spoke' (see **Figure 8.9**). This form is typical for HCI but is not found in HAI. Meronts of *H. canis* can sometimes be detected in tissues with little or no apparent host inflammatory response (**Figure 8.22**). This

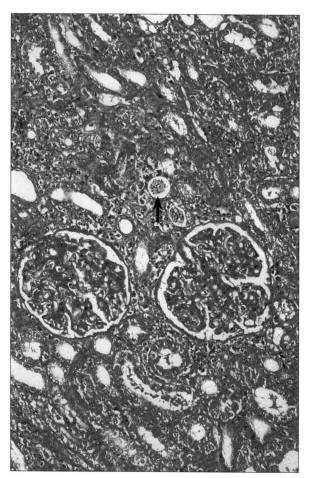

Fig. 8.22 *H. canis* meront in kidney tissue. An arrow indicates the location of the meront. Meronts are often found with little or no surrounding inflammatory response.

is possibly associated with the ability of the parasite to cause chronic subclinical infections and avoid an extreme immune response.

Cachexia and muscle atrophy are consistent gross findings on necropsy examination of dogs infected chronically with *H. americanum*. Roughening and thickening of bone surfaces may be apparent. Grossly, pyogranulomas may appear as multiple, 1–2 mm diameter, white-to-tan foci scattered diffusely throughout muscle and various other tissues. Microscopically, the cysts, meronts and pyogranulomas are found predominantly in skeletal and cardiac muscle, but they may also be found sporadically in other tissues including adipose tissue, lymph node, intestinal smooth muscle, spleen, skin, kidney, salivary gland, liver, pancreas and lung. Vascular changes in various organs include fibrinoid degeneration of vessel walls, mineralization and proliferation of vascular intima and pyogranulomatous vasculitis. Renal lesions are frequently present and include focal pyogranulomatous inflammation with mild glomerulonephritis, lymphoplasmacytic interstitial nephritis, mesangioproliferative glomerulonephritis and, occasionally, amyloidosis. Amyloid deposits may also be found in spleen, lymph nodes, small intestine and liver. Occasional findings include pulmonary congestion, splenic coagulative necrosis, lymphadenopathy and congestion of the gastric mucosa.

Treatment and control

H. canis infection is treated with imidocarb dipropionate (5–6 mg/kg IM every 14 days) until gamonts are no longer present in blood smears. The elimination of *H. canis* gamonts from the peripheral blood may require 8 weeks, and a haematological evaluation every 2 weeks is indicated. Studies have also evaluated treatment with the combination of imidocarb dipropionate, toltrazuril and clindamycin, but sensitive PCR has shown that complete elimination of *H. canis* may not be possible by use of the currently available drugs. Treatment is recommended for all infected dogs, including those with a mild disease, because parasitaemia may increase over time and develop into a severe infection. Generally, the survival rate of dogs with a low *H. canis* parasitaemia is good. It is often dependent on the prognosis of any concurrent disease conditions. The prognosis for dogs with a high parasitaemia is less favourable. Seven of 15 dogs (47%) with a high parasitaemia included in a case-controlled study survived only 2 months after presentation despite specific treatment.

Both specific therapy using antiprotozoal drugs and palliative therapy using a non-steroidal anti-inflammatory drug (NSAID) have been used in the treatment of HAI. The best results occur when both are used together initially. An NSAID at standard doses can provide immediate relief from fever and pain during the first days of therapy before the effects of the antiprotozoal drug become evident.

Currently, it appears there is no drug capable of eliminating all stages of *H. americanum*. Remission of clinical signs can usually be obtained quickly by administering either a combination of trimethoprim–sulphadiazine, clindamycin and pyrimethamine (TCP) for 14 days or ponazuril for 14–28 days (**Table 8.2**). Although the clinical response is dramatic, it is often short-lived and most dogs relapse within 2–6 months following treatment. In the USA, ponazuril

---

Table 8.2 Treatment of *H. americanum* infection.

DRUG	DOSE RATE	FREQUENCY OF ADMINISTRATION
TCP protocol		
Trimethoprim–sulphadiazine	15 mg/kg PO	q12h
Clindamycin	10 mg/kg PO	q8h
Pyrimethamine	0.25 mg/kg PO	q24h
Alternative protocol		
Ponazuril	10 mg/kg PO	q12h for 14–28 days

The TCP (trimethoprim–sulphadiazine, clindamycin and pyrimethamine) combination is given in combination for 14 days and followed by long-term treatment with decoquinate. Alternatively, ponazuril can be administered and similarly followed with decoquinate.

is commercially available in a paste formulation for equine use (Marquis®, Bayer Healthcare); it must be diluted in water or another carrier for administration to dogs.

The anticoccidial drug decoquinate helps prevent relapses when given daily to *H. americanum*-infected dogs after completion of TCP or ponazuril therapy. It likely arrests development of parasites released from mature meronts, thereby interrupting the repeated cycles of asexual reproduction. Decoquinate does not clear gamonts from the dog's circulation nor is it effective in reducing clinical signs associated with acute relapse. This drug must be given every day to be effective. Although not approved for use in dogs, decoquinate has been proven to be safe in this species at both high dosages and prolonged administration. The drug is available in the USA as a cornmeal-based premix for livestock at a concentration of 60 grams of decoquinate per kilogram of premix (Deccox®, Zoetis). The powder is given at a rate of 0.5–1.0 teaspoonful per 10 kg body weight, mixed with moist dog food and fed twice daily. This amount corresponds to a decoquinate dosage of 10–20 mg/kg every 12 hours. It appears that the drug must be given long term (1–2 years and possibly longer) to prevent relapses.

In a study comparing treatment protocols, the 2-year survival rate for dogs receiving only TCP was 12.5% compared with a 2-year survival rate of >84% when TCP was followed by long-term daily decoquinate therapy. Most dogs that received TCP alone had a very good initial response, followed by periodical relapses, resulting in chronic wasting and debilitation and ending in renal failure, euthanasia or death, with a median survival time of approximately 12 months.

Control and prevention

Prevention of both HCI and HAI consists primarily of good tick control using an effective acaricide and close examination of dogs after hunting or outdoor activity. Dogs must be prevented from ingesting ticks. Because dogs can become infected from ingesting cystozoites from wildlife hosts, dogs should also be prevented from scavenging or eating prey, raw meat or organs from wildlife.

FELINE HEPATOZOONOSIS

Feline hepatozoonosis was first described in a domestic cat in 1908 in India, and has since been reported from several countries in Europe, Asia, Africa and North and South America. Feline hepatozoonosis infections are caused mostly by *Hepatozoon felis*; however, feline infection by *H. canis* has also been documented. *H. felis* is associated with infection of muscle tissues and *H. felis* meronts have been identified in the myocardium and skeletal muscles of cats with hepatozoonosis. In addition, elevated activities of the muscle enzyme CK were found in the majority of cats with hepatozoonosis in a retrospective study of this disease. The level of parasitaemia is usually low in cats, with <1% of the neutrophils containing gamonts **(Figure 8.23)**. In comparison with *H. canis* gamonts from dog blood, gamonts of *H. felis* are different due to their generally round nucleus, which is dissimilar to the more elongated horse-shoe shaped *H. canis* nucleus. The *H. felis* meront is round to oval with a mean size of 34.5–39 μm and surrounded by a thick membrane separating it from the surrounding tissues **(Figure 8.24)**. The early *H. felis* meronts contain amorphous material without obvious zoites and as they mature they form nuclei, which develop further into distinct long merozoites. The *H. felis* merozoites are dispersed within the meront without an obvious pattern of arrangement and do not form the typical wheel spoke shape of the *H. canis* meront with merozoites arranged in a circle along the meront circumference around a central core. The vector of *H. felis* is currently unknown. Feline hepatozoonosis is associated commonly with immunosuppressive viral disease caused by feline immunodeficiency virus or feline leukaemia virus.

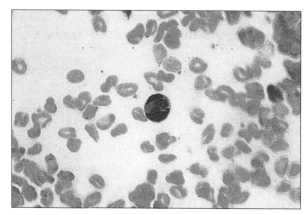

Fig. 8.23 Gamont of *Hepatozoon* spp. in a neutrophil of a naturally infected domestic cat.

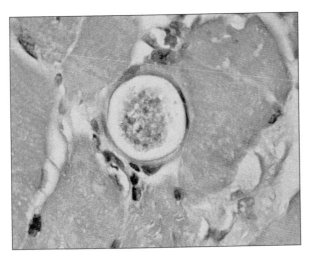

Fig. 8.24 *H. felis* meront in the semimembranosus muscle of the hindlimb of a cat from Israel. Note the thick membrane surrounding the developing meronts in the striated muscle tissue.

ZOONOTIC POTENTIAL/PUBLIC HEALTH SIGNIFICANCE

There is only one report of human infection with a *Hepatozoon* species. Gamonts were found in the blood of a male patient from the Philippines on two different occasions, but liver and bone marrow biopsy samples failed to reveal any parasites. Because canine hepatozoonosis occurs as a result of ingestion of a tick or cystozoites in wild animal carcasses, transmission of *H. canis* or *H. americanum* to humans is unlikely except perhaps in small children inclined to put foreign objects into their mouths. Since other tick-borne diseases may be transmitted through the bite of a tick, all ticks should be removed promptly from any human or animal.

CASE STUDY

Signalment

Roxie, a 14-month-old, neutered female Rottweiler from La Grange, Georgia, USA (see **Figure 8.14**).

History

For the previous 6 weeks, Roxie had been reluctant to move and exhibited a very stiff gait with difficulty rising from a recumbent position. She also had intermittent fever and ocular discharge. Although Roxie had maintained her appetite, she had lost weight and muscle mass. The owner noticed that Roxie also had developed increased thirst and an increased volume of urine. Her clinical signs were unresponsive to antibiotic therapy prescribed by the referring veterinarian, including a course of amoxicillin/clavulanic acid and a course of doxycycline. The owner reported that during the past 2 years his other two Rottweilers had died from an undiagnosed illness after exhibiting similar clinical signs.

Roxie was fed a high-quality commercial dog food, was up to date on all vaccinations and received a monthly heartworm preventive. Although a house dog, she also spent time outdoors in the backyard and hiking with the owner. She had not travelled beyond the local area.

Clinical examination

Vital signs: body weight 34.5 kg; temperature 40.1°C; heart rate 84 beats/min; respiration rate 36 breaths per minute; mucous membranes are pink with a capillary refill time of <2 seconds. The dog is quiet, alert and responsive.

Roxie has marked mucopurulent ocular discharge with negative fluorescein stain test and normal Schirmer tear test results. Her body condition score is 3/9 and there is moderate generalized muscle atrophy. Roxie shows hyperesthesia on palpation of the trunk, limbs and neck. She is reluctant to stand and walk with a stiff gait.

Table 8.3 Haematology findings.

PARAMETER	VALUE	REFERENCE RANGE
PCV	32%	37–55
RBC	$4.90 \times 10^{12}/l$	5.50–8.50
MCV	67.5 fl	60–77
MCHC	35.6 g/dl	32–36
WBC	$56.3 \times 10^9/l$	6.0–17.0
Neutrophils	$49.8 \times 10^9/l$	3.0–11.4
Lymphocytes	$2.53 \times 10^9/l$	1.0–4.0
Monocytes	$3.2 \times 10^9/l$	0.15–1.2
Eosinophils	$0.72 \times 10^9/l$	0.1–0.75
Platelets	$640 \times 10^9/l$	200–400

Table 8.4 Serum biochemistry findings.

PARAMETER	VALUE	REFERENCE RANGE
BUN	3.2 mmol/l	3.57–8.92
Creatinine	70.7 μmol/l	26.5–88.4
ALP	252 U/l	19–50
ALT	54 U/l	17–66
Creatine kinase	167 U/l	92–357
Total bilirubin	5.13 μmol/l	1.71–5.13
Glucose	2.66 mmol/l	4.44 –5.55
Sodium	149 mmol/l	146–160
Potassium	4.0 mmol/l	3.5–5.9
Chloride	110 mmol/l	108–125
Calcium	2.24 mmol/l	2.37–2.94
Phosphorus	1.35 mmol/l	1.06–2.38
Total protein	63 g/l	51–73
Albumin	21 g/l	26–35
Globulin	42 g/l	36–50
Total CO_2	20.0 mmol/l	13.9–31.5

Table 8.5 Urinalysis findings.

PARAMETER	VALUE/COMMENT
Specific gravity	1.023
pH	6.5
Protein	4+
Blood	Negative
Bilirubin	Negative
Glucose	Negative
Sediment	No significant findings
Urine protein	14 g/l
Urine creatinine	733 μmol/l
Urine protein:creatinine ratio	16.8

Laboratory diagnostic findings

Radiography
Smooth periosteal bone proliferation bilaterally on the femurs and pelvic bones.

Muscle biopsy
Numerous 'onion skin' cysts, rare pyogranulomas and a moderate infiltration of inflammatory cells present between muscle fibres was diagnostic for *H. americanum* infection.

Cytology
No organisms were identified on examination of blood smears at the time of hospital admission, but detailed examination of multiple blood smears and buffy coat smears performed in subsequent days revealed jelly-bean shaped inclusions in <0.1% of the neutrophils and monocytes. These were gamonts of *H. americanum*.

Diagnosis
American canine hepatozoonosis (*H. americanum* infection) with protein-losing nephropathy. Renal pathology ranging from mild glomerulonephritis to amyloidosis are occasional sequelae of hepatozoonosis.

Treatment
Combination therapy of trimethoprim–sulphonamide (15 mg/kg PO q24h) together with clindamycin (10 mg/kg PO q8h) and pyrimethamine (0.25 mg/kg PO q24h) for 14 days. On completion of the combination therapy, Roxie was placed on long-term decoquinate treatment (15 mg/kg PO q12h to be continued for 2 years).

Outcome
The fever, pain, mucopurulent ocular discharge and other clinical signs resolved within 72 hours of initiating the combination therapy. The white blood cell count also normalized within days. However, severe proteinuria continued despite treatment. Roxie was clinically normal until 4 months after the diagnosis of American canine hepatozoonosis when she died suddenly. Necropsy examination revealed renal amyloidosis and that the cause of death was thromboembolism. Small numbers of quiescent 'onion skin' cysts were identified in skeletal muscle.

Glomerulonephritis and amyloidosis are occasional complications of *H. americanum* infection. In this case, renal amyloidosis caused severe proteinuria and subsequent depletion of antithrombin III levels, which led to the thromboembolism and Roxie's death.

FURTHER READING

Allen LE, Li Y, Kaltenboeck B *et al*. (2008) Diversity of *Hepatozoon* species in naturally infected dogs in the southern United States. *Veterinary Parasitology* **154**:220–225.

Allen KE, Little EM, Hostettler J *et al*. (2010) Treatment of *Hepatozoon americanum* infection: review of the literature and experimental evaluation of efficacy. *Veterinary Therapeutics* **11**:E1–E8.

Allen K, Yabsley M, Johnson E *et al*. (2011) Novel *Hepatozoon* in vertebrates from the southern United States. *Journal of Parasitology* **97**:648–653.

Allen KE, Johnson EM, Little SE (2011) *Hepatozoon spp.* infections in the United States. *Veterinary Clinics of North America: Small Animal Practice* **41**:1221–1238.

Baneth G (2011) Perspectives on canine and feline hepatozoonosis. *Veterinary Parasitology* **181**:3–11.

Baneth G, Sheiner A, Eyal O *et al*. (2013) Redescription of *Hepatozoon felis* (Apicomplexa: Hepatozoidae) based on phylogenetic analysis, tissue and blood form morphology, and possible transplacental transmission. *Parasites and Vectors* **6**:102.

Companion Animal Parasite Council Current Advice on Parasite Control: Vector-borne Diseases: American Hepatozoonosis (2013) http://www.capcvet.org/capc-recommendations/american-canine-hepatozoonosis.

Cummings CA, Panciera RJ, Kocan KM *et al*. (2005) Characterization of stages of *Hepatozoon americanum* and of parasitized canine host cells. *Veterinary Pathology* **42**:788-796.

De Tommasi AS, Giannelli A, de Caprariis D *et al*. (2014) Failure of imidocarb dipropionate and toltrazuril/emodepside plus clindamycin in treating *Hepatozoon canis* infection. *Veterinary Parasitology* **200**:242–245.

Florin DA, Brinkerhoff RJ, Gaff H *et al*. (2014) Additional US collections of the Gulf Coast tick, *Amblyomma maculatum* (Acari: Ixodidae), from the State of Delaware, the first reported field collections of adult specimens from the State of Maryland, and data regarding this tick from surveillance of migratory songbirds in Maryland. *Systematic and Applied Acarology* **19**:257–262.

Giannelli A, Ramos RA, Di Paola G *et al*. (2013) Transstadial transmission of *Hepatozoon canis* from larvae to nymphs of *Rhipicephalus sanguineus*. *Veterinary Parasitology* **196**:1–5.

Johnson EM, Allen KE, Panciera RJ *et al*. (2008) Infectivity of *Hepatozoon americanum* cystozoites for a dog. *Veterinary Parasitology* **154**:148–150.

Johnson EM, Allen KE, Breshears MA *et al*. (2008) Experimental transmission of *Hepatozoon americanum* to rodents. *Veterinary Parasitology* **151**:164–169.

Johnson EM, Allen KE, Panciera RJ *et al*. (2009) Experimental transmission of *Hepatozoon americanum* to New Zealand white rabbits (*Oryctolagus cuniculus*) and infectivity of cystozoites for a dog. *Veterinary Parasitology* **164**:162–166.

Johnson EM, Panciera RJ, Allen KE *et al*. (2009) Alternate pathway of infection with *Hepatozoon americanum* and the epidemiologic importance of predation. *Journal of Veterinary Internal Medicine* **23**:1315–1318.

Kistler WM, Brown JD, Allison AB *et al*. (2014) First report of *Angiostrongylus vasorum* and *Hepatozoon* from a red fox (*Vulpes vulpes*) from West Virginia, USA. *Veterinary Parasitology* **200**, 216–220.

Li Y, Wang C, Allen KE *et al*. (2008) Diagnosis of canine *Hepatozoon* spp. infection by quantitative PCR. *Veterinary Parasitology* **157**:50–58.

Little SE, Allen, KE, Johnson EM *et al*. (2009) New developments in canine hepatozoonosis in North America: a review. *Parasites and Vectors* **2(Suppl. 1)**:S5.

Mazuz LM, Wolkomirsky R, Sherman A *et al*. (2015) Concurrent neosporosis and hepatozoonosis in a litter of pups. *Israeli Journal of Veterinary Medicine* **70**:53–55.

Rubini AS, Paduan KS, Martins TF *et al*. (2009) Acquisition and transmission of *Hepatozoon canis* (Apicomplexa: Hepatozoidae) by the tick *Amblyomma ovale* (Acari: Ixodidae). *Veterinary Parasitology* **164**:324–327.

Starkey LA, Panciera RJ, Paras K *et al*. (2013) Genetic diversity of *Hepatozoon* spp. in coyotes from the south-central United States. *Journal of Parasitology* **99**:375–378.

DISCLAIMER

The views expressed in this chapter are those of the authors and do not reflect the official policy or position of the Department of the Army, the Department of Defense, or the US Government.

Chapter 9

Leishmaniosis

Laia Solano–Gallego
Xavier Roura
Gad Baneth

BACKGROUND, AETIOLOGY AND EPIDEMIOLOGY

Canine leishmaniosis due to *Leishmania infantum* is an important, potentially fatal disease that is also infectious to people. It is a part of a broad spectrum of diseases caused in man and animals by several species of the intracellular protozoan genus *Leishmania* and is transmitted by sand flies. The diseases caused by *Leishmania* species in people are cutaneous, mucocutaneous and visceral leishmaniosis, the last being the most severe form. Visceral leishmaniosis is further divided into zoonotic leishmaniosis, in which dogs are reservoirs of the disease for people, and anthroponotic leishmaniosis, in which man is the reservoir of infection for other humans and transmission by sand flies occurs without apparent involvement of an animal reservoir. *Leishmania infantum* causes a zoonotic infection, while anthroponotic infection is caused by *Leishmania donovani*, mostly in India and East

Africa. The two main groups of human patients at risk for *L. infantum* infection are young children, human immunodeficiency virus (HIV)-positive patients and other immunocompromised patients. The domestic dog is considered the main reservoir for *L. infantum* infection. Infection among populations of wild mammals such as black rats, hares, foxes and jackals has been reported in the Mediterranean basin and South America and may also play a role in the epidemiology of *L. infantum* infection in these regions. This chapter focuses on *L. infantum* infection in dogs and cats.

L. infantum transmission occurs in tropical, subtropical and temperate regions of the world including southern Europe, North and Central Africa, the Middle East, China and South and Central America (**Figure 9.1**). Canine leishmaniosis caused by *L. infantum* has also been reported from multiple kennels in the eastern USA, where the patterns of transmission are currently unknown. An additional *Leishmania* species, *L. tropica*, which is an agent

Fig. 9.1 The global distribution of canine leishmaniosis.

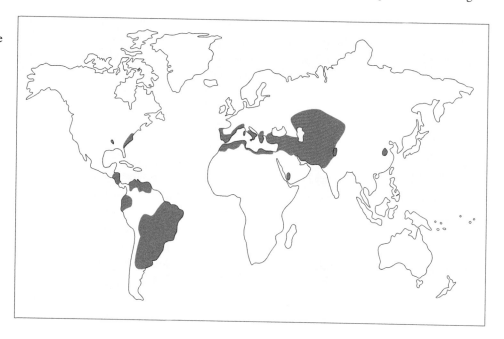

of cutaneous leishmaniosis in the Old World that can visceralize in people, has been reported as a rare cause of canine leishmaniosis in North Africa and the Middle East, and more *Leishmania* species that cause cutaneous leishmaniosis in people in the American continent, such as *L. braziliensis* and *L. amazonensis*, have been reported in dogs.

The prevalence rates of canine leishmaniosis in endemic areas vary depending on the environmental conditions required for transmission and the methods used for detecting infection. Seroprevalence rates in the Mediterranean basin range between 10% and 37% of the dogs in endemic foci. Surveys employing methods for the detection of leishmanial DNA in canine tissues, or combining serology and DNA detection, have revealed even higher infection rates, approaching 70% in some foci. It is probable that the majority of dogs living in endemic foci of leishmaniosis are exposed to infection and will develop either disease or subclinical chronic infection.

Leishmaniosis is now diagnosed frequently in countries where no sand fly transmission occurs in dogs; it is related to increased mobility of dogs and their owners. In Europe, many dogs travel to and from *Leishmania*-endemic areas and re-homing of stray animals from endemic areas by welfare groups is increasing the number of clinical cases seen in non-endemic areas. In addition, leishmaniosis is seen in non-travelled animals resident in non-endemic areas of both Europe and the USA. The most likely mechanisms of transmission in these cases are vertical transmission and sexual contact.

Natural infection in domestic cats caused by *L. infantum* appears to be less frequent than in dogs. Subclinical feline infections are common in areas endemic for canine leishmaniosis, but clinical illness due to *L. infantum* in cats is rare. The prevalence rates of feline infection with *L. infantum* in serological or molecular-based surveys range from 0% to 68%. A higher degree of natural resistance is suspected in cats compared with dogs. It has been shown that cats are relatively resistant to experimental infection with *L. infantum* and *L. donovani*. Cutaneous lesions alone have been reported in association with *L. venezuelensis*, *L. mexicana* and *L. braziliensis* in South America and in the southern USA.

Transmission and life cycle

Leishmania are diphasic parasites that complete their life cycle in two hosts: a vertebrate, where the intracellular amastigote parasite forms are found, and a sand fly, which harbours the flagellated extracellular promastigotes. Sand flies of the genus *Phlebotomus* are vectors in the Old World, while the vectors in the New World are sand flies of the genus *Lutzomyia*. The life cycle in both the reservoir host and vector is illustrated (**Figure 9.2**).

Although transmission of *L. infantum* occurs naturally by the bite of sand flies, vertical transmission *in utero* from dam to offspring and coital sexual transmission have been documented. Direct transmission without involvement of a haematophagous vector has been suspected in some cases of infection in areas where vectors of the disease are absent. Transmission of *L. infantum* by infected blood transfusion has been reported in dogs in North America and in human intravenous drug users sharing syringes in Spain.

PATHOGENESIS

Leishmaniosis is the classical example of a disease where the clinical signs and underlying pathology are intrinsically related to the interaction between the microbe, arthropod vector and host immune system. These interactions have been widely studied in both experimentally induced and spontaneously arising disease in a number of host species, and much of the current knowledge concerning the functional interactions between different T lymphocyte subpopulations was first established using murine models of this infection.

In susceptible animals, motile *Leishmania* promastigotes inoculated percutaneously by sand flies adhere rapidly to resident or recruited mononuclear phagocytes in the skin, using complement receptors. This is followed by rapid internalization of the parasite by phagocytosis and the transformation of promastigotes to non-motile amastigotes that are protected within the phagolysosome by low pH and the proteolytic activity of the parasite's gp63 (**Figure 9.3**). Initially, a granulocytic infiltrate dominates the local cutaneous inflammatory response, but this is followed by a macrophage and natural killer cell response. Later, lymphocytes appear and progression to a local granulomatous response occurs. Spread from the localized cutaneous lesion is a major event in the pathogenesis of leishmaniosis. In susceptible dogs, dissemination of infected macrophages to the local lymph node, spleen and bone marrow occurs within a few hours of inoculation. Susceptible dogs, once infected, may remain sub-

Fig. 9.2 The life cycle of *Leishmania infantum* in the sand fly vector and its mammalian hosts (canines and man). (1) During a blood meal taken by the female sand fly, promastigotes are injected with saliva into the skin of the vertebrate host. (2, 3) Promastigotes are phagocytosed by macrophages in the skin and multiply by binary fission to amastigotes. (4) The macrophage ruptures and free amastigotes penetrate adjacent host cells and disseminate to the visceral organs. (5) Cells containing amastigotes are taken up by the sand fly during a blood meal. (6) Amastigotes are released from host cells, transform to promastigotes and multiply. (7) Promastigotes attach to the gut wall of the sand fly where they continue to multiply and eventually reach the proboscis before infecting a naïve host.

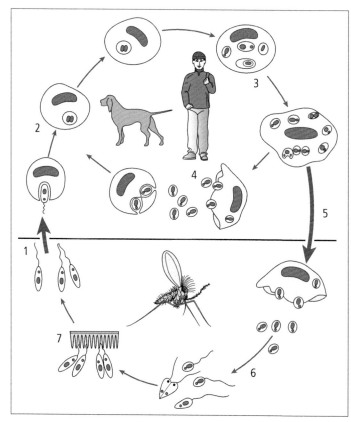

clinically infected for months to years, or even for their lifetime, and incubation periods as long as 7 years have been reported. In resistant dogs, parasites might remain localized in the skin or restricted to a local lymph node.

Immunopathogenesis

Leishmaniosis provides the single best example of polarization of the immune response to an infectious agent (see Chapter 3). A wide spectrum of clinical manifestations and immune responses to *Leishmania* infection exist in man and dogs. The clinical manifestations of this infection in man, dogs and cats include subclinical infection, self-limiting disease and progressive non-self-limiting disease. Mice, humans and dogs generally develop chronic, progressive disease (a 'non-healing' phenotype) when the immune response is dominated by type 2 helper (Th2) immunity. In contrast, where immunity is dominated by a type 1 helper (Th1) response, dogs may become infected without developing clinical disease or develop disease that is mild and self-limiting. The mechanisms underlying this polarization remain unclear. However, there is a clear genetic influence on the disease

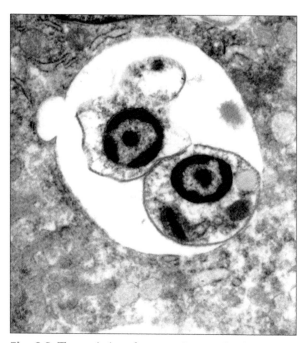

Fig. 9.3 Transmission electron micrograph of a macrophage showing amastigote forms of *Leishmania* within a cytoplasmic compartment.

resistant, 'self-healing' phenotype. This has been shown in murine models and also likely holds true for the dog; for example, Ibizian Hounds have been shown to be relatively disease resistant. Resistance may relate to the early interactions between the organism (e.g. pattern recognition molecules) and particular molecules expressed by antigen presenting cells of the immune system such as Toll-like receptors. An association between disease resistance and expression of a particular form of the gene encoding the NRAMP1 (S1c11a1) protein has been investigated in mice, humans and dogs. The protein encoded by this gene is an ion transporter involved in both macrophage activation and control of *Leishmania* replication within the cytoplasmic phagosome. The gene has been implicated in determining resistance or susceptibility to leishmaniosis in mice, and mutations in this gene resulting in genetic polymorphism may contribute to susceptibility or resistance to the development of clinical canine leishmaniosis. An association between susceptibility to leishmaniosis and specific allotypes of canine major histocompatibility complex (MHC) class II (DLA) genes has also been defined. No single gene was found responsible for the progression from infection to clinical leishmaniosis in the dog, and it is has been estimated that multiple genes and loci affect this trait.

Studies have suggested a role for populations of regulatory T lymphocytes (e.g. interleukin [IL]-10-producing regulatory T cells [Tregs]) in the pathogenesis of leishmaniosis. These Tregs may inhibit the function of effector Th1 cells, thereby preventing complete elimination of the organisms and establishing persistent infection.

There is clear evidence in dogs of susceptible and resistant phenotypes with polarized immune responses. Susceptible animals mount significant antibody responses but have weak cell-mediated immunity. The reverse holds true for resistant dogs. These have reduced serological responses, but strong intradermal responses to leishmanin and production of Th1-related cytokines (e.g. interferon [IFN]-γ) in response to antigen stimulation of lymphocyte cultures. Neutrophils and macrophages derived from *Leishmania*-infected dogs have reduced *in-vitro* killing function. However, lymphocytes from resistant dogs co-cultured with infected macrophages exhibit strong intracellular killing of parasites. This killing is MHC class II restricted and is mediated by CD8+ and CD4+ T lymphocytes that produce IFN-γ. Immunohistochemical

investigations of cutaneous lesions have shown reduced expression of MHC class II by epidermal Langerhans cells and keratinocytes and fewer infiltrating T lymphocytes within severe generalized nodular lesions, compared with milder alopecic dermatitis.

The little information on the immunological response to *Leishmania* infection in the cat is mainly related to humoral response. One cat with cutaneous leishmaniosis in southern Texas failed to respond to intradermal leishmanin injection, although other parameters of immune competence were reported as normal. Studies of cellular immunity in cats with leishmaniosis are lacking.

This immunological background helps explain the clinicopathological features of overt leishmaniosis as it presents in the dog. In animals that develop disseminated infection, lesions and clinical signs develop over a period of 3 months to several years after infection. Parasite-laden macrophages accumulate in various sites of the body, producing mainly granulomatous inflammation. Extension of the disease process commonly leads to the development of granulomatous dermatitis, uveitis and infiltration of the bone marrow with infected macrophages. Case reports of leishmanial granulomatous lesions in a range of other sites (e.g. meninges, pericardium, intestine and muscle) have been published. In addition, other types of inflammatory reactions, including lymphoplasmacytic and neutrophilic or neutrophil and macrophage infiltrates, are also seen in sick dogs.

The dominance of humoral immunity in susceptible animals also has a role in the immunopathogenesis of disease. Lymphadenomegaly and splenomegaly are common findings due to reactive lymphoid hyperplasia induced by the response to the parasite. A massive non-specific polyclonal activation of B lymphocytes and serum polyclonal hypergammaglobulinaemia are observed in susceptible dogs that develop disease. Occasionally, monoclonal gammopathy occurs, suggesting a more restricted activation of B cell clones. This excessive antibody production produces cellular and tissue damage by evoking classical type II and type III hypersensitivity mechanisms, and the end effect mimics the clinical signs of multisystemic autoimmune disease. For example, immune-mediated haemolytic anaemia (Coombs test positive) and thrombocytopenia may occur in infected dogs as a consequence of aberrant antibody production. Infected dogs may also be positive for serum antinuclear antibodies (ANA). Low ANA titres may simply reflect tissue damage in this disease, but the occasional occurrence of high titres makes the distinction of canine leishmaniosis from systemic lupus erythematosus important.

Leishmaniosis is an excellent example of an infectious disease that induces circulating immune complexes (type III hypersensitivity reaction). The detection of glomerulonephritis, uveitis and synovitis, which characterize systemic infection with *Leishmania*, is attributed at least partially to vascular deposition of these complexes. For example, granular and diffuse IgG deposition has been recorded within granulomatous uveal tract lesions of infected dogs, together with evidence of vasculitis and thrombosis. In addition, immunohistochemical studies have demonstrated immunoglobulin deposition within the glomerular lesions of infected dogs. The antigenic content of these complexes has not been sufficiently investigated in the canine disease.

The complex immunopathological mechanisms that underlie the clinical features of *Leishmania* infection may be further complicated in cases of co-infection with other arthropod-borne agents such as *Babesia* or *Ehrlichia* species or other concomitant diseases.

CLINICOPATHOLOGICAL FINDINGS

Dogs

A wide spectrum of clinical disease presentations and degrees of severity is found in dogs, ranging from mild to severe fatal disease with different clinical outcomes, prognosis and treatment options. Four clinical stages of disease have been described by the Leishvet group based on clinicopathological findings and serology, with different treatments and prognosis for each stage (**Table 9.1**).

Table 9.1 **LeishVet staging of clinical canine leishmaniosis.**

PROGNOSIS	CLINICAL SIGNS, LABORATORY ABNORMALITIES AND SEROLOGICAL STATUS	STAGE OF DISEASE
Good	Mild clinical signs including peripheral lymphadenomegaly or papular dermatitis. Usually no clinicopathological abnormalities. Negative to low anti-*Leishmania* antibody levels.	I: mild disease
Good to guarded	Clinical signs listed in stage I and diffuse or symmetrical cutaneous lesions such as exfoliative dermatitis, onychogryposis, ulceration, anorexia, weight loss, fever and epistaxis. Clinicopathological abnormalities include mild non-regenerative anaemia, hyperglobulinaemia and hypoalbuminaemia and serum hyperviscosity syndrome. Levels of anti-*Leishmania* antibodies are low to high. **Two sub-stages:** Stage IIa: • Renal profile is normal with creatinine <123.8 µmol/l. • The dog is not proteinuric. • Urine protein:creatinine (UPC) ratio <0.5. Stage IIb: • Creatinine is <123.8 µmol/l. • UPC ratio is 0.5–1.	II: moderate disease
Guarded to poor	In addition to the clinical signs listed for stages I and II, dogs may present with signs caused by immune complex deposition with lesions due to vasculitis, arthritis, uveitis and glomerulonephritis. Clinicopathological abnormalities are listed in stage II except for chronic kidney disease (CKD) of International Renal Interest Society (IRIS) stage I with UPC ratio >1 or stage II with creatinine of 123.8–176.8 µmol/l. Levels of anti-*Leishmania* antibodies are medium to high.	III: severe disease
Poor	In addition to the clinical conditions listed for stage III, pulmonary thromboembolism or nephrotic syndrome or end-stage renal disease. Clinicopathological abnormalities listed in stage II and in addition CKD of IRIS stage III (creatinine 177–442 µmol/l) or stage IV (creatinine >442 µmol/l). The nephrotic syndrome includes a marked proteinuria with UPC ratio >5. The levels of anti-*Leishmania* antibodies are medium to high.	IV: very severe disease

From Solano-Gallego *et al.*, 2009 (see Further Reading).

Classical clinical canine leishmaniosis has a chronic course. Commonly, there is a history of non-specific illness combined with lymphadenomegaly, cutaneous signs, weight loss, splenomegaly and pale mucous membranes (**Table 9.2**). Cutaneous signs are of major importance in this disease and include exfoliative dermatitis, which produces a characteristic silvery scale that is prominent on the face, periocular region and pinnae; periocular alopecia; and abnormal growth of claws (**Table 9.3**) (**Figures 9.4–9.7**). Ulcerative,

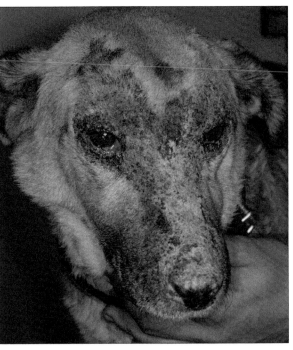

Fig. 9.4 Crossbred dog showing facial alopecia, crusting and ulceration. In addition, there is depigmentation and ulceration of the nasal planum.

Table 9.2 **Frequency of clinical signs occurring in canine leishmaniosis.**

CLINICAL SIGNS	RELATIVE FREQUENCY OF OCCURRENCE (%)
Lymphadenomegaly	65.2–88.7
Cutaneous involvement	56.0–81.0
Pale mucous membranes	58.0
Splenomegaly	9.5–53.3
Weight loss	25.3–32.0
Abnormal claws	24.0–30.5
Ocular involvement	16.0–24.1
Anorexia	16.5–18.0
Epistaxis	3.8–10.0
Lameness	3.3
Diarrhoea	3.0–3.8

Data from >100 animals from Italy and Greece. From Ciaramella *et al.*, 1997; Koutinas *et al.*, 1999 (see Further Reading).

Table 9.3 **Frequency of cutaneous findings in canine leishmaniosis.**

DERMATOLOGICAL SIGNS	RELATIVE FREQUENCY OF OCCURRENCE (%)
Exfoliative dermatitis	90.9
Ulceration	63.6
Generalized hypotrichosis, especially face and pinnae	59.1
Abnormal claws	54.5
Focal alopecia (pinnae and face)	50.0
Mild to moderate pruritus	18.2
Paronychia	13.6

Data based on 22 cases from Greece. From Koutinas *et al.*, 1993 (see Further Reading).

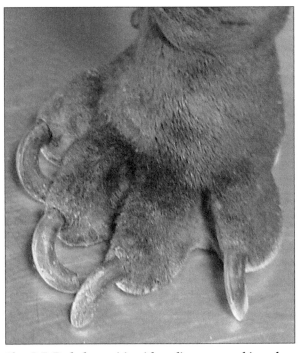

Fig. 9.5 Pododermatitis with scaling, paronychia and onychogryphosis in a dog with leishmaniosis.

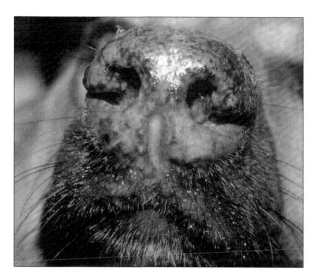

Fig. 9.6 Depigmentation, erosion, ulceration and loss of the normal cobblestone pattern of the planum nasale in a dog with leishmaniosis.

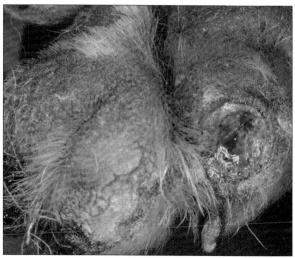

Fig. 9.7 Central foot pad ulceration secondary to granulomatous dermatitis and/or vasculitis in a dog with leishmaniosis.

Table 9.4 **Frequency of ocular and periocular findings in canine leishmaniosis.**	
OPHTHALMOLOGICAL SIGNS	RELATIVE FREQUENCY OF OCCURRENCE (%)
Anterior uveitis	42.8
Conjunctivitis	31.4
Keratoconjunctivitis	31.4
Blepharitis	29.5
Periocular alopecia	26.7
Posterior uveitis	3.8
Keratoconjunctivitis sicca	2.8
Orbital cellulitis	1.9
Based on 105 cases from Spain. From Peña *et al.*, 2000 (see Further Reading).	

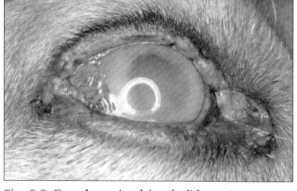

Fig. 9.8 Granulomas involving the lid margins, granulomatous bulbar conjunctivitis and corneal opacity in a dog with leishmaniosis.

nodular and papular dermatitis may occur, secondary to vasculitis and granulomatous inflammation.

Ocular and periocular signs are frequently seen in canine leishmaniosis (**Table 9.4**) (**Figures 9.8, 9.9**). Less commonly, lameness due to arthropathies, diarrhoea and epistaxis are reported (**Table 9.2**) (**Figure**

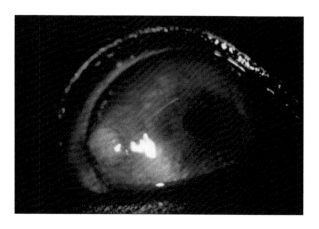

Fig. 9.9 Corneal granulomatous infiltrate with uveitis in a dog with leishmaniosis.

9.10). Although multisystemic disease is characteristic of leishmaniosis, affected dogs may present with clinical signs referable to one body system only. There are reports of infections associated with colitis, myositis, osteomyelitis and arthrosynovitis, as well as isolated ocular disease.

Clinical laboratory findings are dominated by high globulin levels due to massive polyclonal gammaglobulin production (**Table 9.5**) (**Figure 9.11**). Hypoalbuminaemia, predominantly due to protein-losing glomerulonephropathy, is also a common finding. Mild to moderate normocytic–normochromic non-regenerative anaemia is identified frequently. Affected dogs can be ANA positive. Thrombocytopenia has been described with varying frequency in cases of canine leishmaniosis. Both antibody-mediated destruction and disseminated intravascular coagulation have been suggested as underlying mechanisms. In addition, co-infection with *Ehrlichia* and *Anaplasma* species should be ruled out in cases with bleeding tendencies. Concurrent *Ehrlichia canis* seropositivity was found in 14% of 150 Italian cases of leishmaniosis.

Cats

The pathogenesis of the disease in cats has not been investigated. The clinical presentation is similar to that seen in dogs, although the small number of cases makes the association of infection and clinical signs difficult to interpret. Cutaneous lesions include diffuse areas of alopecia and granulomatous dermatitis of the head, scaling and pinnal dermatitis, ulceration and nodules. Systemic involvement with *L. infantum* has been reported in association with lymphadenomegaly, jaundice, vomiting, hepatomegaly, splenomegaly, membranous glomerulonephritis and granulomatous gastroenteritis. An association with feline leukaemia virus and feline immunodeficiency virus infections has been described.

DIAGNOSIS

Confirming a diagnosis of leishmaniosis in an individual case may be difficult, particularly if the clinical signs are not specific. In addition, longitudinal studies of *Leishmania* infection show that relative predictive values for diagnostic tests vary depending on the stage of infection. Consequently, a diagnostic approach that

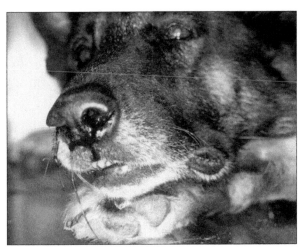

Fig. 9.10 Epistaxis in a German Shepherd Dog with leishmaniosis.

Table 9.5 **Frequency of clinical laboratory findings in canine leishmaniosis.**

CLINICAL LABORATORY SIGNS	RELATIVE FREQUENCY OF OCCURRENCE (%)
Hyperglobulinaemia	70.6
Hypoalbuminaemia	68.0
Anaemia	58.0
Positive ANA	52.8
Neutrophilia	24.0
Thrombocytopenia	29.3
Positive Coombs test	20.8
Azotemia	16.0
Elevated liver enzymes	16.0

Based on 150 cases from Italy. From Ciaramella *et al.,* 1997 (see Further Reading).

involves multiple testing modalities is recommended and no single diagnostic technique identifies all infected animals.

Microscopical identification of organisms or their DNA

Intracellular or extracellular *Leishmania* amastigotes can be identified in Giemsa- or other Romanowsky-type-stained tissue aspirates and impressions or biopsy samples from lymph node, conjunctiva, bone marrow (**Figure 9.12**), spleen and lesional skin (**Figures 9.13,**

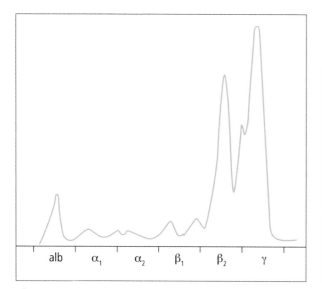

Fig. 9.11 Serum protein electrophoresis from a dog with leishmaniosis showing a biclonal gammopathy.

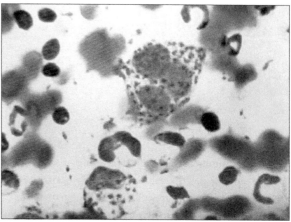

Fig. 9.12 Bone marrow aspirate from a dog with leishmaniosis showing intracellular *Leishmania* amastigotes.

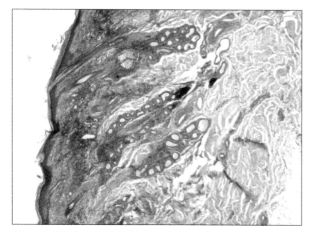

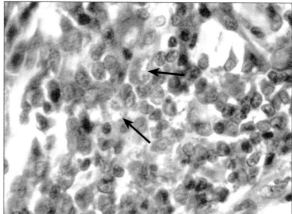

Figs. 9.13, 9.14 Skin biopsy from a dog with leishmaniosis. There are numerous infiltrating macrophages in the superficial dermis, within which *Leishmania* amastigotes (arrows) can be seen clearly.

9.14). Amastigotes are small round or oval bodies, $1.5-3.0 \times 2.5-3.5$ μm in size and without a free flagellum. The organism has a relatively large nucleus and a kinetoplast. However, the sensitivity of microscopical examination is relatively poor (60%), as more than 50% of lymph node and bone marrow samples have low parasite density. Polymerase chain reaction (PCR) targeting kinetoplast DNA, and immunohistochemical techniques for increasing sensitivity and specificity of *Leishmania* detection, have been developed for use in fresh and frozen bone marrow, lymph node and skin biopsy specimens (**Figure 9.15**). On such samples, the sensitivity of PCR approaches 95–100%. However, the sensitivity of PCR on peripheral blood samples is lower.

Serology

Most dogs with leishmaniosis develop a specific humoral immune response and serodiagnostic testing is widely used. The sensitivity of serology is lowest (41%) early in *Leishmania* infection (first few months),

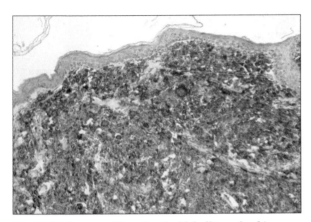

Fig. 9.15 Immunohistochemical labelling of a skin biopsy from a dog with leishmaniosis to demonstrate the presence of amastigotes. (Courtesy Department of Pathology, Veterinary Faculty, Universitat Autònoma de Barcelona)

but high with progressive infection (93–100%). Sensitivity may also be limited in cases of mild diseases such as localized cutaneous leishmanial infection. A wide variety of serological assays are available, utilizing indirect immunofluorescence antibody testing, direct agglutination, conventional enzyme-linked immunosorbent assay (ELISA), dot-ELISA, competitive ELISA and western blotting. Although there is some variation in specificity, sensitivity and predictive values, most such tests are acceptable. At present, most tests employ crude *Leishmania* antigen, although a recombinant *Leishmania* K39 ELISA has been validated. Several rapid immunochromatographic test kits have also been produced for canine leishmaniosis, but although most are relatively specific, sensitivity ranges from 35–76%.

In dogs that have not been vaccinated against leishmaniosis, high antibody levels are usually associated with disease and a high parasite density and, for this reason, they are conclusive of a diagnosis of leishmaniosis. However, the presence of lower antibody levels is not necessarily indicative of patent disease and needs to be confirmed by other diagnostic methods such as PCR, cytology or histology. The challenges of interpreting serology results include cross-reactivity with other pathogens and antibodies elicited by vaccination. Serological cross-reactivity with different pathogens is possible with some serological tests, especially those based on whole parasite antigen. Cross-reactivity has

been reported with other species of *Leishmania* and with *Trypanosoma cruzi*. Therefore, the specificity of serology may be decreased in Central and South America due to cross-reactivity with *Trypanosoma* species infection. Because there are currently no serological techniques that discriminate between antibodies formed after infection and those elicited by vaccination, knowledge about the kinetics of antibodies to vaccination is crucial. The maximum peak of antibodies elicited by vaccination with the CaniLeish® vaccine is 2 weeks after the third vaccination of the initial vaccination protocol. A decrease in antibody levels is observed over time and the majority of vaccinated dogs do not have antibody detectable by IFAT 6 months post vaccination.

Culture and species characterization

Culture can be used for diagnosis of canine *Leishmania* infection, but it requires access to a laboratory with technical expertise and appropriate containment facilities. In addition, multiple samples are required from several sites to achieve appropriate sensitivity. It is, however, the basis for species characterization using traditional isoenzyme analysis and molecular techniques such as multilocus sequence typing and microsatellite identification. However, as primer sequences for differentiation of New and Old World species are now available, PCR and sequencing are commonly used.

TREATMENT AND PREVENTION

Chemotherapeutic treatment of canine leishmaniosis

Several drugs are currently used for the treatment of canine leishmaniosis (**Table 9.6**). In dogs, the objectives of treatment are typically to induce a general reduction of the parasite load, to treat organ damage caused by the parasite, to restore efficient immune responses, to stabilize a drug-induced clinical improvement and to treat clinical relapse.

Treatment will depend on the degree of severity of disease and the clinical classification of dogs. Antimonials have been used for the therapy of leishmaniosis since the early 20th century, when tartar emetic (antimony potassium tartrate) was adapted for the treatment of human leishmaniosis in South America after proving effective against African trypanosomiasis. Pentavalent antimonials are still widely used against the different forms of leishmaniosis in both human and veterinary medicine. The antimonials selectively inhibit leishmanial enzymes that are required for glycolytic and fatty acid oxidation. Meglumine antimonate is the principal antimonial used for the treatment of dogs, usually in combination with allopurinol.

Allopurinol is an orally administered purine analogue that is metabolized by *Leishmania* parasites and incorporated into RNA, causing an interruption in protein synthesis. The relative non-toxicity, clinical efficacy, low cost and convenience of oral administration have made allopurinol a popular choice for the treatment of canine leishmaniosis. It is recommended as daily treatment for a long period of time and is commonly administered in combination with meglumine antimoniate or miltefosine. In addition, long-term therapy with allopurinol decreases the rate of relapse after meglumine antimoniate or miltefosine treatment.

The most widely used treatment protocol for dogs with leishmaniosis is the combination of meglumine antimoniate and allopurinol. Meglumine antimoniate (100 mg/kg SC q24h for 4 weeks) is administered in combination with allopurinol (10 mg/kg PO q12h for at least 1 year). The dose of meglumine antimoniate can be divided into two equal doses of 50 mg/kg (q12h) and administered for a period ranging from 4–8 weeks.

The second most used protocol is the combination of miltefosine, an alkylphosphocholine, and allopurinol. Miltefosine (2 mg/kg PO q24h for 28 days) is administered in combination with allopurinol (10 mg/kg PO q12 h) as described above.

The use of allopurinol alone is employed when administration of meglumine antimoniate or miltefosine are not desirable due to their potential toxicities, when these two drugs are not available or in dogs with mild disease. Short-term treatment is administered only in dogs with rare mild disease that carries a good prognosis (clinical stage I), such as dogs with papular dermatitis.

In one limited study, treatment with domperidone, a dopamine D2 receptor antagonist (0.5 mg/kg PO q24h for 4 weeks), led to reduction in clinical signs and antibody titres in dogs with very mild leishmaniosis.

Diagnosis and treatment of concurrent diseases such as ehrlichiosis and babesiosis may be required, as these infections are common in endemic areas of *L. infantum*.

The prognosis for canine leishmaniosis is currently more favourable than in the past, and should not always be considered poor, especially in the absence of severe renal disease and if dogs are correctly treated and monitored. Prognosis depends on the clinical stage and in sick dogs mostly depends on the severity of clinicopathological alterations and in particular on renal damage, as well as treatment response. Unfortunately, it is not easy to predict outcome in dogs with leishmaniosis due to the limited information available and the lack of controlled studies evaluating prognostic factors. However, as mentioned previously, there are no treatment protocols published that result in parasitological

Table 9.6 **Drugs used for treatment of canine leishmaniosis.**

DRUG	COMMON TRADE NAME	CLASS	MODE OF ACTION	THERAPEUTIC PROTOCOL	ADVERSE EFFECTS
Meglumine antimoniate	Glucantime	Pentavalent antimonial	Inhibition of enzymes active in glycolysis and fatty acid oxidation	100 mg/kg SC q24h or 50 mg/kg SC q12h for 4–8 weeks, always together with allopurinol	Potential nephrotoxicity; muscle fibrosis, abscess and pain at the site of injection
Allopurinol	Zyloric	Pyrazolpyrimidine	Incorporation into RNA and inhibition of protein synthesis	10 mg/kg PO q12h for at least 6 months (frequently 12 months and sometimes longer)	Xanthine crystals and urolith formation
Miltefosine	Milteforan	Alkylphosphocholine	Impairment of signalling pathways and cell membrane synthesis	2 mg/kg PO q24h (with food) for 4 weeks, always together with allopurinol	Gastrointestinal disorders (vomiting and diarrhoea)

cure. Consequently, monitoring of sick dogs should be carried out both during and after leishmaniosis treatment in order to assess clinical and clinicopathological remission, adequacy of response to treatment and possible occurrence of clinical relapse.

Prevention

Two main prevention strategies of canine leishmaniosis have been shown to be effective in the dog: the use of topical insecticides/repellents (pyrethroids) by spot-on or collar, which is the most effective mean of protection, and vaccination. Commercial vaccines against canine leishmaniosis have been approved in Brazil and Europe; they do not completely prevent infection, but rather decrease the occurrence of clinical disease. The only commercial vaccine currently available in Europe is CaniLeish® (Virbac), which consists of excreted–secreted products obtained by *in-vitro* culture of *L. infantum* promastigotes with the QA-21 saponin adjuvant. The first immunization consists of three subcutaneous injections at 3-week intervals in dogs over 6 months of age, and booster vaccinations are recommended every year. The vaccines marketed in Brazil include Leishmune® (Zoetis), which is also an excreted–secreted product based on a purified fucose–mannose compound of *L. donovani* with QuilA saponin adjuvant, and Leishtec® (Hertape Calier) based on the *L. donovani* A2 recombinant protein with a saponin adjuvant. At the time of writing, the Leishmune® vaccine is not available on the market. However, the protection of each single dog, although high, is not 100% guaranteed with any of these two methods. The preventive efficacy of pyrethroids is 86–98% in the individual dog and 100% at the population level. Domperidone (Leishguard®; Esteve), has been registered for use as a prophylactic medication against canine leishmaniosis. The drug is a dopamine D2 receptor antagonist, which has been reported to have immunostimulant properties via the stimulation of prolactin secretion, which in turn acts to induce pro-inflammatory cytokines and Th1 immune response with IFN-γ production. A statistically significant protective effect of the drug against the appearance of clinical disease was observed in one study, but further assessments are required to evaluate its prophylactic efficacy against infection and disease. The various existing preventive strategies can be combined to increase their efficacy; however, no data are available confirming that this approach increases the degree of protection compared with single use. The use of topical insecticides is recommended in any healthy, infected or sick (whether under treatment or not) dog as an effective strategy to reduce the risk of infecting dogs and, indirectly, humans.

ZOONOTIC POTENTIAL/PUBLIC HEALTH SIGNIFICANCE

Visceral leishmaniosis is a potentially fatal disease. A World Health Organization report from 2014 indicates that there are approximately 200,000–400,000 new human cases of visceral leishmaniosis annually, with 20,000 to 30,000 deaths. The population at risk globally is about 200 million people. Anthroponotic visceral leishmaniosis caused by *L. donovani*, mainly in India and Sudan, is responsible for a large proportion of the fatalities in people. However, zoonotic canine leishmaniosis, with the dog as a major reservoir for the parasite, is a main concern in other parts of the world including South America, the Mediterranean basin, the Middle East, Central Asia and China. The link between canine and human infections probably differs between regions and according to life style and could depend on factors such as human nutrition, time spent outdoors, the density of dogs and the behaviour of local sand fly vectors. The major risk group for human disease caused by *L. infantum* has traditionally been infants and children. Malnutrition has long been recognized as a risk factor for infantile leishmaniosis and this may explain why the disease is more prevalent among children in poor countries, compared with children in more affluent areas, where there is a similar high prevalence rate in the dog population.

With the appearance of the acquired immunodeficiency syndrome epidemic, HIV-positive patients became the predominant group of patients in southern Europe. Co-infection of HIV and leishmaniosis is reported from more than 33 countries where these infections overlap geographically. HIV-positive patients are sensitive to new infection or a reactivation of a dormant infection. The presence of large numbers of parasites in their tissues and blood makes them highly infectious to sand flies. However, the development of successful anti-retroviral drugs for treatment of HIV has considerably decreased the number of severe HIV–leishmaniosis co-infection patients in countries where this treatment is available.

The treatment of infected dogs in areas where suitable vectors are found should be presented realistically to owners, by veterinarians, because of the potential risk of transmission to other people and pets in the community. Before deciding on therapy, owners must receive a thorough explanation about the disease, its zoonotic potential and the prognosis for their dog and what should be expected from treatment.

CASE STUDY

Signalment

Zoe, a 3-year-old, neutered female Boxer from a farm in Israel (**Figure 9.16**). Lives mostly outdoors with indoor access.

History

For the previous 8 weeks, the owners have noticed that the dog is losing weight and has become less active than before. She had developed lesions on her ears with hair loss and crusts. The owners also noticed occasional bleeding from the ears for the past month.

Clinical examination

Body weight 29 kg; temperature 38.4°C; heart rate 64 beats/min; respiration rate 20 breaths per minute; mucous membranes are pink with a capillary refill time of <2 seconds. The dog is alert and responsive.

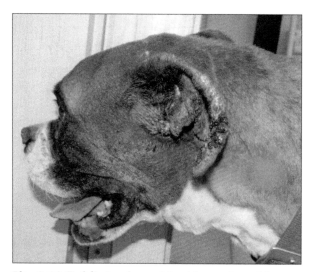

Fig. 9.16 Exfoliative dermatitis with crusting of the ear.

Zoe has exfoliative dermatitis with skin thickening and crusting over both ears. She also has fine exfoliation of skin over the fore- and hindlimbs. Her body condition score is 4/9 and there is moderate generalized muscle atrophy. Her submandibular, prescapular and popliteal lymph nodes are enlarged (about double their normal size) and the spleen feels enlarged on abdominal palpation.

Laboratory diagnostic findings

Table 9.7 **Haematological examination.**

PARAMETER	VALUE	REFERENCE RANGE
WBC	$5.15 \times 10^9/l$	5.2–13.9
RBC	$4.6 \times 10^{12}/l$	5.7–8.8
Hct	29.0%	37.1–57
MCV	63.1 fl	58.8–71.2
MCHC	33.6 g/dl	31–36.2
Neutrophils	$3.81 \times 10^9/l$	3.9–8.0
Lymphocytes	$0.88 \times 10^9/l$	1.3–4.1
Monocytes	$0.31 \times 10^9/l$	0.2–1.1
Eosinophils	$0.15 \times 10^9/l$	0.0–0.6
Platelets	$189 \times 10^9/l$	160–400

Table 9.8 **Serum biochemistry.**

PARAMETER	VALUE	REFERENCE RANGE
Total protein	89 g/l	54–75
Globulin	69 g/l	27–44
Albumin	20 g/l	26–40
ALP	22 U/l	19–50
ALT	54 U/l	17–66
Amylase	1,373 U/l	200–1,480
BUN	5.2 mmol/l	3.57–8.92
Cholesterol	145 mg/dl	135–180
Creatinine	60.2 µmol/l	26.5–88.4
Creatine kinase	145 U/l	92–357
Total bilirubin	2.53 µmol/l	1.71–5.13
Glucose	4.8 mmol/l	4.44–5.55
Sodium	145 mmol/l	142–159
Potassium	5.1 mmol/l	3.8–5.6
Chloride	112 mmol/l	102–117
Calcium	2.34 mmol/l	2.37–2.94
Phosphorus	1.35 mmol/l	1.06–2.38

Table 9.9 Urinalysis.

PARAMETER	VALUE/COMMENT
Specific gravity	1.030
pH	7.5
Protein	+
Blood	Negative
Bilirubin	Negative
Glucose	Negative
Sediment	None
Urine protein:creatinine ratio	0.25

Summary of hematological and serum biochemistry abnormalities

Moderate normocytic–normochromic anaemia with mild leucopenia consisting of mild neutropenia and lymphopenia. Hypoalbuminaemia with hyperglobulinaemia with mild hypocalcaemia; probably due to hypoalbuminaemia.

Lymph node cytology

Reactive lymph node with large numbers of plasma cells, an occasional mitotic figure and macrophages containing *Leishmania* amastigotes (**Figure 9.17**).

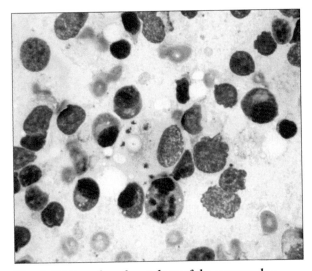

Fig. 9.17 Lymph node cytology of the prescapular lymph node (×1,000, May–Grünwald–Giemsa stain). Note the abundant plasma cells, a macrophage with *Leishmania* amastigotes and a mitotic figure.

Serology

Leishmania serology by crude *L. infantum* promastigote ELISA is positive with an optical density of 1.45 (positive from 0.5).

PCR

PCR of a lymph node aspirate was positive for *Leishmania* kDNA.

Diagnosis

Canine leishmaniosis stage IIa.

Treatment

Combination therapy of meglumine antimoniate (100 mg/kg SC q24h SC for 4 weeks) with allopurinol (10 mg/kg PO q12h PO continued for 18 months).

Outcome

The skin disease started to improve within 4 weeks of treatment. Haematology and serum biochemistry normalized within 6 months of the start of treatment. Serum anti-*Leishmania* antibodies dropped continuously during the follow-up period until they were below the cut-off level at 18 months from the start of treatment. Urine remained normal with no proteinuria and the dog gained weight (4 kg). Although allopurinol treatment was stopped at 18 months, the dog continues to be monitored for anti-*Leishmania* antibodies and wears an insecticide collar to protect against sand flies.

FURTHER READING

Baneth G, Koutinas AF, Solano-Gallego L *et al.* (2008) Canine leishmaniosis – new concepts and insights on an expanding zoonosis: part one. *Trends in Parasitology* **24**:324–330.

Baneth G, Shaw SE (2002) Chemotherapy of canine leishmaniasis. *Veterinary Parasitology* **106**:315–324.

Baneth G, Zivotofsky D, Nachum-Biala Y *et al.* (2014) Mucocutaneous *Leishmania tropica* infection in a dog from a human cutaneous leishmaniasis focus. *Parasites and Vectors* **7**:118.

Barbosa-De-Deus R, Dos Mares-Guia ML *et al.* (2002) *Leishmania major*-like antigen for specific and sensitive serodiagnosis of human and canine visceral leishmaniasis. *Clinical and Diagnostic Laboratory Immunology* **9**:1361–1366.

Boggiatto PM, Gibson-Corley KN, Metz K *et al.* (2011) Transplacental transmission of *Leishmania infantum* as a means for continued disease incidence in North America. *PLoS Neglected Tropical Diseases* **5**:e1019.

Ciaramella P, Oliva G, de Luna R *et al.* (1997) A retrospective clinical study of canine leishmaniasis in 150 dogs naturally infected by *Leishmania infantum. Veterinary Record* **141**:539–543.

GarciaAlonso M, Blanco A, Reina D *et al.* (1996) Immunopathology of the uveitis in canine leishmaniasis. *Parasite Immunology* **18**:617–623.

Gómez-Ochoa P, Castillo JA, Gascón M *et al.* (2009) Use of domperidone in the treatment of canine visceral leishmaniasis: a clinical trial. *Veterinary Journal* **179**:259–263.

Koutinas AF, Polizopoulou ZS, Saridomichelakis MN *et al.* (1999) Clinical considerations on canine visceral leishmaniasis in Greece: a retrospective study of 158 cases (1989–1996). *Journal of the American Animal Hospital Association* **35**:376–383.

Koutinas AF, Scott DW, Kantos V *et al.* (1993) Skin lesions in canine leishmaniasis (Kala-Azar): a clinical and histopathological study on 22 spontaneous cases in Greece. *Veterinary Dermatology* **3**:121–131.

Lombardo G, Pennisi MG, Lupo T *et al.* (2014) Papular dermatitis due to *Leishmania infantum* infection in seventeen dogs: diagnostic features, extent of the infection and treatment outcome. *Parasites and Vectors* **7**:120.

Millán J, Ferroglio E, Solano-Gallego L (2014) Role of wildlife in the epidemiology of *Leishmania infantum* infection in Europe. *Parasitology Research* **113**:2005–2014.

Monge-Maillo B, Norman FF, Cruz I *et al.* (2014) Visceral leishmaniasis and HIV coinfection in the Mediterranean region. *PLoS Neglected Tropical Diseases* **8**:e3021.

Moreno J, Vouldoukis I, Martin V *et al.* (2012) Use of a LiESP/QA-21 vaccine (CaniLeish) stimulates an appropriate Th1-dominated cell-mediated immune response in dogs. *PLoS Neglected Tropical Diseases* **6**:e1683.

Moreno J, Vouldoukis I, Schreiber P *et al.* (2014) Primary vaccination with the LiESP/QA-21 vaccine (CaniLeish) produces a cell-mediated immune response which is still present 1 year later. *Veterinary Immunology and Immunopathology* **158**:199–207.

Nieto CG, Navarrete I, Habela MA *et al.* (1992) Pathological changes in kidneys of dogs with natural *Leishmania* infection. *Veterinary Parasitology* **45**:33–47.

Oliva G, Nieto J, Foglia Manzillo V *et al.* (2014) A randomised, double-blind, controlled efficacy trial of the LiESP/QA-21 vaccine in naïve dogs exposed to two *Leishmania infantum* transmission seasons. *PLoS Neglected Tropical Diseases* **8**:e3213.

Pena MT, Roura X, Davidson MG (2000) Ocular and periocular manifestations of leishmaniasis in dogs: 105 cases (1993–1998). *Veterinary Ophthalmology* **3**:35–41.

Porrozzi R, Santos da Costa MV, Teva A *et al.* (2007) Comparative evaluation of enzyme-linked immunosorbent assays based on crude and recombinant leishmanial antigens for serodiagnosis of symptomatic and asymptomatic *Leishmania infantum* visceral infections in dogs. *Clinical and Vaccine Immunology* **14**:544–548.

Quilez J, Martínez V, Woolliams JA *et al.* (2012) Genetic control of canine leishmaniasis: genome-wide association study and genomic selection analysis. *PLoS One* **7**:e35349.

Quinnell RJ, Courtney O, Davidson S *et al.* (2001) Detection of *Leishmania infantum* by PCR, serology and cellular immune response in a cohort study of Brazilian dogs. *Parasitology* **122**:253–261.

Quinnell RJ, Kennedy LJ, Barnes A *et al.* (2003) Susceptibility to visceral leishmaniasis in the domestic dog is associated with MHC class II polymorphism. *Immunogenetics* **55**:23–28.

Ready PD (2014) Epidemiology of visceral leishmaniasis. *Clinical Epidemiology* **6**:147-154.

Reis AB, Teixeira-Carvalho A, Vale AM *et al.* (2006) Isotype patterns of immunoglobulins: hallmarks for clinical status and tissue parasite density in Brazilian dogs naturally infected by *Leishmania (Leishmania) chagasi. Veterinary Immunology and Immunopathology* **112**:102–116.

Roura X, Fondati A, Lubas G *et al.* (2013) Prognosis and monitoring of leishmaniasis in dogs: a working group report. *Veterinary Journal* **198**:43–47.

Sabaté D, Llinás J, Homedes J *et al.* (2014) A single-centre, open-label, controlled, randomized clinical trial to assess the preventive efficacy of a domperidone-based treatment programme against clinical canine leishmaniasis in a high prevalence area. *Preventive Veterinary Medicine* **115**:56–63.

Sanchez-Robert E, Altet L, Utzet-Sadurni M *et al.* (2008) Slc11a1 (formerly Nramp1) and susceptibility to canine visceral leishmaniasis. *Veterinary Research* **39**:36.

Sherry K, Miró G, Trotta M *et al.* (2011) A serological and molecular study of *Leishmania infantum* infection in cats from the Island of Ibiza (Spain). *Vector Borne Zoonotic Diseases* **11**:239–245.

Silva FL, Oliveira RG, Silva TM *et al.* (2009) Venereal transmission of canine visceral leishmaniasis. *Veterinary Parasitology* **160**:55–59.

Silva KL, de Andrade MM, Melo LM *et al.* (2014) CD4+FOXP3+ cells produce IL-10 in the spleens of dogs with visceral leishmaniasis. *Veterinary Parasitology* **202**:313–318.

Sobrinho LS, Rossi CN, Vides JP *et al.* (2012) Coinfection of *Leishmania chagasi* with *Toxoplasma gondii*, feline immunodeficiency virus (FIV) and feline leukemia virus (FeLV) in cats from an endemic area of zoonotic visceral leishmaniasis. *Veterinary Parasitology* **187**:302–306.

Solano-Gallego L, Koutinas A, Miro G *et al.* (2009) Directions for the diagnosis, clinical staging, treatment and prevention of canine leishmaniosis. *Veterinary Parasitology* **165**:1–18.

Solano-Gallego L, Llull J, Ramos G *et al.* (2000) The Ibizian hound presents a predominantly cellular immune response against natural *Leishmania* infection. *Veterinary Parasitology* **90**:37–45.

Solano-Gallego L, Miro G, Koutinas A *et al.* (2011). LeishVet guidelines for the practical management of canine leishmaniosis. *Parasites and Vectors* **4**:86.

Solano-Gallego L, Morell P, Arboix M *et al.* (2001) Prevalence of *Leishmania infantum* infection in dogs living in an area of canine leishmaniasis endemicity using PCR on several tissues and serology. *Journal of Clinical Microbiology* **39**:560–563.

Solano-Gallego L, Villanueva-Saz S, Carbonell M *et al.* (2014) Serological diagnosis of canine leishmaniosis: comparison of three commercial ELISA tests (Leiscan, ID Screen and Leishmania 96), a rapid test (Speed Leish K) and an in-house IFAT. *Parasites and Vectors* **7**:111.

Turchetti AP, Souza TD, Paixão TA *et al.* (2014) Sexual and vertical transmission of visceral leishmaniasis. *Journal of Infection in Developing Countries* **8**:403–407.

Vélez ID, Carrillo LM, López L *et al.* (2012) An epidemic outbreak of canine cutaneous leishmaniasis in Colombia caused by *Leishmania braziliensis* and *Leishmania panamensis*. *American Journal for Tropical Medicine and Hygiene* **86**:807–811.

World Health Organization (2015) http://www.who.int/mediacentre/factsheets/fs375/en/

Borreliosis

Reinhard K. Straubinger

AETIOLOGY AND EPIDEMIOLOGY

Aetiology

Spirochaetes comprising the genus *Borrelia* are vector-transmitted bacteria of the order Spirochaetales. Endoflagella, around which the protoplasmic cylinder of the bacterium is wound, create a spiral, elongated structure, which enables an undulating motility in environments of high viscosity such as the intercellular matrix of skin (**Figure 10.1**). Nineteen known genospecies of the *Borrelia burgdorferi* complex are transmitted by hard-shelled ticks of the genus *Ixodes* (**Table 10.1**). Several *Borrelia* species (especially *B. burgdorferi* sensu stricto,

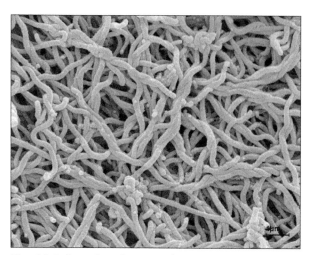

Fig. 10.1 Scanning electron microscope image of *Borrelia burgdorferi* organisms. The image shows typical clustering of spirochaetes in Barbour–Stoenner–Kelly (BSK II) liquid culture medium. The unique bipolar orientated flagellum of the spirochaetes is encapsulated by the outer surface envelope, enabling the slender protoplasmic cylinder to coil. (Courtesy of Dr R. Straubinger, Dr S. Al-Robaiy, Professor J. Seeger and Dr J. Kacza)

B. afzelii, *B. bavariensis* and *B. garinii*; www.eucalb.com) are important in terms of infections for humans and animals, particularly for dogs, cats and horses. The other *Borrelia* species of the *B. burgdorferi* complex (e.g. *B. valaisiana*, *B. lusitaniae*) are not of great veterinary clinical importance. A second group of *Borrelia* species is the cause of relapsing fever in humans and animals. For example, *B. recurrentis* is a louse-borne agent, while *B. hermsii* is transmitted by soft ticks of the genus *Ornithodorus*. Both can cause relapsing fever in man. Likewise, *B. persica* is transmitted by *Ornithodorus tholozani* and causes relapsing fever in humans, cats and dogs. It seems that a third group of *Borrelia* species is emerging from the vast diversity of spiral-shaped bacteria; *Borrelia* transmitted by hard-shelled ticks, but exhibiting characteristics of relapsing fever-causing spirochaetes (e.g. *B. miyamotoi* transmitted by *Ixodes* ticks; *B. theileri* transmitted by *Boophilus/Rhipicephalus* tick species)

Epidemiology of the *Borrelia burgdorferi* complex

Many wild mammals and birds are known reservoirs for *B. burgdorferi* species. The range of these is discussed fully in Chapter 2 and summarized in **Figure 10.2**.

European *Ixodes* species ticks may harbour up to four different *Borrelia* species simultaneously. Generally, *B. afzelii* and *B. bavariensis/B. garinii* appear to be most prevalent. However, a competitive interaction occurs among *B. burgdorferi* strains within a host and the order of appearance of the strains is the main determinant of the competitive outcome. The first strain to infect a host shows an absolute fitness advantage over the later strains. Nevertheless, where strain variation exists, one tick bite may result in heterogeneous infection.

Dogs are capable of maintaining *Borrelia* infection; however, their role in the sylvatic cycle is limited. The reservoir competency of cats is currently unknown. Serological surveys of dogs for *B. burgdorferi* complex

Table 10.1 Distribution, vectors and clinical relevance of the major *Borrelia* species.

ORGANISM	MAIN VECTOR	MAIN RESERVOIRS	DISTRIBUTION	HUMAN DISEASE	CANINE INFECTION	CANINE DISEASE
B. burgdorferi sensu stricto	*I. ricinus*, *I. scapularis*, *I. pacificus*	Rodents/birds	North America/ western Europe	North America/ western Europe	North America/ western Europe	North America/ western Europe
B. afzelii	*I. ricinus*, *I. persulcatus*, *I. hexagonus*	Mainly rodents	Eurasia	Europe	Europe	Europe
B. bavarienis	*I. ricinus*, *I. persulcatus*	Mainly rodents	Eurasia	Europe	Europe	Europe
B. garinii	*I. ricinus*, *I. persulcatus*, *I. uriae*	Mainly birds	Eurasia	Europe	Europe/Japan	Europe/Japan
B. valaisiana	*I. ricinus*, *I. columnae*	Mainly birds	Eurasia	Uncertain	Europe	No
B. lusitaniae	*I. ricinus*, *I. persulcatus*	Not well known	South-central Europe	No	No	No
B. bisettii	*I. pacificus*, *I. scapularis*	Rodents	USA	No	No	No
B. andersonii	*I. dentatus*	Lizards	USA	No	No	No
B. japonica	*I. ovatus*	Rodents	Japan	No	Japan	Japan
B. sinica	*I. ovatus*	Rodents	South China	Unknown	Unknown	Unknown
B. tanukii	*I. tanuki*	Birds	Japan	No	No	No
B. turdae	*I. turdus*	Birds	Japan	No	No	No

B. burgdorferi sensu stricto is the main species present in the USA. Its distribution is mainly in the northeastern and mid-western states, where it is transmitted by *I. scapularis*, and in the south-east where it is transmitted by *I. pacificus*. In Europe, *B. burgdorferi* sensu stricto is transmitted by *I. ricinus*. *B. burgdorferi* sensu stricto does not survive in *I. persulcatus* and therefore is not found in Asia. *B. garinii* is probably the most widespread species, with a range extending from western Europe to Japan. It is transported by migratory thrushes through European and Asian countries, and has great strain diversity. It is also carried from the northern to the southern hemisphere by sea birds carrying *I. uriae*. However, *B. garinii* is not detected in humans or in domestic animal species from the southern hemisphere. More species are being identified

have been used as an indicator for infection rates in the local tick and wild animal populations and, thus, as an indication of risk for human infection. In Europe, 20–40% of questing, unfed ticks collected from the coat of dogs or from vegetation contain *Borrelia* DNA, yet seroprevalence rates for European dogs range between 1.9% and 10.3%. In Westchester County, New York, USA, 80% of questing ticks may contain borreliae and surveys of dogs in the north-eastern USA reveal extremely high levels of seropositivity (30–90%).

In North America, *B. burgdorferi* sensu stricto is the only pathogenic species found in dogs. In Japan, dogs are probably infected with *B. japonica* and *B. garinii*. In Europe, dogs are mainly infected with *B. burgdorferi* sensu stricto and probably with *B. afzelii*, *B. bavariensis* and *B. garinii*, chiefly in areas where ticks carry mul-

tiple *Borrelia* species. Species differences may imply differences in infectivity and tissue invasiveness. The differential tissue tropism that the major three species are supposed to exhibit in the human host – *B. afzelii* to skin, *B. garinii* to the central nervous system and *B. burgdorferi* sensu stricto to synovial tissues – suggests that differences in tissue affinity might also be expected in the canine host.

Not all infected dogs develop clinical signs. The fraction of infected dogs under field conditions that go on to succumb to disease is not determined. Consequently, persistence of specific serum antibody against *Borrelia* species is not necessarily associated with clinical disease. However, dogs that harbour co-infections with other tick-transmitted pathogens (e.g. *Ehrlichia* species, *Anaplasma* species, *Bartonella* species, *Babesia*

Fig. 10.2 The cycle of *Borrelia* spirochaetes through the tick vector and vertebrate hosts. The European situation with four *Borrelia* species is depicted, emphasizing the central role of the nymph. During the 2-year tick life cycle the successive stages acquire or transmit spirochaetes by feeding on successively larger hosts. Birds are reservoirs for *B. garinii* and *B. valaisiana*. Small mammals are the reservoir animals for *B. burgdorferi* sensu stricto, *B. afzelii* and *B. bavariensis*.

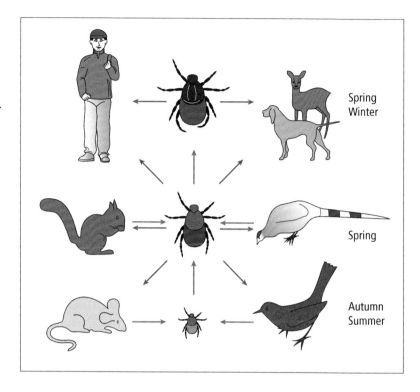

species and/or *Rickettsia* species) may be more likely to develop clinically apparent disease than dogs infected with a single organism.

Information on feline *Borrelia* infection is sparse. In a serological survey of cats in the northeastern USA, 20–47% of cats showed specific antibodies against *B. burgdorferi*. In a study from the UK, 4.2% of cats were positive compared with more than 20% of dogs.

PATHOGENESIS

Different mechanisms are exploited by borreliae to avoid clearance by the immune system, resulting in a persistent infection and possibly chronic disease (**Figure 10.3**). The *Borrelia* genome is unusual compared with that of other bacteria, as it has a linear chromosome and a large number (21) of circular and linear plasmids. The chromosome has been completely sequenced and is thought to contain only around 800 genes encoding molecules with metabolic functions. Many genes encoding molecules with metabolic functions normally present in bacterial genomes are missing, suggesting that borreliae are highly dependent on the host for metabolism. *Borrelia* species do not depend on iron, which is possibly an adaptation

to localization within tissue with limited access to the bloodstream. A large portion of the genome encodes molecules involved in motility, indicating the importance of migration in pathogenesis.

The plasmids encode around 100 proteins, of which the majority consists of lipoproteins located on the outer surface envelope in direct contact with the host. Several surface proteins (e.g. OspA to OspF, decorin binding proteins, complement regulator-acquiring surface proteins) have been characterized, and these are highly immunogenic and to some extent antigenically variable. OspA (31–34 kDa) has been typed serologically, and seven serotypes are defined and assigned to three groups corresponding to the major pathogenic *B. burgdorferi* species. The change in expression from OspA to OspC on the outer envelope (the 'OspA/OspC switch') is mandatory for infection of the vertebrate host. This occurs within the first 24–48 hours of tick attachment. The expression of OspA is downregulated by contact with blood combined with the elevated surface temperature of the new host (~33°C) and OspC is expressed as *Borrelia* organisms migrate from the tick midgut to the tick salivary gland. Subsequently, spirochaetes expressing OspC on their surface and coated with numerous tick salivary proteins are injected into

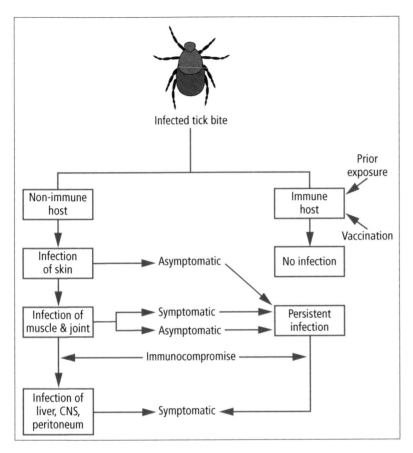

Fig. 10.3 Possible outcome of *Borrelia* infection. If an infected tick bites an immune host, infection will not establish and the animal will remain asymptomatic. Transmission of borreliae to a non-immune host will allow the establishment of progressive infection in skin and then muscle and joints. This infection may be either symptomatic or asymptomatic and is likely to be persistent. Immunocompromise is likely to result in further spread of the infection, with the development of progressive clinical signs.

the skin of the new host. Consequently, OspC is one of the first antigens encountered by the host immune system; antibodies are produced and these antibodies are detected in the early phase of infection in man and animals.

The enormous potential for antigenic variation and immune evasion within the *Borrelia* species is even more evident when recombination of numerous redundant gene copies found in the variable major protein-like sequence, expressed (VlsE) encoding for the VlsE surface lipoprotein is considered. The VlsE antigen is hypervariable and still it contains fixed invariant regions that are conserved within the *Borrelia* species, making the invariant regions useful targets for serodiagnosis (VlsE protein- and C6 peptide-based tests).

The 41 kDa flagellin protein of the *Borrelia* flagellum is highly immunogenic. Antibody directed against flagellin cross-reacts with similar antigen of other flagellated bacteria such as *Treponema* and *Leptospira* species. Antibodies directed at certain domains of the flagellin molecule may also cross-react with neuroaxonal proteins, contributing to the development of neuroborreliosis.

Although large quantities of specific antibodies against borreliae are produced during infection, immunocompetent host species studied, including rats, mice, hamsters, dogs and humans, tend to develop a persistent infection without clinical manifestations. For example, experimental infection of hamsters results in persistent cardiac and urinary tract infection without clinical signs or histological changes. Immunosuppression is required for persistently infected animals to develop clinical disease. Susceptibility of laboratory mice to borreliosis is mouse strain-dependent and related to the nature of the CD4[+] T cell response to the organism (see Chapter 3).

In experimental canine infection, a single exposure to infected ticks results in active disease in very young animals only. In one study, Beagle puppies (6–12 weeks of age) were infected by ticks harbouring *B. burgdor-*

Table 10.2 Presence of *Borrelia burgdorferi* in the tissues of symptomatic dogs.

TISSUE	PERCENTAGE POSITIVE TISSUES IN SYMPTOMATIC DOGS BY:			
	CULTURE (APPEL *et al.*, 1993)	CULTURE (STRAUBINGER *et al.*, 2000)	PCR (CHANG *et al.*, 1996)	PCR (HOVIUS *et al.*, 1999)
	n = 17	n = 42	n = 6	n = 10
Skin	30	85	85	50
Lymph node	0	75	65	0
Joint capsule	25	70	95	60
Fascia	NT	70	90	NT
Muscle	50	65	100	0
Peritoneum	25	65	50	25
Pericardium	NT	80	65	NT
Heart	5	75	85	25
Meninges	NT	30	50	NT
CNS	5	NT	NT	35
Liver	0	NT	NT	60
Spleen	0	0	35	0
Kidney	5	0	0	0

NT, not tested

B. burgdorferi sensu stricto as a single agent in experimental infection (first three columns) may have a different tissue tropism (fibrous tissues) compared with *B. garinii* (liver) given as a co-infection with *B. burgdorferi* sensu stricto to European dogs (final column). Skin, lymph node, fascia, muscle and joint capsule consistently become infected by active migration along connective tissue planes. It is possible that this migratory route extends through the thoracic and abdominal wall and reaches the peritoneum and pericardial tissues, which in experimental infections frequently contain *Borrelia*. Parenchymatous tissues, supposedly infected by the circulatory route, contain fewer *Borrelia*. This likely reflects the fact that the organisms are more easily eliminated by the immune system in these sites. Difference in sampling technique may explain the discrepancy in results for muscle tissue between the naturally and experimentally infected dogs. Viable *Borrelia* organisms were not detected in the kidney

feri sensu stricto. Two to 5 months after tick exposure, the pups developed mild clinical disease characterized by transient fever and lameness. Approximately 75% of the animals had recurrent episodes of disease. After 4–6 months clinical signs abated, but infection and high serum antibody levels persisted. By contrast, adult dogs did not develop apparent clinical disease after a single exposure to *Borrelia*-infected ticks under experimental settings. Affected joint capsules, however, contained spirochaetes and there was interleukin-8 production within the synovial membrane and chemotactic attraction of neutrophils into the joint. After several months of persistent infection, a mild subclinical polysynovitis occurred, with lymphoplasmacytic infiltration of the synovial membrane.

Quantitative PCR has been used to monitor infectious load in the tissues of dogs infected experimentally with *B. burgdorferi* sensu stricto (**Table 10.2**). Skin and joint capsule taken from symptomatic dogs 4 months after infection contained many more spirochaetes than those from infected asymptomatic dogs. Symptomatic dogs also had higher serum antibody levels. In this model, disease is self-limiting and the convalescent stage is characterized by a delicate balance achieved between the spirochaete and the host immune system. When this balance is disturbed, spirochaete numbers increase in tissue again, antibody titres rise and clinical signs may recur. If the symptomatic dogs are treated with appropriate antibiotics, spirochaete numbers decrease more rapidly than when convalescent. However, in some cases, several months post antibiotic therapy (especially when glucocorticoids are used concurrently), *Borrelia* DNA can again be detected, indicating survival of the agent despite therapy.

CLINICAL SIGNS

Borreliosis in dogs

Between 1975 and 1985, novel human and canine infections were described from Old Lyme and other areas in Connecticut and from the lower Hudson Valley in New York State, USA. Dogs were described with overt lameness and swollen joints, mostly combined with fever. Although the lameness spontaneously resolved in four days, 33% of dogs relapsed. Similarities with human Lyme disease were recognized. In one dog, spirochaetes were visualized microscopically within the synoviae and identified by immunofluorescence as *B.*

burgdorferi. Lameness was associated with fever and was described as intermittent and shifting, with involvement of several joints.

In clinical practice, confirmation of the aetiological agent by detection of live spirochaetes is uncommon. However, in experimental and some clinical cases the spirochaete is most often detected in skin and joints, although there is only mild pathology in these tissues (**Figures 10.4A–D**). More often, a presumptive diagnosis is made based on compatible clinical signs of acute malaise (i.e. fatigue, anorexia and fever) followed by recurrent lameness (i.e. stiff gait, joint swelling and arthralgia), and on the exclusion of other differential

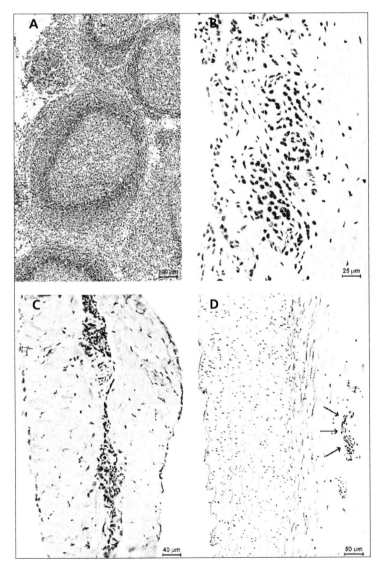

Figs.10.4A–D Histopathological lesions in borreliosis. Lesions occur in many organ systems and are characterized by an infiltration of plasma cells and lymphocytes, as seen in experimental infection. (A) Severe follicular hyperplasia of the lymph node adjacent to the location of tick bite (infection). (B) Accumulation of plasma cells in the synovial membrane of the joint near the site of tick bite. (C) Mild non-suppurative pericarditis. A naturally infected case in the USA presented with a complete heart block, showing plasmacytic interstitial myocarditis with macrophage infiltration and focal fibre necrosis. (D) Periarteritis, visible as small cuffs of mononuclear cells around the vasa vasorum in an artery walls, is frequently seen in experimental infection. (Reprinted with permission of Elsevier Science from Straubinger RK, Rao TD, Davidson E *et al.* (2001) Protection against tick-transmitted Lyme disease in dogs vaccinated with a multiantigenic vaccine. *Vaccine* 20:181–93)

diagnoses (**Figure 10.5**). The period of malaise may precede lameness by days to weeks and its severity varies from listlessness to high fever (pyrexia occurs in 60–70% of cases).

Clinical signs relate not only to joint disease, but also to multiple organ involvement. The skin is seldom visibly affected and the easily recognizable erythema migrans (EM) lesion seen in human infections does not occur in dogs. There is some evidence suggesting that mild localized excoriation and alopecia may be associated with infection, but this is difficult to distinguish from acute dermatitis initiated by the tick bite. Cardiac involvement has rarely been observed clinically, but is described in the literature. Renal involvement may occur and is considered to be an immunopathological sequela to the infection, since *Borrelia* antigen complexed with specific antibodies can be detected in the kidney tissues (**Table 10.2**). Severe renal disease with membranoproliferative glomerulonephritis ('canine Lyme nephritis') has been reported in the USA, most frequently in Golden and Labrador Retrievers. This is characterized by azotaemia, haematuria and urinary casts, with progression to irreversible uraemia. In Europe, a familial glomerulopathy preceded by fever and lameness has been described in Bernese Mountain Dogs, with a similar clinical and pathological progression.

Involvement of the peripheral nervous system in canine borreliosis has been described in single cases showing loss of proprioception, hyperaesthesia, posterior paresis or unilateral facial paralysis. Generally, mild to severe inflammatory infiltrates are seen in the nervous system and spirochaetes can be detected in 30–50% of clinical cases in the meninges (**Table 10.2**).

Borreliosis in cats

Reports of naturally occurring feline borreliosis are rare. In one UK study, positive *Borrelia* serology was not associated with clinical signs of lameness or fever, and clinical signs seen in seropositive cats were not attributable to the spirochaete. Experimentally infected cats exhibited recurrent lymphocytosis and eosinophilia every 2–3 months, with concurrent hyperplasia of lymphoid tissue. Despite minimal clinical signs (a minority of cats exhibited slight lameness), infected cats had histopathological lesions that paralleled those of natural canine infection. Lesions included perivascular lymphocytic infiltration of joint capsules, cerebrum, meninges, kidney and liver, and mild multifocal pneumonia.

DIAGNOSIS

Clinical diagnosis

The clinical signs described above are not pathognomonic and dogs lack a clinical marker as in EM in humans. Consequently, making a definitive diagnosis based on clinical signs alone is not possible. As the onset of *Borrelia*-associated lameness often occurs after the period of fever and malaise, it may be difficult to make a diagnosis on the basis of a single consultation. *Borrelia* species or strain variation, or co-infection with other arthropod-borne pathogens, may also alter clinical presentation.

A presumptive diagnosis of borreliosis is based on a history of tick exposure, compatible clinical signs, including a history of recurrence, and exclusion of other causes of non-degenerative arthropathy and fever of unknown origin. In particular, other immune-mediated causes of fever and shifting limb lameness should be considered (e.g. osteochondrosis dissecans). A definitive diagnosis of borreliosis always requires the addition of appropriate serological and, sometimes, molecular tests.

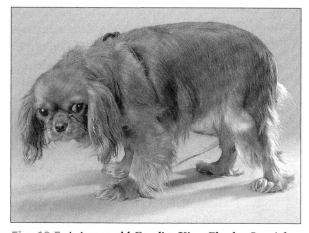

Fig. 10.5 **A 4-year-old Cavalier King Charles Spaniel with a history of recurrent malaise, pyrexia, generalized musculoskeletal pain and polyarthritis. The dog is both serologically positive (rising titre) and PCR positive for *B. burgdorferi* complex.**

Laboratory detection of infection and disease

Confirmation of the clinical diagnosis of borreliosis is difficult and requires correlation and realistic interpretation of multiple laboratory investigations. Results from a European reference laboratory show that only 4.3% of sera from dogs clinically diagnosed as having borreliosis have significantly high *B. burgdorferi* antibody levels. Very high antibody levels were found in 24.6% of sera from Bernese Mountain Dogs with suspected borreliosis, a dog breed known to produce and maintain high antibody levels (**Figure 10.6**). It is evident that disease due to *Borrelia* infection would be overdiagnosed if based on positive serological results alone.

Serologic testing for borreliosis

The presence of specific elevated antibody levels to *B. burgdorferi* signifies exposure to *Borrelia* species, but does not prove that a current clinical illness is caused by the spirochaetes. The diagnosis of borreliosis has become a serological diagnosis, because culture and genetic detection of the organism from tissue samples are uncommon and are regularly negative from body fluids. Serological studies should be viewed as determining 'seroreactivity to *B. burgdorferi*' rather than providing definitive evidence of the disease.

Dogs develop detectable IgG antibodies by 4–6 weeks after tick exposure. Antibody levels are at their highest by 3 months after tick exposure and last for years. Specific antibody levels against *Borrelia* often decline after antibiotic treatment and patients become clinically healthy, but measurable IgG levels often remain for months to years. Because of shortcomings of antibody measurements with whole-cell antigens (e.g. inadequate specificity), serological tests of this type have been largely discontinued. Instead, recombinant proteins are now widely used as test antigens.

Enzyme-linked immunosorbent assay and immunofluorescent antibody test

Enzyme-linked immunosorbent assay (ELISA) and immunofluorescent antibody test (IFAT) based on whole-cell antigens (lysates of *Borrelia* cultures) are usually used for initial screening, because the tests are inexpensive, easy to perform and highly sensitive. However, these whole-cell antigen ELISAs and IFATs show inadequate specificities, requiring an additional confirmatory test, and cannot distinguish between antibodies induced by natural infection or vaccination.

Immunoblotting (western blotting)

Rarely used for initial screening, immunoblotting, where the spirochaete proteins are separated in an electric field, has been employed as a second phase of diagnosis to help confirm positive results from other serological tests. It is a helpful tool to exclude false-positive results due to cross-reactive antibodies and to differentiate infected from vaccinated animals. The pattern of antibody reactivity

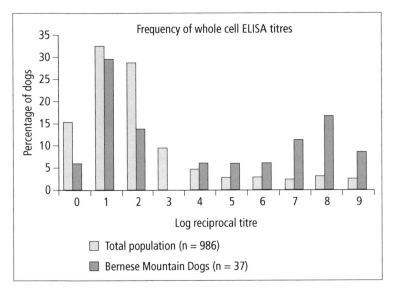

Fig. 10.6 Frequency distribution of the antibody titres of sera from dogs with a putative clinical diagnosis of borreliosis submitted to the referral laboratory of Utrecht University, the Netherlands. Around 4% of these dogs have a very high IgG antibody titre in whole cell ELISA (log reciprocal 8 and higher) and may thus be suspected of having borreliosis. Referral sera from Bernese Mountain Dogs have an even greater fraction (around 25%) of very high titres and this breed may have high susceptibility for borreliosis. The data would suggest that borreliosis is clinically overdiagnosed.

after natural tick infection differs from that produced by vaccination. Sera from dogs that are vaccinated with any current vaccine on the market exhibit reactivity predominantly to the OspA antigen, which is expressed only on the surface of *B. burgdorferi* organisms in ticks. Hence, reactivity to OspA occurs in vaccinated dogs, but is absent in naturally infected dogs. After natural exposure to *B. burgdorferi*, dogs produce antibodies against proteins in the range of 100/83, 75, 66, 60, 58, 43, 41 (flagellin), 39, 30, 23 (OspC) and 21 kDa. Reactivity against the VlsE surface protein can be observed when recombinant VlsE antigen is contained within western blot strips. When, finally, all antigens are produced with recombinant techniques and are incorporated into carrier membranes, a line immunoassay (LIA) is created. Due to the standardized quality and amounts of the antigens used for the test, LIA is currently the most reliable assay for antibody detection.

Antibodies to specific outer surface proteins – VlsE and C6

As outlined above, variation in the genes that encode the immunodominant VlsE surface protein helps the spirochaete to escape the host immune response. One immunodominant region of VlsE, known as IR6, is highly conserved among many *B. burgdorferi* strains and genospecies. A recombinant peptide known as C6 is encoded by the *IR6* gene sequence. The C6 test can differentiate accurately between vaccinated and infected dogs. Again, as for all other serological tests, the C6 antibody response does not always correlate with clinical illness in dogs.

Molecular diagnosis

The detection of *Borrelia* DNA in tissue can be attempted using PCR analyses that target *Borrelia* genes encoding molecules such as flagellin or OspA, or the intergenic spacer region of ribosomal 5S and 23S RNA genes and many additional genetic targets. PCR positivity has been correlated with the presence of clinical signs; however, because of the low spirochaete density in tissues, false-negative PCR results are common and do not rule out infection. Only positive PCR results are confirmative.

Bacterial culture

Isolation of *B. burgdorferi* by culture is difficult and is only successful when liquid media are employed (e.g. Barbour–Stoenner–Kelly medium; modified Kelly–Pettenkofer medium). During culture, media are inspected weekly for 2 months for the presence of spirochaetes by dark-field microscopy. Cultures of skin biopsies taken from the edge of an EM lesion in infected humans are a sensitive method for confirming the presence of borreliae and are used as the 'gold standard' for diagnosis. Blood is not considered the sample of choice since *B. burgdorferi* migration is in general not haematogenous. Although spirochaetes were recovered by culture in 100% of skin biopsy samples taken 2 weeks after experimental infection of dogs, a positive skin culture of naturally infected dogs can only occasionally be achieved, because the location of the infecting tick bite is usually not known.

TREATMENT AND CONTROL

Antibiotic therapy

Recovery from infection is ultimately dependent on activation of specific cell-mediated immunity and production of specific antibodies against *Borrelia* (**Figure 10.7**). In contrast, disease can be induced if immunity is disrupted by administration of high-dose corticosteroids. The effect of antibiotic therapy on the course of infection is difficult to evaluate clinically, as the episodes of lameness and fever usually resolve spontaneously after 4 days without treatment. Antibiotic therapy is most effective when administered during the early episodes of the disease; the spirochaete load is greatly reduced and *Borrelia*-specific antibody levels decline in parallel. However, in experimentally infected dogs and in some naturally infected dogs with chronic infection, spirochaetes can still be detected by PCR more than 500 days after treatment. It is hypothesized that spirochaetes evade antibiotic therapy within tissue cysts or 'privileged sites', such as fibroblasts.

Doxycycline (10 mg/kg PO q12h for 28 days) is the antibiotic of choice for borreliosis because of its intracellular penetration and concurrent effects on co-infecting *Anaplasma* and *Ehrlichia* species. Amoxicillin (20 mg/kg PO q8h for 28 days) may be a better choice in very young animals because of the negative effects of tetracyclines (not doxycycline) on enamel formation.

Vaccination

Whole cell bacterin vaccines (lysate vaccines) and a recombinant OspA vaccine are licensed and widely used in the

Fig. 10.7 (A) Antibody dynamics of a Golden Retriever acutely developing fever and lameness in its fourth year in association with a steep rising titre in whole cell ELISA. The dog was treated with antibiotics and the disease resolved, while the titre declined and remained low. **(B)** Western blots were performed before, during and after disease.

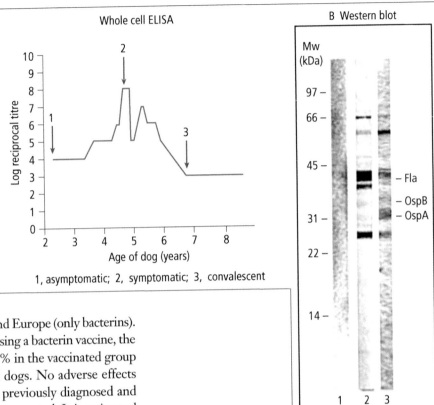

USA (bacterins and rOspA) and Europe (only bacterins). In a large field efficacy study using a bacterin vaccine, the incidence of borreliosis was 1% in the vaccinated group and 4.7% in non-vaccinated dogs. No adverse effects of vaccination, even on dogs previously diagnosed and recovered from borreliosis, were noted. It is estimated that around 75% of dogs in northeastern USA have been vaccinated and it has been suggested that the prevalence of canine Lyme arthritis has decreased as a consequence. The antibody response of vaccinated dogs is directed predominantly against OspA. The vaccinal antibodies are protective by immobilizing the spirochaetes in the gut of the feeding tick. Active immunization with recombinant OspA renders the same protection against infection. Mixtures of antigens from different *Borrelia* species may confer a broad enough protection in areas where different *Borrelia* species occur. Recombinant OspC vaccines have been shown to protect gerbils and mice from infection by inhibiting the colonization of the tick salivary gland and thus blocking transmission to the vertebrate host. It is feasible that vaccines containing OspC (lysate vaccines) antigens may also protect against chronic infection.

Prevention

Dogs with naturally occurring borreliosis generally have a history of severe tick infestation and in experimental infections, only dogs with high infectious loads develop fever and lameness. Consequently, prevention of heavy tick infestations by regular use of long-acting topical acaricides and/or repellents in collars, sprays, spot-ons or in orally administered tablets is key to the prevention of disease. In addition, removing ticks within 1 day of attachment, before spirochaetes reach the tick salivary glands and the host's skin, will minimize transmission and lower infectious load. Avoidance of areas known to have a high density of ticks should be considered. It is probable that owner awareness and widespread use of effective acaricides/repellents has played a role in decreasing the prevalence of canine borreliosis in the last decade.

PUBLIC HEALTH SIGNIFICANCE

Borreliosis in humans is a serious and debilitating disease with high morbidity in endemic areas. Clinical signs relate to the skin, neurological and/or musculoskeletal systems, depending on the *Borrelia* species involved. EM typically develops within 3–30 days after an infectious tick bite. This expanding rash was first described in 1910, and is thought to indicate intradermal multiplication of spirochaetes accompanied by a vigorous attempt by the host's innate immune response to fight the infection. The rash disperses through the skin from the point of inoculation. The major *Borrelia* species pathogenic for man can be cultured from or detected by PCR in these lesions. In humans the presence of IgM antibodies confirms the diagnosis in this initial stage of borreliosis; this is not possible in dogs because EM does not develop in canines. The second phase of the disease in humans is marked by dissemination to multiple organ systems. In Europe, neurological disease is a more common presenting complaint than chronic arthritis. This is probably due to the high infection rate of European ticks with *B. bavariensis/B. garinii* and their tropism for the neurological system. Although *B. bavariensis/B. garinii* are the major species involved in neuroborreliosis, *B. afzelii* and *B. burgdorferi* sensu stricto are also isolated from skin and to a lesser extent from nervous tissue, and co-infections involving all pathogenic species can occur. *B. afzelii* is almost exclusively isolated from the skin of chronically infected human patients with acrodermatitis chronica atrophicans, and arthritis is supposed to be the main clinical sign of a *B. burgdorferi* sensu stricto infection. Consequently, this species is isolated particularly from synovial tissue samples, but rarely from synovial fluid.

Serological surveillance of dogs in an area endemic for borreliosis may provide information on the risk for human infection. In this respect, dogs function as sentinels. Pet dogs and cats are 'accidental hosts' for *Borrelia* and do not interface to a major degree with sylvatic wildlife cycles of *Borrelia* infection. Consequently, they pose no direct threat to human beings. However, dogs and cats may carry infected ticks into the peri-domestic environment, where there is a small risk that an infected unattached tick may be dislodged. It is unlikely that this would represent any more of a risk than exposure to infected nymphs derived from small rodents or deer with access to the garden. There is anecdotal evidence of direct transfer of infected ticks from animals to humans but no confirmed reports of disease transmission. There are no reports of humans becoming infected by canine bodily fluids.

Precautions should be taken when removing ticks attached to dogs or cats to prevent the possibility of exposure to borreliae released from crushed tick bodies, which might infect small wounds on the hand, although this has never been documented. Humans may develop disease following a single tick bite and therefore should also take precautions, such as wearing protective clothing, when entering areas of high tick density.

FURTHER READING

Devevey G, Dang T, Graves CJ *et al.* (2015) First arrived takes all: inhibitory priority effects dominate competition between co-infecting *Borrelia burgdorferi* strains. *BMC Microbiology* **15**:61.

Eschner AK, Mugnai K (2015) Immunization with a recombinant subunit OspA vaccine markedly impacts the rate of newly acquired *Borrelia burgdorferi* infections in client-owned dogs living in a coastal community in Maine, USA. *Parasites & Vectors* **8**:92.

Kelly AL, Raffel SJ, Fischer RJ *et al.* (2014) First isolation of the relapsing fever spirochete, *Borrelia hermsii*, from a domestic dog. *Ticks and Tick-Borne Diseases* **5**:95–99.

Krupka I, Pantchev N, Lorentzen L *et al.* (2007) Durch Zecken übertragbare bakterielle Infektionen bei Hunden: Seroprävalenzen von *Anaplasma phagocytophilum, Borrelia burgdorferi* sensu lato und *Ehrlichia canis* in Deutschland. *Der Praktische Tierarzt* **88**:776–788.

Magnarelli LA, Bushmich SL, IJdo JW *et al.* (2005) Seroprevalence of antibodies against *Borrelia burgdorferi* and *Anaplasma phagocytophilum* in cats. *American Journal of Veterinary Research* **66**:1895–1899.

Mannelli A, Bertolotti L, Gern L *et al.* (2012) Ecology of *Borrelia burgdorferi* sensu lato in Europe: transmission dynamics in multi-host systems, influence of molecular processes and effects of climate change. *FEMS Microbiology Reviews* **36**:837–861.

Margos G, Wilske B, Sing A *et al.* (2013) *Borrelia bavariensis* sp. nov. is widely distributed in Europe and Asia. *International Journal of Systematic and Evolutionary Microbiology* **63**:4284–4288.

Rauter C, Hartung T (2005) Prevalence of *Borrelia burgdorferi* sensu lato genospecies in *Ixodes ricinus* ticks in Europe: a metaanalysis. *Applied Environmental Microbiology* **71**:7203–7216.

ACKNOWLEDGMENT

In the first edition of this book, this chapter was prepared by K Emil Hovius. This revised and updated chapter is based on that original content and Dr Straubinger acknowledges this earlier work and Dr Hovius as the source of the illustrative material used in the chapter.

Chapter 11

Bartonellosis

Richard Birtles

BACKGROUND, AETIOLOGY AND EPIDEMIOLOGY

Bartonellosis is the generic name given to a wide range of infections caused by members of the genus *Bartonella*, a group of fastidious, facultatively intracellular, gram-negative bacteria that are most closely related to the *Brucella* genus and members of the plant-associated taxa *Agrobacterium* and *Rhizobium*.

To date, 34 taxa have been described in association with a wide range of mammalian hosts (**Table 11.1**). Although not proven for all species, a general natural

Table 11.1 Identity of currently recognized *Bartonella* species and details of their likely maintenance host species.

BARTONELLA TAXON	LIKELY MAINTENANCE HOST	CAT/DOG ASSOCIATION
B. acomydis	Rodents	No
B. alsatica	Rabbits	No
B. ancashensis	Unknown	No
B. bacilliformis	Man	No
B. birtlesii	Rodents	No
B. bovis	Cattle	No
B. callosciuri	Rodents	No
B. capreoli	Deer	No
B. chomelii	Cattle	No
B. clarridgeiae	Felines	Yes
B. coopersplainsensis	Rodents	No
B. doshiae	Rodents	No
B. elizabethae	Rodents	Yes
B. florencae	Shrews	No
B. grahamii	Rodents	No
B. henselae	Felines	Yes
B. jaculi	Rodents	No
B. japonica	Rodents	No
B. koehlerae	Felines	Yes
B. pachyuromydis	Rodents	No
B. peromysci	Rodents	No
B. queenslandensis	Rodents	No
B. quintana	Man	No
B. rattaustraliani	Rodents	No
B. rochalimae	Unknown	No
B. schoenbuchensis	Deer	No
B. senegalensis	Unknown	No
B. silvatica	Rodents	No
B. talpae	Moles	No
B. taylorii	Rodents	No
B. tribocorum	Rodents	No
B. vinsonii subsp. *arupensis*	Rodents	No
B. vinsonii subsp. *berkhoffii*	Canines	Yes
B. vinsonii subsp. *vinsonii*	Rodents	No

cycle for *Bartonella* species involves a mammalian maintenance host, in which infection is usually chronic and asymptomatic, and a haematophagous arthropod vector that transmits infection between maintenance hosts. However, outside this cycle, the occurrence of infections in non-maintenance hosts following accidental exposure to the bacteria has long been recognized. Although little is known about the relative ease with which *Bartonella* species are able to infect accidental hosts, once established, infections can lead to overt clinical manifestations ranging from mild and self-limiting to life threatening disease. However, bartonellae may not just be opportunistic pathogens. The results of studies investigating the effects of parasitism on maintenance hosts have suggested that these infections may also be detrimental to host well-being.

The nature of bartonellosis in cats is considered different from that in dogs. Cats are recognized as maintenance hosts for *Bartonella henselae*, the species most often implicated in human infections in the USA and Europe, and they are also likely maintenance hosts for two other species, *B. clarridgeiae* and *B. koehlerae*. There has been no direct demonstration of naturally occurring disease in cats caused by *B. henselae*. However, there is experimental evidence that in certain circumstances *B. henselae* infection can provoke clinical manifestations, and there is increasing speculation about the role of *B. henselae* as a cause or co-factor in chronic diseases of cats. In contrast, domestic dogs have not been clearly implicated as maintenance hosts for any *Bartonella* species, although the possibility that they may fulfil such a role cannot be ruled out. Dogs are known to be prone to infections by *Bartonella vinsonii* subspecies *berkhoffii* that may be asymptomatic or may provoke overt disease. Whether such infections are transmissible and, therefore, whether dogs serve as truly competent reservoirs, remains unknown, but experimental studies suggest this may be so; for example, dogs inoculated with *B. vinsonii* subsp. *berkhoffii* develop chronic bacteraemia akin to those observed for other *Bartonella* species in their respective reservoir hosts, and the species is capable of *in-vitro* invasion of canine erythrocytes.

Arthropods as vectors of *Bartonella* species

Although the role of arthropods as vectors for *Bartonella* species is widely accepted, there is very limited evidence relating to transmission of this bacterium. Experimen-

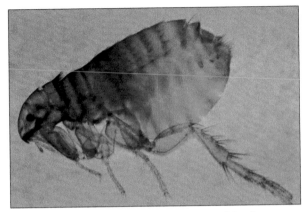

Fig. 11.1 Photograph of *Ctenocephalides felis*, the cat flea. (Photo courtesy Merial Animal Health UK)

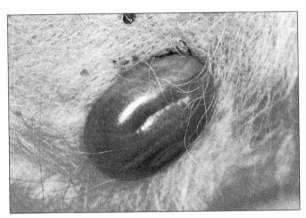

Fig. 11.2 An engorged adult *Ixodes* species tick attached to the skin of a dog.

tal transmission of *B. henselae* has been achieved by the transfer of cat fleas (*Ctenocephalides felis*) (**Figure 11.1**) from bacteraemic cats to specific pathogen-free (SPF) cats. Bartonellae have also been observed in the midgut of infected fleas and they can be cultured from infected flea faeces for up to 9 days post feeding. Furthermore, intradermal inoculation of SPF cats with flea faeces has been shown to induce bacteraemia. Thus, it appears that the transmission of *B. henselae* between cats involves the uptake of infected blood by fleas, followed by multiplication of bacteria in the flea midgut, then excretion and persistence in flea faeces and finally infection of a new host by the cutaneous inoculation of infected faeces via a scratch or abrasion.

Although experimental studies into the transmission of *B. vinsonii* subspecies *berkhoffii* have yet to be reported, epidemiological evidence suggests that ticks may be involved in this process. Evaluation of the risk factors associated with exposure to this species identified that seropositive dogs were 14 times more likely to have a history of heavy tick exposure than control animals. In addition, there appears to be a high frequency of co-infections between *B. vinsonii* subspecies *berkhoffii* and other tick-borne pathogens. Finally, surveys of questing ixodid ticks (**Figure 11.2**) in the USA and Europe using PCR-based methods have yielded gene sequences that are very similar to those from several *Bartonella* species, including some for which other arthropods have been established as vectors.

Bartonella henselae and *Bartonella clarridgeiae* infection of domestic cats

The role of cats as reservoir hosts for *B. henselae* and *B. clarridgeiae* has been established on the basis of extensive surveys of domestic cat populations and experimental studies of laboratory animals. **Table 11.2** summarizes these surveys, which have been carried out in over 30 countries and have included more than 13,000 animals. Overall, these data indicate that worldwide, 13% of cats tested have ongoing infection and 30% have evidence of past infection.

Table 11.2 **National estimates of prevalence of infection and exposure among domestic cats.**

COUNTRY	YEAR OF SURVEY/S	PREVALENCE OF INFECTION	PREVALENCE OF EXPOSURE	SPECIES IDENTIFIED*
Algeria	2012	36/211, 17%	NT	BH
Argentina	2014	8/101, 8%	NT	BH
Australia	1996	27/77, 35%	NT	BH
Austria	1995	NT	32/96, 33%	
Brazil	2011	NT	19/40, 48%	
Canada	2008	14/896, 2%	NT	BH
China	2011	26/356, 7%	NT	BH
Czech Republic	2003	5/61, 8%	NT	BH
Denmark	2002, 2004	32/118, 27%	42/92, 47%	BH
Egypt	1995	NT	8/42, 19%	
France	1995,1997, 2001, 2004	138/693, 20%	202/500, 40%	BH, BC
Germany	1997, 1999, 2001, 2011, 2012	44/800, 6%	198/958, 21%	BH, BC
Indonesia	1999	9/14, 64%	40/74, 54%	BH, BC
Iraq	2013	9/207, 4%	31/207, 15%	BH
Israel	1996, 2013	30/334, 9%	45/114, 39%	BH, BC, BK
Italy	2002 × 2, 2004 × 2, 2009	525/2618, 20%	875/2462, 36%	BH
Jamaica	2005	12/62, 19%	NT	BH
Japan	1995, 1996, 1998, 2000, 2003	181/2170, 8%	73/670, 11%	BH, BC
Netherlands	1997	25/113, 22%	85/163, 52%	BH, BC
New Caledonia	2011	4/8, 50%		BH
New Zealand	1997	8/48, 18%	NT	BH
Norway	2002	0/100, 0%	1/100, 1%	
Philippines	1999	19/31, 61%	73/107, 68%	BH, BC
Portugal	1995	NT	2/14, 14%	
Singapore	1999	NT	38/80, 47%	
Spain	2005, 2013	33/262, 13%	193/795, 24%	BH
South Africa	1996, 1999, 2012	6/129, 5%	35/154, 23%	BH
Sweden	2002, 2003	1/100, 1%	73/292, 25%	BH
Switzerland	1997	NT	61/728, 8%	
Thailand	2001, 2009	123/563, 22%	NT	BH, BC
Turkey	2009, 2011	29/256, 11%	83/298, 28%	BH, BC
UK	2000, 2002, 2011	139/2142, 6%	61/148, 41%	BH
USA	1994 × 2, 1995 × 4, 1996, 1998, 2004, 2010, 2011	168/724, 23%	1072/3086, 35%	BH, BC
Zimbabwe	1996	NT	28/119, 24%	

* by culture-based assessment only.

NT, not tested; BH, *Bartonella henselae*; BC, *Bartonella clarridgeiae*; BK, *Bartonella koehlerae*.

Significant differences in the prevalence of *B. henselae* infection among subsets of the cat population have been reported, leading to the recognition of a number of predisposing factors. Risk factors associated with bacteraemia include flea infestation, young age and being stray or housed in cat shelters. Among pet cats, risk factors include ownership for less than 6 months, adoption from a shelter/found as a stray and cohabitation with one or more cats. It has also been suggested that the prevalence of infection/exposure is inversely related to latitude. The seroprevalence of *B. henselae* is higher in cat populations living in the southern USA than in those living in the north, and surveys of cats in central and northern Scandinavia have found little evidence of *B. henselae* infections. This correlation may be related to warmer, more humid regions favouring *Ct. felis* infestation, but may also reflect differences in the age profile or numbers of stray/feral cats in local populations.

Feline *B. clarridgeiae* and *B. koehlerae* infections appear to be less common than those due to *B. henselae*. Less than half of the surveys that encountered *B. henselae* also encountered *B. clarridgeiae*, and when both species were encountered, the prevalence of *B. henselae* was always the greater, with over 80% of culture-positive cats yielding *B. henselae* and only about 25% yielding *B. clarridgeiae*. However, as currently used sampling methods have been optimized for the recovery of *B. henselae*, the recovery of *B. clarridgeiae* may be compromised. The geographical distribution of *B. clarridgeiae* may also be more limited than that of *B. henselae*. The species is rarely encountered in the USA, but appears more common in Europe and the Far East. Within Europe, the species is relatively widely distributed. To date, *B. koehlerae* has only been isolated from a very small number of cats in Israel, although PCR-based methods have suggested its distribution may be more widespread.

B. vinsonii subspecies *berkhoffii* infection of dogs

There is now strong evidence that *B. vinsonii* subspecies *berkhoffii* exploits canids in the same manner as *B. henselae* exploits felids. Early studies identified coyotes (*Canis latrans*) as a major reservoir for *B. vinsonii* subspecies *berkhoffii* and subsequently other wild-living canids have also been implicated. Although asymptomatic infections in domestic dogs appear less common, surveys have revealed a higher prevalence in shelter and/or feral dog populations. For example, a study in Turkey failed to isolate *B. vinsonii* subspecies *berkhoffii* from 40 pet dogs, but recovered 25 isolates from 210 shelter or feral dogs. Serological surveys of domestic dog populations around the world suggest that a significant proportion of dogs have been exposed to *B. vinsonii* subspecies *berkhoffii*.

B. henselae, *B. clarridgeiae* and other *Bartonella* species infection of dogs

In many parts of the world dogs are as prone to infestation with the cat flea as cats themselves, so it is surprising that *B. henselae* infections of dogs, either clinical or subclinical, appear to be rare. Surveys of healthy dogs have occasionally yielded isolates of *B. henselae* and, more frequently, *B. clarridgeiae*, and numerous serosurveys have yielded evidence of exposure in apparently healthy dog populations, although the accuracy of a serological approach as a species-specific indicator of *Bartonella* species infection is debatable. There is also some evidence that asymptomatic infections of a recently described *Bartonella* species, *B. rochalimae*, may occur in canids. In one study, this species was isolated from three of 182 dogs and 22 of 53 grey foxes (*Urocyon cinereoargenteus*). Furthermore, PCR-based studies have reported the presence of DNA from several other *Bartonella* species in either clinical samples or ectoparasites collected from dogs.

There is some circumstantial evidence that dogs can transmit *B. henselae* and *B. clarridgeiae*. Reports from Japan and Israel have suggested that human cases of *B. henselae* infection may result from contact with dogs, possibly acting as vehicles for infected fleas.

Molecular epidemiology of *Bartonella* species associated with cats and dogs

Delineation of *B. henselae* isolates into one of two genogroups on the basis of differences in 16S ribosomal RNA gene sequences has long been recognized, and descriptions of isolates as type I and type II are commonplace. However, the distribution of these two types among isolates does not appear to be entirely congruent with lineages allocated using a multilocus sequence typing (MLST) approach to assess the *B. henselae* population structure. It therefore appears that distinguishing strains solely on a type I/type II basis is not a sensitive indicator of clonal divisions within the species. The population structure proposed by MLST is supported by other means of assessing inter-strain genetic relatedness, including pulsed field gel electrophoresis (PFGE).

PFGE, together with other pan-genomic sampling methods such as amplified fragment length polymorphism analysis, enterobacterial repetitive intergenic consensus-PCR and arbitrarily primed-PCR, has been used to delineate *B. henselae* isolates, but these methods have been superseded by comparison of sequence data derived from single (e.g. 16S/23S rRNA intergenic spacer region, *groEL* and *pap31*) or multiple genetic loci (e.g. MLST or multiple loci variable number tandem repeat (VNTR)

analysis. The freely accessible online MLST database (http://bhenselae.mlst.net/) contains data for almost 350 *B. henselae* isolates obtained in over 15 different countries. The 30+ distinct MLST genotypes obtained to date have been used to define a population structure for the species, which consists of three divergent clonal complexes. In an epidemiological setting, VNTR has proven to possess very high discriminatory power; the online database for this scheme (http://mlva.u-psud.fr/) contains almost 400 entries from 10 different countries that have been delineated into over 200 distinct profiles (**Figure 11.3**). There is some suggestion that certain MLST or VNTR types may be more or less frequent in different parts of the world, but there is no evidence

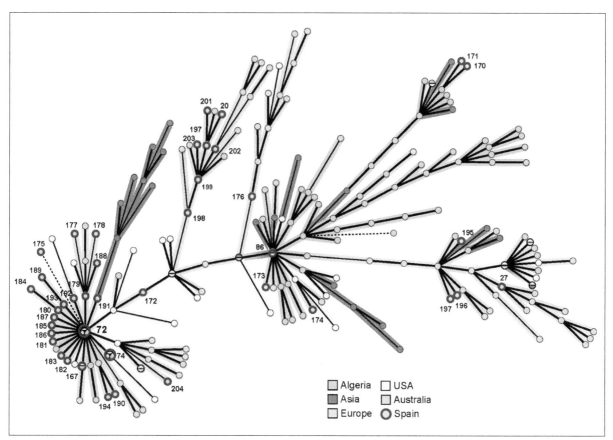

Fig. 11.3 Minimum spanning tree of *B. henselae* multiple loci VNTR analysis profiles. Profiles connected by a shaded background differ by a maximum of one of the five VNTR markers; regular connecting lines represent two marker differences; thick interrupted lines represent three differences. The length of each branch is also proportional to the number of differences. The colours of the branches and circles are related to the geographical origin of the detected profile. All the isolates from Spain used to build this diagram are labelled with a thick red circle and their own profile number according to the public database (http://mlva.u-psud.fr/). VNTR, variable number tandem repeat. (Reproduced with permission from *Plos One* 2013, 8:e68248)

that MLST or VNTR type has any clinical relevance in veterinary medicine.

Genotyping of *B. vinsonii* subspecies *berkhoffii* and other canine or feline-associated bartonellae is far less advanced, and is primarily based on comparison of sequence data derived from single genetic loci such as the 16S rDNA gene or the intergenic spacer region separating the 16S rDNA and 23S rDNA genes.

PATHOGENESIS

B. henselae infection in cats

Experimental infections have demonstrated that cats are prone to protracted bacteraemia of at least 8 weeks, during which time the bacteria associate with, then (probably) invade, erythrocytes. The concentration of bacteria in blood rises rapidly to reach a peak within 1 week of inoculation, after which it gradually subsides. Although in most experiments this resulted in disappearance of bacteraemia after about 3 months, in some animals infection was more protracted and in others, recurrent periods of bacteraemia were observed (**Figure 11.4**).

Cats elicit a strong humoral response against inoculated bartonellae. Significant titres of IgG and IgM can be detected in animals within 2 weeks of inoculation and antibodies persist for several months. However, the evolution of immunoglobulin titres varies between individuals (**Figure 11.5**). Western blot analysis has allowed the identification of at least 24 *Bartonella*-specific antigens recognized by experimentally infected cats, with the kinetics of antibody appearance during infection varying with individual antigens. A large-scale survey of naturally infected cats has demonstrated that the spectrum of *B. henselae* immunogenic antigens varies between individual animals, but that a subset of the antigens recognized by experimentally infected cats is encountered consistently.

There is conflicting evidence regarding the role played by the humoral immune response in the abrogation of *B. henselae* bacteraemia. Experimental infection of B-cell deficient mice has demonstrated that the cessation of bacteraemia due to *Bartonella grahamii* (a species associated with woodland rodents) is antibody-mediated, as persistent bacteraemia was converted to a transient course by transfer of immune serum. However, infected cats with or without serum IgG antibodies to *B. henselae* may become blood-culture negative simultaneously, suggesting that IgG is not required to clear bacteraemia. There is no doubt that infected cats are prone to recurrent *B. henselae* bacteraemia despite the presence of circulating antibodies. However, as yet there is no evidence for the emergence of antigenic variants to explain this phenomenon, and the potential for intracellular survival of *Bartonella* in cells other than erythrocytes has not been fully investigated.

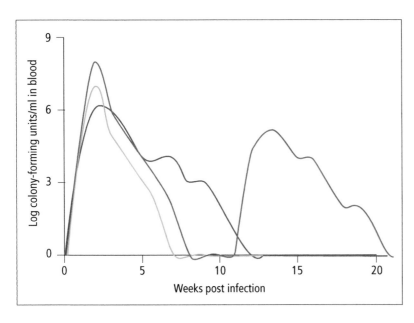

Fig. 11.4 Examples of different types of bacteraemias detected in cats infected experimentally with *B. henselae*. The green curve represents the most commonly observed, shortest infections; the blue curve represents a more protracted infection; while the red curve represents recurrent bacteraemia.

There has been very little study of the *Bartonella*-specific cell-mediated immune response. Positive cutaneous delayed hypersensitivity reactions in cats following exposure and challenge with live *B. henselae* have been reported. However, experimentally infected cats failed to make a similar response following intradermal administration of the cat scratch disease (CSD) antigen that is comprised of heat-treated pus collected from the lymph nodes of human CSD patients. The nature of the *Bartonella*-specific *in-vitro* lymphocyte proliferative response has also been examined.

Other *Bartonella* infections in cats

Experimental infections of cats with *B. clarridgeiae, B. koehlerae* and *B. rochalimae*, but not *B. vinsonii* subspecies *berkhoffii, Bartonella quintana* or *Bartonella bovis* resulted in a subclinical chronic bacteraemia similar to that seen with *B. henselae*. Comparison of infection kinetics indicated that cats inoculated with *B. koehlerae* have a shorter duration of bacteraemia than those inoculated with *B. clarridgeiae*, and none developed relapsing bacteraemia. All infected cats mounted a humoral response against the specific inoculum. There were no apparent differences in the course of infection between cats inoculated with blood co-infected with *B. henselae* and *B. clarridgeiae* and those inoculated with *B. henselae* alone.

B. vinsonii subspecies *berkhoffii* infection in dogs

Current understanding of the pathogenesis of *B. vinsonii* subspecies *berkhoffii* infection in dogs is very limited. However, an immunopathological study of the species in experimentally infected dogs found that despite production of substantial levels of specific antibody, *B. vinsonii* subspecies *berkhoffii* was able to establish chronic infection. This resulted in immune suppression characterized by defects in monocytic phagocytosis, decreased numbers of peripheral blood CD8+ T lymphocytes, together with phenotypic alteration of their cell surface, and an increase in CD4+ lymphocytes in the peripheral lymph nodes. More recently, experimental infections of dogs with strains of *B. vinsonii* subspecies *berkhoffii* and *B. rochalimae*, but not *B. henselae*, resulted in subclinical bacteraemias comparable to those observed in the earlier experiment.

Demonstration of microscopic lesions in cardiac tissue from naturally infected dogs has been used to infer *B. vinsonii* subspecies *berkhoffii* pathogenicity. Multiple foci of myocarditis and endocarditis have been observed, leading to the suggestion that bartonellae may preferentially colonize previously damaged tissue and that once colonization is established a progressive inflammatory response develops to the organisms.

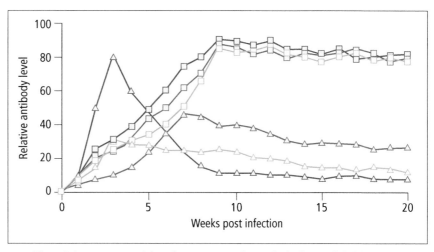

Fig. 11.5 Examples of different types of antibody kinetics in cats infected experimentally with *B. henselae*. The relative antibody levels for IgM (Δ) and IgG (□) are shown. Type 1 (blue curves) involves an acute, strong, but short-lived IgM peak, followed by a strong and protracted IgG response. Type 2 (red curves) involves a far weaker and delayed IgM response, closely followed by a strong and protracted IgG response. Type 3 (green curves) involves an acute but relatively weak IgM response, followed by a strong and protracted IgG response.

CLINICOPATHOLOGICAL SIGNS OF FELINE BARTONELLOSIS

It is generally believed that the cost of *B. henselae* parasitism to the feline host is minimal. However, there is evidence that some strains of *B. henselae* may provoke overt clinical signs in cats, and that hosting chronic *Bartonella* infection is detrimental.

Experimental infection with *B. henselae*

Clinical and pathological evaluations of experimentally infected cats have yielded inconsistent results, which may reflect differences in experimental procedure between different studies. Although in most animals clinical signs were minimal and gross necropsy findings were unremarkable, histopathological findings have included inflammatory foci in the kidneys, heart, liver and spleen and in the peripheral lymph nodes. Less commonly, overt clinical signs have been described including fever, lethargy, transient anaemia, lymphadenomegaly and neurological dysfunction. Some cats infected experimentally with *B. henselae* developed delayed conception or lack of conception, or fetal involution or resorption.

Only one group of researchers has consistently reported clinical disease resulting from experimental inoculation of laboratory cats, including the development of injection site reactions followed by fever and

lethargy. It was proposed that the isolate of *B. henselae* associated with the atypical clinical observations was a more 'virulent' strain, implying that the virulence of *B. henselae* in cats is strain dependent. This hypothesis has not yet been tested elsewhere.

Disease association in natural feline *B. henselae* infection

Disease association with naturally occurring *B. henselae* infection is difficult to determine because of its high prevalence in asymptomatic cats. In Japan, one survey demonstrated that seropositivity for *B. henselae* and feline immunodeficiency virus was significantly associated with a history of lymphadenomegaly and gingivitis. Similarly, a survey of cats from the USA and the Caribbean found that seropositivity was significantly associated with fevers of unknown origin, gingivitis, stomatitis, lymphadenomegaly and uveitis (**Figure 11.6**). In support of this final finding, a further survey in the USA demonstrated that 14% of cats suffering from uveitis, but no healthy cats, had detectable *Bartonella* antibodies in their aqueous humour. In a Swiss survey of over 700 cats, there was significant correlation between high *B. henselae* antibody titres and a range of renal and urinary tract abnormalities. Furthermore, all sick cats over 7 years old in this survey were seropositive.

Individual case reports supporting these associations are almost entirely lacking. In one cat with anterior

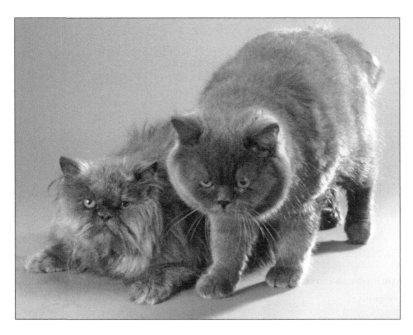

Fig. 11.6 Two 1-year-old, littermate Persian cats, one of which has a febrile syndrome with pyogranulomatous lymphadenitis. Blood from the cat was PCR positive for *B. henselae*. The histopathological appearance of a lymph node biopsy sample from this cat is shown in Figures 11.9 and 11.10.

uveitis, significant ocular production of *Bartonella*-specific antibodies was demonstrated, supporting this as the aetiological agent. *B. henselae* has also been unconvincingly associated with vegetative endocarditis in a small number of cats. Postmortem evidence of pyogranulomatous myocarditis and diaphragmatic myositis has been forthcoming for two cats.

CLINICOPATHOLOGICAL SIGNS OF CANINE BARTONELLOSIS

Most *Bartonella*-associated disease in dogs has been associated with *B. vinsonii* subspecies *berkhoffii* infection. However, as only a small number of cases have been recognized, the true spectrum of clinical manifestations induced by *Bartonella* species in dogs must be considered virtually unknown. The most frequently reported clinical presentation is endocarditis. However, case studies suggesting the involvement of *Bartonella* in the aetiologies of numerous other syndromes has also been published, including granulomatous disease, anterior uveitis and choroiditisepistaxis, lymphadenitis, vasoproliferative haemangiopericytomas, bacillary angiomatosis, polyarthritis, trauma-associated seroma and a dog with idiopathic cavitary effusion (**Figures 11.7, 11.8**).

Both *B. clarridgeiae* and *B. henselae* have been associated with rare clinical disease in dogs. *B. clarridgeiae* was identified in blood culture from a fatal case of canine endocarditis. In addition, *B. clarridgeiae* DNA was detected in the deformed aortic valve and the dog was also seropositive for *Bartonella* species. *B. clarridgeiae* DNA has also been detected in a dog with lymphocytic hepatitis. *B. henselae* has been implicated as a causative agent in a case of canine peliosis hepatis following the detection of species DNA in affected hepatic tissue. *B. henselae* has also been associated with chronic illness in three dogs. Although each animal presented with varying clinical manifestations, severe weight loss, protracted lethargy and anorexia were common to all three. All three dogs also possessed similar haematological and biochemical abnormalities that included eosinophilia, monocytosis, alterations in platelet numbers and elevated serum amylase. *B. henselae* was implicated in the pathogenesis by the detection of DNA in peripheral blood samples. The clinical relevance of these microbiological findings is difficult to infer from such a small case number, particularly given the degree of variation in clinical, haematological and biochemical abnormalities observed. Furthermore, two of the dogs had other concurrent disease. However, the fact that several features were shared among the animals, and that all responded well to appropriate antibiosis, may support a pathogenic role for *B. henselae*. More recently, and primarily on the basis of PCR-based diagnostics, *B. henselae* has been linked to canine cases of endocarditis,

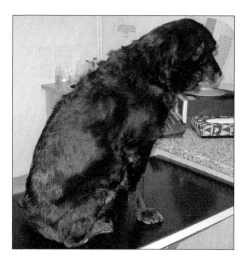
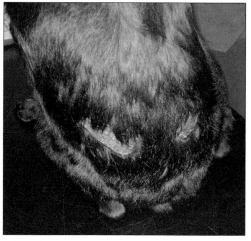

Figs. 11.7, 11.8 A 10-year-old, neutered female Labrador Retriever-cross dog with a history of generalized lymphadenomegaly, pyrexia, lethargy, grade III cardiac murmur and localized areas of ulceration over the gluteal region. Histopathology revealed pyogranulomatous dermatitis and necrotizing lymphadenitis, and Warthin–Starry staining of the lymph node revealed the presence of organisms consistent with *Bartonella* species. Blood from the dog was PCR positive for *Bartonella* species. The dog had been previously treated with glucocorticoids for polyarthritis.

pyogranulomatous and granulomatous lymphadenitis, polyarthritis, prostatitis, steatitis, diarrhoea, panniculitis and fever. *B. henselae* DNA was also detected in a dog with idiopathic cavitary effusion.

Various epidemiological studies have helped determine the relative importance of *Bartonella* species infections in specific clinical syndromes. For example, bartonellae were implicated as an infrequent cause of canine endocarditis in a retrospective study of 71 dogs (although bartonellae were relatively frequently diagnosed [20%] in cases of culture-negative endocarditis). Furthermore, a matched case-control study of 102 *Bartonella* species-seropositive and 203 *Bartonella* species-seronegative dogs revealed that *Bartonella* species-seropositive dogs were more likely to be lame or have arthritis-related lameness, nasal discharge or epistaxis or splenomegaly than *Bartonella* species-seronegative dogs.

DIAGNOSIS

Difficulties in interpreting the significance of positive blood cultures and serology, particularly in cats, necessitate the use of multiple diagnostic methods. Although isolation of a *Bartonella* species by blood culture from a non-reservoir host (e.g. *B. henselae* or *B. clarridgeiae* from an ill dog) is supportive of its role as a causative agent, diagnosis of bartonellosis is best confirmed by demonstration of bartonellae in infected tissues using histological, immunohistochemical or molecular methods (**Figures 11.9, 11.10**).

Histology and immunohistochemistry

The value of histopathology in the diagnosis of naturally occurring *Bartonella* infections has only really been explored in dogs. The histopathological presentation of endocarditis and myocarditis due to infection with *B. vinsonii* subspecies *berkhoffii* is quite characteristic. In one of the two reports of granulomatous disease in dogs associated with *B. vinsonii* subspecies *berkhoffii*, Warthin–Starry (WS) silver staining of tissue sections revealed the presence of clusters of rod-like organisms within and between cells. However, in the second report the stain failed to detect any organisms. A similar degree of inconsistency was apparent during diagnosis of *B. vinsonii* subspecies *berkhoffii*-associated endocarditis. In the first case report, WS and Gram staining revealed intense bacterial colonization of the margins of the infected valves, while in a subsequent case, no organisms were apparent. Transmission electron microscopy has also been used to demonstrate the presence of gram-negative bacteria in tissue sections (**Figure 11.11**).

Isolation of *Bartonella* species

The recovery of bartonellae from the blood of naturally infected reservoirs is relatively straightforward, while their recovery from non-reservoir (accidental)

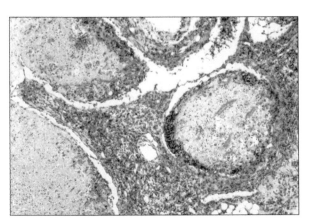

Fig. 11.9 Section of lymph node from the cat in Figure 11.6 with bartonellosis. Within the medullary area there are foci of necrosis associated with mixed mononuclear cell inflammation.

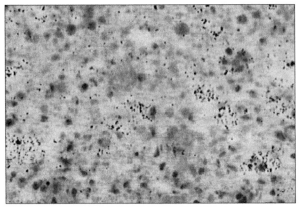

Fig. 11.10 Section of lymph node from the cat in Figure 11.6 with bartonellosis stained by the Warthin–Starry method. The darkly stained aggregates are consistent with the expected appearance of *Bartonella* colonies.

hosts is extremely difficult. The cultivation of *B. hense-lae* and *B. clarridgeiae* from the blood of cats untreated with antibiotics is, therefore, relatively simple, requiring prolonged incubation of inoculated blood-rich agar plates at 35–37°C in a moist, 5% CO_2 atmosphere. Colonies of bartonellae become visible between 5 and 15 days and are usually small, cauliflower-like, dry and of an off-white colour (**Figure 11.12**), although often a 'wetter' phenotype occurs, with colonies appearing smoother and shiny. There is some evidence to suggest that the manner in which blood samples are handled may influence the success of culture. Two procedures that enhance recovery of *B. henselae* from infected cat blood are: (1) freezing samples to –80°C for 24 hours prior to testing; and (2) collection of blood into isolator blood lysis tubes rather than EDTA tubes.

The isolation of *B. vinsonii* subspecies *berkhoffii* from wild canids has been achieved using methods similar to those described for the isolation of *B. henselae* from cats. However, using these methods, the recovery of isolates from the tissues of infected domestic dogs appears to be far less efficient.

A novel liquid medium, termed BAPGM, has been developed and extensively employed by one laboratory to enhance the recovery of bartonellae from clinical samples. This medium has been used not only to obtain bacterial isolates, but also to promote the growth of bartonellae to a level at which, while still uncultivable, they are detectable by PCR.

Serological methods

Detection of circulating antibodies to *Bartonella* species has been performed using several different assay formats including immunofluorescent antibody tests, enzyme-linked immunosorbent assays and western blotting. Antigens for use in these assays are usually

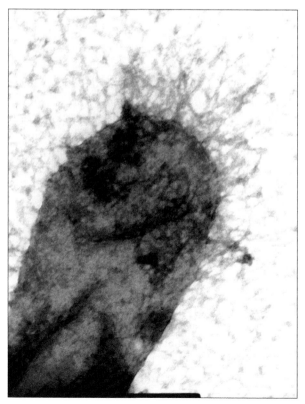

Fig. 11.11 Transmission electron microscopic image of *Bartonella henselae*. The outer surface of the bacterium is pilated. (×146,000) (Courtesy Dr J. Iredell)

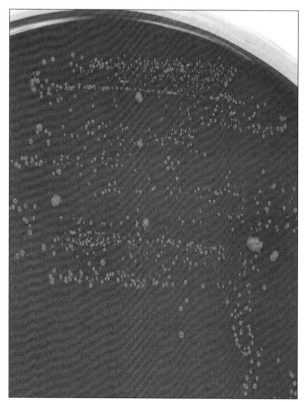

Fig. 11.12 *Bartonella henselae* colonies growing on blood agar 8 days after the plate was inoculated with the blood of an infected cat. The plate was incubated at 35°C in a 5% CO_2 atmosphere.

whole bacteria that have been cultivated either on agar plates or, more often, in association with eukaryotic cell cultures. Serology is most commonly performed on serum/plasma samples, but most body fluid samples, including aqueous humour, can be used.

In cats, serum IgG is very persistent, which limits the diagnostic usefulness of elevated antibody levels as an indicator of ongoing infection. Investigation of the relationship between infection status and seropositivity, using a convenience sample of about 200 cats in the USA, revealed that antibody titres were higher in bacteraemic cats than in non-bacteraemic cats, and that younger age and seropositivity to *B. henselae* were associated with bacteraemia. However, as expected, the estimated positive predictive value of seropositivity as an indicator of bacteraemia was found to be less than 50%, underlining the limited value of the assay.

In the canine cases reported to date for which serological data are available, significant antibody levels were detected. However, as several surveys have demonstrated significant antibody titres in apparently healthy dogs, the predictive value of serology for diagnosing clinical disease due to *B. vinsonii* subspecies *berkhoffii* is likely to be limited.

The interpretation of *Bartonella* serological results has also been compromised by presumed cross-reactivity. Certainly there is marked cross-reaction among *Bartonella* species, although not with antigens derived from close relatives of the Bartonellaceae (i.e. *Brucella canis*, *Ehrlichia canis* and *Rickettsia rickettsii*). However, cross-reactivity between *Bartonella* antigens and the antisera of dogs with molecular evidence of infection due to non-*Bartonella* alpha-subgroup Proteobacteria has been reported.

Molecular methods

A number of molecular methodologies have been developed for the diagnosis of human *Bartonella* infections and some have been successfully applied to veterinary medicine. PCR-based methods have been described, targeting a range of DNA fragments. However, the sensitivity of these methods for the detection of *Bartonella* DNA in infected blood appears limited and in several comparative surveys they have not performed as well as culture. Nonetheless, as tools for the detection of *Bartonella* DNA in the tissues of diseased animals,

PCR-based methods have proven useful additions to histological and serological methods. Genomic targets for PCRs include fragments of the 16S rRNA-encoding gene or the 16S/23S intergenic spacer region, and the citrate synthase-encoding gene (*gltA*).

TREATMENT AND CONTROL

Antibiotic therapy

Treatment of *B. henselae* bacteraemia in cats is problematic. Doxycycline, amoxicillin and amoxicillin/clavulanate used at higher than recommended dose rates have been reported to be successful in suppressing bacteraemia in experimental infections. However, more detailed study suggested that although enrofloxacin was more efficacious than doxycycline for the treatment of *B. henselae* or *B. clarridgeiae*, neither drug eliminated the infection in all animals, even when administered for 4 weeks. Data relating to the treatment of naturally infected animals are scant. However, because of the difficulty in eliminating bacteraemia, antibiotic therapy is only recommended for those cats that have confirmed *Bartonella*-associated disease or those in contact with immunosuppressed owners.

Treatment of canine endocarditis due to *B. vinsonii* subspecies *berkhoffii* is also difficult. There has been no clinical response reported to therapeutic protocols incorporating amoxicillin, enrofloxacin, cephalexin, doxycycline and amikacin in combination with diuretics and various combinations of cardiovascular drugs. Two dogs with granulomatous disease due to *B. vinsonii* subspecies *berkhoffii* appeared to respond well to antibiotics: a 3-week course of enrofloxacin (12.5 mg/kg PO q12h) in the first case and a 30-day course of doxycycline (5.4 mg/kg PO q12h) in the second.

Ectoparasite control

Ectoparasitic control should be of great prophylactic benefit in preventing transmission of *B. henselae* and *B. clarridgeiae* infection between cats. However, despite the availability and use of effective flea adulticide treatments, *Bartonella* species infections remain common, even in the domestic cat populations of the industrialized, affluent countries of Europe and North America. As yet no studies have been carried out examining the efficacy of different ectoparasiticides in the prevention of *B. henselae* transmission. Until proven otherwise, it is feasible that fleas introduced to ectoparasite-treated animals have the capacity to transmit infection before being affected.

ZOONOTIC POTENTIAL/PUBLIC HEALTH SIGNIFICANCE

The zoonotic potential of *B. henselae* is enormous. For example, in the UK, 4.5 million households (or more than 1 in 4) house over 7.5 million cats, of which about 10% are *B. henselae* bacteraemic. The potential threat of this reservoir is reflected in the frequency with which humans acquire *B. henselae* infections, most commonly manifesting as CSD. In the USA, about 24,000 cases of CSD are reported each year, of which about 2,000 require hospitalization. Fortunately, this syndrome is usually benign and self-limiting, manifesting as a regional lymphadenomegaly and affecting mainly children and young adults (**Figure 11.13**). However, systemic complications may arise, leading to more profound diseases. Accurate diagnosis of CSD is important as it requires differentiation from other potentially more serious causes of lymphadenitis such as abscesses, lymphoma, mycobacterial infections, toxoplasmosis and Kawasaki disease.

When first characterized in the late 1980s, *B. henselae* was specifically associated with opportunistic infections in acquired immunodeficiency syndrome patients. The advent of more effective prophylactic therapy for these patients has seen the incidence of these infections decline in the USA and Europe, although they are likely to remain a significant health burden in Africa and other developing parts of the world where therapies are not currently affordable. However, medical interest in zoonotic bartonellae continues today, as an increasing spectrum of syndromes among immunocompetent individuals is encountered. Perhaps of most relevance currently is the emergence of *B. henselae* in the aetiologies of ocular syndromes such as uveitis and neuroretinitis. *B. clarridgeiae* has also been implicated as an agent of CSD and *B. vinsonii* subspecies *berkhoffii* has also been identified as the aetiological agent of endocarditis.

Intriguingly, there is some evidence to suggest that cryptic *Bartonella* species infections may be an occupational hazard for veterinarians and veterinary technicians. A recent study reported PCR-based detection of *Bartonella* species DNA in the blood of 32 of 114 veterinary subjects surveyed. Correlation of these results with clinical symptoms indicated that *Bartonella* species DNA-positive subjects were more likely to report headaches and irritability than *Bartonella* species DNA-negative subjects.

Fig. 11.13 **Cutaneous lesion and inguinal lymphadenomegaly in a boy following a cat scratch on his right leg. (Courtesy Dr C. Wilkinson)**

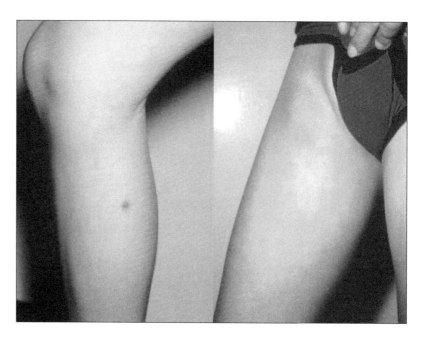

FURTHER READING

Beerlage C, Varanat M, Linder K *et al.* (2012) *Bartonella vinsonii* subsp. *berkhoffii* and *Bartonella henselae* as potential causes of proliferative vascular diseases in animals. *Medical Microbiology and Immunology* **201**:319–326.

Breitschwerdt EB, Lappin MR (2012) Feline bartonellosis: we're just scratching the surface. *Journal of Feline Medicine and Surgery* **14**:609–610.

Breitschwerdt EB, Linder KL, Day MJ *et al.* (2013) Koch's postulates and the pathogenesis of comparative infectious disease causation associated with *Bartonella* species. *Journal of Comparative Pathology* **148**:115–125.

Chomel BB, Kasten RW (2010) Bartonellosis, an increasingly recognized zoonosis. *Journal of Applied Microbiology* **109**:743–750.

Henn JB, Gabriel MW, Kasten RW *et al.* (2009) Infective endocarditis in a dog and the phylogenetic relationship of the associated *Bartonella rochalimae* strain with isolates from dogs, gray foxes, and a human. *Journal of Clinical Microbiology* **47**:787–790.

Lantos PM, Maggi RG, Ferguson B *et al.* (2014) Detection of *Bartonella* species in the blood of veterinarians and veterinary technicians: a newly recognized occupational hazard? *Vector Borne and Zoonotic Diseases* **14**:563–570.

Pennisi MG, Marsilio F, Hartmann K *et al.* (2013) *Bartonella* species infection in cats: ABCD guidelines on prevention and management. *Journal of Feline Medicine and Surgery* **15**:563–569.

Sykes JE, Kittleson MD, Pesavento PA *et al.* (2006) Evaluation of the relationship between causative organisms and clinical characteristics of infective endocarditis in dogs: 71 cases (1992–2005). *Journal of the American Veterinary Medicine Association* **228**:1723–1734.

Chapter 12

Ehrlichiosis and Anaplasmosis

Shimon Harrus
Trevor Waner
Anneli Bjöersdorff

INTRODUCTION

Based on phylogenetic analysis of the family Rickettsiaceae, the following three genera are recognized as pathogenic in animals and humans:

- Genus *Ehrlichia* retains the 'type' species *Ehrlichia canis*, the cause of monocytic ehrlichiosis in dogs and other canids. Other species reported to infect dogs, primarily in the USA, include *Ehrlichia chaffeensis* and *Ehrlichia ewingii*.
- Genus *Anaplasma* now includes the 'type' species *Anaplasma phagocytophilum*, the cause of granulocytic anaplasmosis in dogs, cats and many other animals as well as humans, and *Anaplasma platys*, the cause of canine infectious cyclic thrombocytopenia.

- Genus *Neorickettsia* includes the 'type' species *Neorickettsia risticii*, the cause of Potomac horse fever in the USA. There are also species that cause canine infection and disease in the USA. Cats are susceptible to experimental infection with *N. risticii*, and serological evidence of naturally occurring infection has been reported.

Of these, organisms in the genera *Ehrlichia* and *Anaplasma* are tick transmitted and are discussed in this chapter. The relationships of those species causing naturally occurring disease in dogs and cats to the other species in the genera are illustrated (**Figure 12.1**). Members of the genus *Neorickettsia* are non-arthropod transmitted.

Fig. 12.1 Phylogeny of the family Ehrlichiae. (After Dumler JS and Walker DH (2001) *Lancet Infectious Diseases* April, 21–28.)

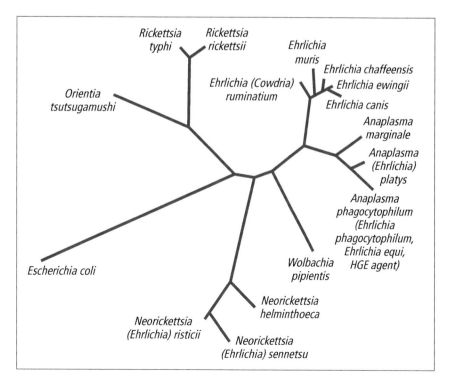

Part 1: Canine Monocytic Ehrlichiosis

Shimon Harrus and Trevor Waner

BACKGROUND, AETIOLOGY AND EPIDEMIOLOGY

Ehrlichia canis, the principal member of the *E. canis* group (**Table 12.1**), is a small, pleomorphic, gram-negative, coccoid, obligatory intracellular bacterium. It is the aetiological agent of canine monocytic ehrlichiosis (CME), a tick-borne disease previously known as tropical canine pancytopenia. *E. canis* parasitizes circulating monocytes intracytoplasmically in clusters of organisms called morulae (**Figures 12.2, 12.3**). It infects dogs and other members of the Canidae family. *E. canis* was first identified by Donatien and Lestoquard in Algeria in 1935, and since then CME has been recognized worldwide as an important canine disease. CME gained much attention when hundreds of American military dogs, many of which were German Shepherd Dogs, died from the disease during the Vietnam War. *E. canis* received further

Table 12.1 **Members of the *Ehrlichia* genus infecting canines*: their geographical distribution, vectors, hosts and target cells.**

EHRLICHIAL SPECIES	GEOGRAPHICAL DISTRIBUTION	PRIMARY VECTOR	PRIMARY HOST	TARGET CELL
E. canis	Worldwide, not Australia	*Rhipicephalus sanguineus*	Canids	Monocyte, macrophage
E. chaffeensis	USA, Brazil Venezuela, Cameroon, South Korea	*Amblyomma americanum*	Humans	Monocyte, macrophage
E. ewingii	USA, Cameroon	*Amblyomma americanum*	Canids	Neutrophil, eosinophil

*The *Ehrlichia canis* clade includes another two members: *Cowdria ruminantium*, which infects ruminants, and *E. muris*, which infects mice. These two members have not been reported to naturally infect dogs or cats.

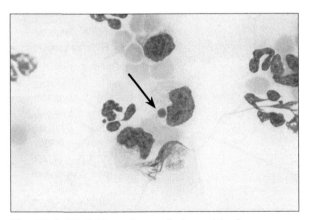

Fig. 12.2 *Ehrlichia canis* morula (arrow) in the cytoplasm of a monocyte as visualized in a blood smear. (Giemsa stain, original magnification ×1,000)

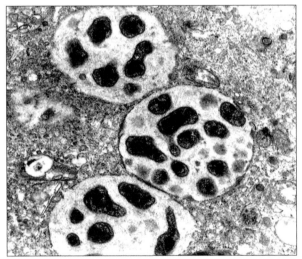

Fig. 12.3 Morulae consisting of many *Ehrlichia canis* organisms in the cytoplasm of tissue culture cells (DH82 macrophages) as visualized by electron microscopy. (Original magnification ×20,000)

Fig. 12.4 A female (A), a male (B) and a nymph (C) of the brown dog tick *Rhipicephalus sanguineus*.

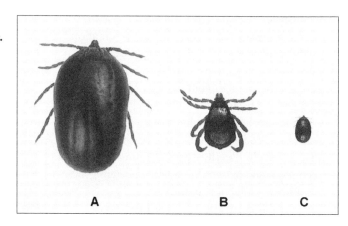

attention in the late 1980s, when the organism was erroneously suspected to infect humans.

Ehrlichia-like morulae have been detected in leucocytes of cats and serum antibodies reactive with *E. canis* antigen have been detected in both domestic and wild cats. In recent years, *E. canis* DNA has been identified in the blood of cats from Canada, Brazil and Portugal, but to date, attempts to culture *E. canis* from suspected feline cases have been unsuccessful. The potential of *E. canis* to infect cats and cause disease has yet to be fully elucidated.

E. canis is transmitted by ticks belonging to the *Rhipicephalus sanguineus* complex (the brown dog tick) (**Figure 12.4**). Experimentally, it has also been transmitted by *Dermacentor variabilis* (the American dog tick), but the biological role of the latter in natural cases seems negligible. Transmission in the tick occurs transstadially but not transovarially. Larvae and nymphs become infected while feeding on bacteraemic dogs and transmit the infection to the host after moulting to nymphs and adults, respectively. A recent experimental study has shown that most *R. sanguineus* ticks, placed on dogs, attach to the dogs within 24 hours and reach full engorgement within 7 days. Moreover, when the ticks were fed on *E. canis*-infected dogs, they reached infection rates of 12–19% by this time period. Throughout feeding, ticks inject *E. canis*-contaminated salivary gland secretions into the feeding site. When infected ticks were placed on naïve dogs, dogs became infected as early as 3 hours post exposure. Adult ticks have been shown to transmit infection for up to 155 days after becoming infected. This phenomenon allows ticks to overwinter and infect hosts in the following spring. The occurrence and geographical distribution of CME are related to the distribution and biology of its vector. *R. sanguineus* ticks are abundant during the warm season; therefore, most acute cases of CME occur during this period. As *R. sanguineus* ticks are cosmopolitan, the disease has a worldwide distribution (Asia, Europe, Africa and America). Dogs living in endemic regions and those travelling to endemic areas should be considered potential candidates for developing CME. Infection with *E. canis* may also occur through infected blood transfusion; therefore screening of blood donors is extremely important.

PATHOGENESIS

The incubation period of CME is 8–20 days. During this period, ehrlichial bacteria enter the bloodstream and lymphatics and localize in macrophages, mainly in the spleen and liver, where they replicate by binary fission. From there, infected macrophages disseminate the infection to other organ systems. The incubation period may be followed consecutively by an acute, a subclinical and a chronic phase:

- The acute phase may last 1–4 weeks; most dogs recover from this phase provided there is adequate treatment.
- Untreated dogs and those treated inappropriately may enter the subclinical phase of the disease. Dogs in this phase may remain persistent carriers of *E. canis* for months or years. Ehrlichial organisms have the ability to evade the immune system by modulation of host cell gene transcription, affecting signalling pathways and resulting in decreased antimicrobial activity. The following

mechanisms have been documented for several *Ehrlichia* species: decreased antigen presentation by downregulation of class II molecules of the major histocompatibility complex on monocytes and macrophages; inhibition of host cell apoptosis; inhibition of bacterial trafficking to lysosomes and lysosomal fusion (to form phagolysosomes); decreased production of reactive oxygen species that are involved in the bacterial killing process; and recombination of outer membrane protein genes, resulting in antigenic variation.

- Some persistently infected dogs may recover spontaneously; however, others may subsequently develop the chronic severe form of the disease. Not all dogs develop the chronic phase of CME, and factors leading to the development of this phase remain unclear. The prognosis at this stage is grave, and death may occur as a consequence of haemorrhage and/or secondary infection.

Immunological mechanisms appear to be involved in the pathogenesis of the disease. Positive Coombs and auto-agglutination tests indicate that infection induces the production of antibodies and complement proteins that bind to the membrane of erythrocytes. Whether these are true autoantibodies (red cell antigen specific) has not been determined. The demonstration of platelet-bound antibodies in infected animals suggests that these play a role in the pathogenesis of thrombocytopenia, causing a shortened platelet life span and thrombocytopathy in CME. Other mechanisms involved in the development of thrombocytopenia in CME include increased platelet consumption, splenic sequestration and decreased production in the chronic phase. Circulating immune complexes were demonstrated in the sera of dogs infected naturally and experimentally with *E. canis*, suggesting that some pathological and clinical manifestations in CME may be immune-complex mediated.

CLINICAL SIGNS

E. canis infects all breeds of dog; however, the German Shepherd Dog appears to be more susceptible to clinical CME. Moreover the disease in this breed appears to be more severe than in other breeds, with a higher mortality rate. There is no predilection for age and both genders are equally affected. The disease is manifested by a wide variety of clinical signs. Factors involved include differences in pathogenicity between *E. canis* strains, breed of dog, co-infections with other arthropod-borne pathogens and the immune status of the host.

Clinical signs in the acute phase range from mild and non-specific to severe and life threatening. Common non-specific signs in this phase include depression, lethargy, anorexia, pyrexia, tachypnoea and weight loss. Specific clinical signs include lymphadenomegaly, splenomegaly, petechiae and ecchymoses of the skin and mucous membranes, and occasional epistaxis (**Figures 12.5, 12.6**). Less commonly reported clinical signs include vomiting, serous to purulent oculonasal discharge and dyspnoea.

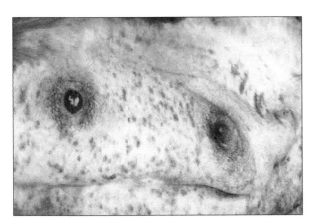
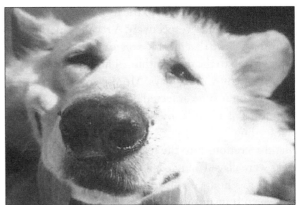

Figs. 12.5, 12.6 Petechiae and ecchymoses (12.5) and epistaxis (12.6) in dogs suffering from canine monocytic ehrlichiosis.

The signs in the chronic severe form of the disease may be similar to those seen in the acute disease, but with greater severity. In addition, pale mucous membranes, emaciation and peripheral oedema, especially of the hindlimbs and scrotum, may also occur. Secondary bacterial and protozoal infections, interstitial pneumonia and renal failure may occur during the chronic severe disease.

Ocular signs are reported to occur during the acute and chronic phases and involve nearly every structure of the eye. Conjunctivitis, conjunctival or iridal petechiae and ecchymoses, corneal oedema, panuveitis and hyphaema have been reported (**Figures 12.7, 12.8**). Subretinal haemorrhage and retinal detachment resulting in blindness may occur due to a monoclonal gammopathy and hyperviscosity.

Neurological signs may occur during both the acute and chronic disease. These signs may include ataxia, seizures, paresis, hyperesthesia, cranial nerve deficits and vestibular (central or peripheral) signs. Neurological signs may be attributed to meningitis or meningoencephalitis, as evidenced by the extensive lymphoplasmacytic and monocytic infiltration, perivascular cuffing and gliosis. On rare occasions, morulae may be detected in the cerebrospinal fluid of dogs with neurological signs.

DIAGNOSIS

Diagnosis of CME is based on a compatible history, clinical presentation and clinical pathological findings in combination with serology, polymerase chain reaction (PCR) or *in-vitro* culture of the organism. Living in an endemic area or travelling to such an area and/or a history of tick infestation should increase the suspicion of infection with *E. canis*. The importance of early diagnosis lies in the relatively good response to treatment before the dog enters the chronic phase.

Haematology and blood smear evaluation

Intracytoplasmic *E. canis* morulae may be visualized in monocytes during the acute phase of the disease in about 4% of cases (see **Figure 12.2**) and their presence

is diagnostic of CME. In order to increase the chance of visualizing morulae, buffy-coat smears should be performed and carefully evaluated (see Chapters 4 and 6).

Thrombocytopenia is the most common and consistent haematological finding in CME. A concurrent increase in the mean platelet volume is usually seen in the acute phase and megaplatelets appear in the blood smear, reflecting active thrombopoiesis. Mild leucopenia and

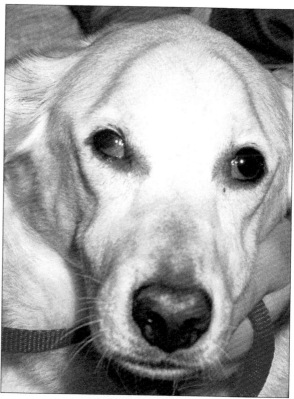

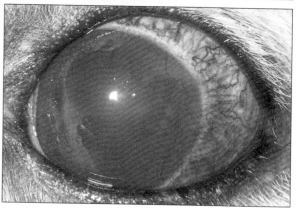

Figs. 12.7, 12.8 A 4-year-old Labrador Retriever with secondary glaucoma, episcleral and conjunctival congestion, corneal neovascularization, corneal oedema and iris bombé secondary to *Ehrlichia canis* infection. (Courtesy Dr. D. Gould) (12.8 from *Journal of Small Animal Practice* (2000) 41:263–265, with permission.)

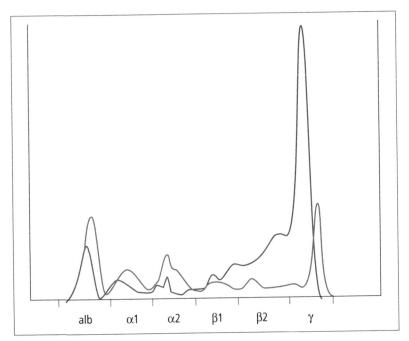

Fig. 12.9 Serum protein electrophoresis from the dog shown in Figures 12.7 and 12.8. At the time of presentation (blue line) there is a monoclonal gammopathy, the severity of which is reduced 6 months post presentation (red line). (From *Journal of Small Animal Practice* (2000) 41:263–265, with permission).

Serum biochemistry

Hypoalbuminaemia and hyperglobulinaemia are the principal biochemical abnormalities in dogs infected with CME. Hyperglobulinaemia is mainly due to hypergammaglobulinaemia, which is usually polyclonal, as determined by serum protein electrophoresis. On rare occasions, monoclonal gammopathy may be noticed and may result in a hyperviscosity syndrome (**Figure 12.9**). Pancytopenic dogs have significantly lower concentrations of total protein, total globulin and gammaglobulin compared with non-pancytopenic dogs. Mild transient increases in serum ALT and ALP activities may also be present.

An antiplatelet antibody test as well as a Coombs test may be positive in infected dogs. Circulating immune complexes may also be demonstrated; however, antinuclear antibodies have not been detected in *E. canis*-infected dogs.

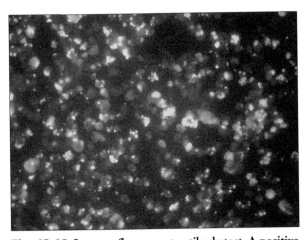

Fig. 12.10 Immunofluorescent antibody test. A positive test result showing *Ehrlichia canis* morulae detected by overlaying seropositive patient serum and fluorescein-conjugated anti-dog IgG.

anaemia may also occur in the acute phase. Absolute monocytosis and the presence of reactive monocytes and large granular lymphocytes are typical findings in acute CME. Mild thrombocytopenia is a common finding in the subclinical phase of the disease, while severe pancytopenia is the hallmark of the chronic severe phase, occurring as a result of a suppressed hypocellular bone marrow.

Specific tests
Serology

The immunofluorescent antibody test (IFAT) is a widely used serological assay for the diagnosis of canine ehrlichiosis (**Figure 12.10**). It is considered the serological 'gold standard' for the detection and titration of *E. canis* antibodies. The presence of *E. canis* antibody titres at equal to or greater than 40 or 80, depending on the reference laboratory, is considered evidence of exposure. Two consecutive tests are recommended, 1–2 weeks apart. A fourfold increase in the antibody titre indicates active infection. In areas that are endemic for other *Ehrlichia* species, serological cross-reactivity may confound the diagnosis. Serological cross-reactivity between *E. canis* and *E. ewingii*, *E. chaffeensis*, *A. phagocytophilum*, *N. risticii* and *N. helminthoeca* has been documented and should be taken into consideration. There is no serological cross-reaction between *E. canis* and *A. platys* (**Table 12.2**).

Table 12.2 **Serological cross-reactivity of ehrlichial organisms with *E. canis* antigen.**

EHRLICHIAL AGENT	SEROLOGICAL IFAT CROSS-REACTIVITY WITH *E. CANIS*
E. chaffeensis	+++
E. ewingii	++/+++
VHE/VDE* agent	+++
A. phagocytophilum	-/+
A. platys	-
N. helminthoeca	++
N. risticii	+

-, no cross-reaction; +, weak cross-reaction; ++, intermediate cross-reaction; +++, strong cross-reaction; *Venezuela human *Ehrlichia*/Venezuela dog *Ehrlichia*.

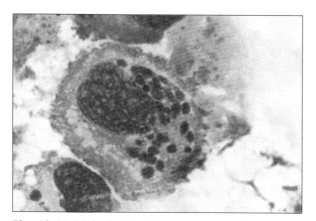

Fig. 12.11 Multiple *Ehrlichia canis* morulae in the cytoplasm of a tissue culture cell (DH82 macrophage). (Giemsa stain, original magnification ×1,000)

Conventional enzyme-linked immunosorbent assays (ELISAs) for *E. canis* IgG antibodies have been developed and are useful in detecting *E. canis* antibodies. Several sensitive and specific commercial dot-ELISA tests for *E. canis* antibodies, designed for rapid in-clinic use, have been developed. These include assays that use the whole cultured organism or specific recombinant *E. canis* proteins (p30 and p30/31) as a source of antigen.

Isolation

E. canis can be cultured on macrophage cell lines (DH82 or J774.A1) (**Figure 12.11**); however, initial culture may take 4–8 weeks. In addition, this method requires expensive equipment and trained staff and therefore is reserved for research rather than diagnostic laboratories.

Polymerase chain reaction

Conventional PCR and sequencing are sensitive methods for detecting and characterizing *E. canis* DNA, respectively. Detection of *E. canis* DNA can be achieved as early as 4–10 days post inoculation. Several assays are based on a variety of different target genes; however, the 16S rRNA and the p30-based PCR assays are used commonly. Splenic samples are considered more sensitive samples for PCR evaluation of ehrlichial elimination. Real-time PCR is a more sensitive assay than conventional PCR, allowing quantitative analysis of specific DNA. It is less prone to contamination than conventional methods and therefore is rapidly becoming the preferred method for diagnosis of *E. canis*.

In recent years, point-of-care loop-mediated isothermal amplification (LAMP)-based methods have been introduced to veterinary diagnosis. A commercial LAMP-based assay for *E. canis* DNA has been developed and made available to veterinarians. This method is simple, specific, sensitive and rapid. It will probably have an important role in future in-clinic diagnosis of canine ehrlichiosis.

Concurrent infections with other tick-borne pathogens such as *Babesia* species and *Hepatozoon canis* are common. Therefore, it is important to examine blood smears of infected dogs microscopically and to consider multiple serological or PCR screening for co-infecting organisms.

TREATMENT AND CONTROL

Doxycycline (10 mg/kg PO q24h or 5 mg/kg PO q12h) for a minimum period of 3 weeks is the treatment of choice for acute CME. Other drugs with known efficacy against *E. canis* include tetracycline hydrochloride (22 mg/kg q8h), oxytetracycline (25 mg/kg q8h), minocycline (20 mg/kg q12h) and chloramphenicol (50 mg/kg q8h). Most acute cases respond to treatment and show clinical improvement within 24–72 hours. One study, using tick acquisition feeding (xenodiagnosis), showed that some dogs treated for 28 days with doxycycline remained positive. Dogs in the subclinical phase may require prolonged treatment. Treatment of dogs suffering from the chronic severe form of the disease is unrewarding.

Imidocarb dipropionate has been used previously in conjunction with doxycycline in the treatment of CME. *In-vivo* and *in-vitro* studies using molecular assays have indicated that this drug is not effective against *E. canis*, therefore the use of imidocarb is indicated only when concurrent infections with other protozoa such as *Babesia* species and/or *Hepatozoon canis* are diagnosed.

After treatment, *E. canis* antibody titres may persist for months or years. The persistence of high antibody titres for extended periods may represent an aberrant immune response or treatment failure, but a progressive decrease in the gammaglobulin concentrations was shown to be associated with elimination of the organism. *E. canis* antibodies do not provide protection against re-challenge, and seropositive dogs remain susceptible to re-infection after successful treatment.

Lower white blood cell (WBC) counts, haematocrit and platelet counts, as well as pronounced pancytopenia, are risk factors for mortality. Severe leucopenia (WBC $<0.93 \times 10^9$/l), severe anemia (packed cell volume [PCV] <11.5 l/l), and prolonged activated partial thromboplastin time (APTT >18.25 seconds) were each found to predict mortality with a probability of 100%. In contrast, WBC counts above 5.18×10^9/l, platelet counts above 89.5×10^9/l, PCV >33.5 l/l and APTT <14.5 seconds each provided 100% prediction for survival. These prognostic indicators can be measured readily at presentation, are inexpensive and may be useful aids when treatment and prognosis are being considered.

To date, no effective commercial anti-*E. canis* vaccine has been developed. An attenuated Israeli strain was found to be effective as a potential vaccine. Its efficacy must still be evaluated against different strains from different geographical regions. Tick control therefore remains the most effective preventive measure against infection. In endemic areas, low-dose oxytetracycline treatment (6.6 mg/kg PO q24h) has been suggested as a prophylactic measure. This method has been used with success by the French army in Senegal, Ivory Coast and Djibouti, where dogs were treated prophylactically with oxytetracycline (250 mg/dog PO q24h). The estimated failure rate of the treatment was found to be 0.9%. This prophylactic method should be reserved for cases where all other prophylactic measures have failed, and should be applied with great caution due to the potential of drug resistance.

ZOONOTIC POTENTIAL/PUBLIC HEALTH SIGNIFICANCE

In the years 1987–1991, *E. canis* was suspected to infect humans, until a closely related organism named *E. chaffeensis* was identified as the cause of human monocytic ehrlichial disease. *E. canis* is not considered a zoonotic agent. However, an *E. canis*-like agent was isolated from a human in Venezuela in 1996, suggesting that the zoonotic potential of *E. canis* has yet to be fully elucidated.

FURTHER READING

Braga Mdo S, André MR, Freschi CR *et al.* (2012) Molecular and serological detection of *Ehrlichia* spp. in cats on São Luís Island, Maranhão, Brazil. *Brazilian Journal of Veterinary Parasitology* **21**:37–41.

Harrus S, Waner T (2011) Diagnosis of canine monocytotropic ehrlichiosis (*Ehrlichia canis*): an overview. *Veterinary Journal* **187**:292–296.

Fourie JJ, Stanneck D, Luus HG *et al.* (2013) Transmission of *Ehrlichia canis* by *Rhipicephalus sanguineus* ticks feeding on dogs and on artificial membranes. *Veterinary Parasitology* **197**:595–603.

Faggion SA, Salvador AR, Jacobino KL *et al.* (2013) Loop-mediated isothermal amplification assay for the detection of *Ehrlichia canis* DNA in blood samples from dogs. *Archivos de Medicina Veterinaria* **45**:197–201.

Liu H, Bao W, Lin M *et al.* (2012) *Ehrlichia* type IV secretion effector ECH0825 is translocated to mitochondria and curbs ROS and apoptosis by upregulating host MnSOD. *Cell Microbiology* **14**:1037–1050.

Maia C1, Ramos C, Coimbra M *et al.* (2014) Bacterial and protozoal agents of feline vector-borne diseases in domestic and stray cats from southern Portugal. *Parasites and Vectors* **8**:138

McBride JW, Walker DH (2011) Molecular and cellular pathobiology of *Ehrlichia* infection: targets for new therapeutics and immunomodulation strategies. *Expert Reviews in Molecular Medicine* doi: 10.1017/S1462399410001730.

McClure JC, Crothers ML, Schaefer JJ *et al.* (2010) Efficacy of a doxycycline treatment regimen initiated during three different phases of experimental ehrlichiosis. *Antimicrobial Agents and Chemotherapy* **54**:5012–5020.

Rikihisa Y (2010) *Anaplasma phagocytophilum* and *Ehrlichia chaffeensis*: subversive manipulators of host cells. *Nature Reviews Microbiology* **8**:328–339.

Rudoler N, Baneth G, Eyal O *et al.* (2012) Evaluation of an attenuated strain of *Ehrlichia canis* as a vaccine for canine monocytic ehrlichiosis. *Vaccine* **31**:226–233.

Shipov A, Klement E, Reuveni-Tager L *et al.* (2008) Prognostic indicators for canine monocytic ehrlichiosis. *Veterinary Parasitology* **153**:131–138.

Waner T, Nachum-Biala Y, Harrus S (2014) Evaluation of a commercial in-clinic point-of-care polymerase chain reaction test for *Ehrlichia canis* DNA in artificially infected dogs. *Veterinary Journal* **202**:618–621.

Part 2: Other Erhlichiae

Shimon Harrus and Trevor Waner

EHRLICHIA CHAFFEENSIS

BACKGROUND, AETIOLOGY AND EPIDEMIOLOGY

Ehrlichia chaffeensis, the cause of human monocytic ehrlichiosis (HME), was first isolated from a human patient in 1991. The organism has been identified from humans, deer, dogs and ticks. Human cases were reported mainly from the USA from the south-central, southeastern and Mid-Atlantic States and California. Sporadic human cases were also reported from Mexico, South America, Africa and Europe. Detection of *E. chaffeensis* DNA by PCR amplification in canine blood provided evidence for natural canine *E. chaffeensis* infection in southeastern Virginia, Oklahoma and North Carolina (USA), Brazil and Venezuela (South America), Cameroon (Africa) and South Korea (Asia).

E. chaffeensis is transmitted by *Amblyomma americanum* (the lone star tick) and, to a lesser extent, by *D. variabilis*. Persistently infected white-tailed deer (*Odocoileus virginianus*) in the USA, Brazilian marsh deer (*Blastocerus dichotomus*) in Brazil, spotted deer (*Cervus nippon*) in Japan and Korea, and possibly canines, serve as reservoirs.

CLINICAL SIGNS

Pups infected experimentally with *E. chaffeensis* have shown pyrexia and no other signs. Only one report has suggested that *E. chaffeensis* may cause clinical signs in dogs. Therefore, the clinical significance of natural canine infection has yet to be determined. The persistence of *E. chaffeensis* infection in the blood of dogs has been documented.

DIAGNOSIS

The IFAT is a good screening test for exposure to rickettsiae; however, it cannot differentiate between *E. canis*, *E. chaffeensis* and *E. ewingii* antibodies. It is possible to discriminate between the three species by western immunoblot analysis and by PCR using species-specific primers.

TREATMENT AND CONTROL

Tetracyclines are considered the drugs of choice. Prophylaxis is based on tick control.

ZOONOTIC POTENTIAL/PUBLIC HEALTH SIGNIFICANCE

E. chaffeensis infects humans and causes HME. Common symptoms are fever, malaise, headache, myalgia, chills, diaphoresis, nausea and anorexia. HME has been documented to be potentially fatal in elderly and immuno-compromised humans.

Deer have been identified as the reservoir host of *E. chaffeensis* while humans, dogs and other vertebrate animals are considered as incidental hosts.

EHRLICHIA EWINGII

BACKGROUND, AETIOLOGY AND EPIDEMIOLOGY

Ehrlichia ewingii, the causative agent of a granulocytic ehrlichiosis in canines, infects granulocytes. Based on 16S rRNA gene sequence, *E. ewingii* is most closely related to *E. chaffeensis* (98.1%) and *E. canis* (98.0%). *E. ewingii* has not yet been cultured *in vitro*.

Canine ehrlichiosis caused by *E. ewingii* has been diagnosed in the USA and Cameroon. It occurs mainly in the spring and early summer. *E. ewingii* DNA has been identified in a large variety of ticks including *R. sanguineus*, *A. americanum*, *D. variabilis*, *Ixodes scapularis*, *I. pacificus* and *Haemaphysalis longicornis*. Of these tick species, *A. americanum* is the only proven vector for *E. ewingii*. The role of the other tick species in transmission of the organism warrants further investigation.

White-tailed deer and probably other deer are potential reservoirs. Although *E. ewingii* DNA has been identified in dogs and striped field mice (*Apodemus agrarius*) from Cameroon and South Korea, respectively, their role as reservoirs has to be elucidated.

CLINICAL SIGNS

The disease is usually an acute mild disease that can lead to polyarthritis in chronically infected dogs. Lameness, joint swelling, stiff gait and pyrexia are common clinical signs. Persistent infections for months or even years have been documented with *E. ewingii* in the blood of dogs.

DIAGNOSIS

Haematological changes in *E. ewingii* infection are mild and include thrombocytopenia and anaemia. Identification of ehrlichial morulae in neutrophils in peripheral blood or joint effusions is diagnostic of granulocytic ehrlichiosis. However, PCR using species-specific primers should be used to determine the *Ehrlichia* species. Species determination is important as *A. phagocytophilium* is also associated with morulae formation within neutrophils and similar clinical signs in dogs. *E. ewingii* has not been cultured *in vitro*, so antigen is not readily available for IFAT development. *E. ewingii* antibodies cross-react strongly with *E. canis* and *E. chaffeensis* and do not (or weakly) react with *A. phagocytophilium*. Therefore, demonstration of granulocytic ehrlichial morulae and negative serology for *A. phagocytophilium* should increase the suspicion of infection with *E. ewingii*. In such situations, PCR for acute cases would be the preferred diagnostic test.

TREATMENT AND CONTROL

Tetracyclines, especially doxycycline, elicit rapid clinical improvement. As for the other ehrlichioses, prophylaxis is based on tick control.

ZOONOTIC POTENTIAL/PUBLIC HEALTH SIGNIFICANCE

E. ewingii is the causative agent of human granulocytic ehrlichiosis. Human cases are seen during the summer months, most commonly in the southeastern and central USA. The role of the dog as a zoonotic reservoir for *E. ewingii* infection is unknown. The potential for persistently infected dogs to serve as a reservoir for the bacterium has to be further elucidated.

FURTHER READING

Chae JS, Kim CM, Kim EH *et al*. (2003) Molecular epidemiological study for tick-borne disease (*Ehrlichia* and *Anaplasma* spp.) surveillance at selected US military training sites/installations in Korea. *Annals of the New York Academy of Sciences* **990**:118–125.

Gongóra-Biachi RA, Zavala-Velázquez J, Castro-Sansores CJ *et al.* (1999) First case of human ehrlichiosis in Mexico. *Emerging Infectious Diseases* **5**:481.

Kocan AA, Levesque GC, Whitworth LC *et al.* (2000) Naturally occurring *Ehrlichia chaffeensis* infection in coyotes from Oklahoma. *Emerging Infectious Diseases* **6**:477–480.

Little SE (2010) Ehrlichiosis and anaplasmosis in dogs and cats. *Veterinary Clinics of North America, Small Animal Practice* **40**:1121–1140.

Martínez MC, Gutiérrez CN, Monger F *et al.* (2008) *Ehrlichia chaffeensis* in child, Venezuela. *Emerging Infectious Diseases* **14**:519–520.

Ndip LM, Ndip RN, Esemu SN *et al.* (2005) Ehrlichial infection in Cameroonian canines by *Ehrlichia canis* and *Ehrlichia ewingii. Veterinary Microbiology* **30**:59–66.

Part 3: Granulocytotropic Anaplasmosis: *Anaplasma phagocytophilum* infection

Anneli Bjöersdorff

BACKGROUND, AETIOLOGY AND EPIDEMIOLOGY

Anaplasma phagocytophilum is a tick-transmitted rickettsial microorganism that primarily infects neutrophils. The microorganisms cause an acute febrile disease, described originally in the early 1930s in Scottish sheep. During the 1950s and 1960s the microorganism was reported from England and Finland, respectively, as a cause of 'pasture fever' in cattle. Anaplasmosis in dogs due to *A. phagocytophilum* was reported from Switzerland, Sweden and North America in the 1980s. Granulocytotropic anaplasmosis in cats was first reported from Sweden in the late 1990s. Numerous case reports have since shown that the infection is present in many countries within the northern temperate zone.

As gene sequencing techniques have developed and been used to analyze the microorganism, it has been reclassified and renamed several times. Former names include *Cytoecetes phagocytophila*, *Ehrlichia phagocytophila*, *Ehrlichia phagocytophilum*, *Ehrlichia equi* and human granulocytic *Ehrlichia* agent.

A. phagocytophilum is a gram-negative, obligate intracellular organism that infects cells of bone marrow derivation. They are internalized in the host cell and appear within the cytoplasm in membrane-bound vacuoles **(Figure 12.12)**. The bacteria multiply by binary fission and eventually form large inclusion bodies (morulae).

In untreated animals the cytoplasmic inclusions can be detected in circulating neutrophils for 1–2 weeks.

Rodents, as well as domestic and wild ruminants (sheep and deer), have been reported as reservoir hosts of *A. phagocytophilum*. The predominant reservoir host varies depending on the local natural and agricultural landscape. The main vectors of *A. phagocytophilum* are *Ixodes* species ticks and the organisms are transmitted transstadially within the tick. *Ixodes* species feed on a

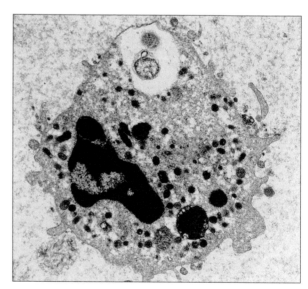

Fig. 12.12 Electron micrograph of an equine neutrophil showing *Anaplasma* organisms inside a cytoplasmic vacuole.

wide range of vertebrate animals and transmission of the infectious agent may take place to multiple host species. Vector-to-host transmission is thought to occur within a window of 24–48 hours of feeding.

PATHOGENESIS

The complete pathogenesis of granulocytotropic anaplasmosis is still unknown. Organisms enter the dermis via tick-bite inoculation. It is not known whether the organisms invade mature cells or precursor myeloid cells for primary replication, but endothelial cells, megakaryocytes as well as haemopoietic cells are suggested targets. In order to infect neutrophils, *A. phagocytophilum* adheres and binds to molecules (e.g. PSGL-1 and sLe^x) on the membrane of the target cell. The organism is then internalized by endocytosis into the neutrophil. *A. phagocytophilum* is seen in mature granulocytes, mainly in neutrophils, but also in eosinophils, of the peripheral blood. After endocytosis, the bacteria multiply within cytoplasmic vacuoles. One virulence factor of *A. phagocytophilum* is their ability to prevent the fusion of lysosomes with *Anaplasma*-containing vacuoles within the cell, thereby evading degradation of the vacuole.

A long lifespan of infected cells in the blood stream is important for the *Anaplasma* organism, as it needs to be ingested by an uninfected tick for further transmission. Factors promoting the lifespan of infected cells include the ability of the *Anaplasma* to inhibit cellular apoptosis and their ability to decrease neutrophil adherence to endothelial cells.

In experimental infections of dogs, the first cytoplasmic inclusions can be detected in peripheral blood granulocytes after 4–14 days. Immunohistological studies have demonstrated the presence of *A. phagocytophilum* in phagocytes in many organs (e.g. spleen, lungs and liver). Endogenous bacterial pyrogens have not been described in experimental infections. It is speculated that the pathogenesis of granulocytotropic anaplasmosis is not entirely caused by the organism itself, but that injury may be in part host-mediated. Severe pulmonary inflammation, alveolar damage and vasculitis of the extremities in the absence of bacterial organisms suggest an immunopathological course of events, such as cytokine-mediated stimulation of host macrophages and non-specific mononuclear phagocyte

activity. The infection may also induce an overactive inflammatory response, such as a septic shock-like syndrome, or diffuse alveolar damage leading to respiratory distress syndrome. Neutrophils infected with *A. phagocytophilum* have a reduced phagocytic capacity and this may result in defective host defence and subsequent secondary infections. Infection with *A. phagocytophilum* has been shown to predispose sheep to disease of increased severity on exposure to parainfluenza type-3 virus or louping ill virus. In addition, concurrent *A. phagocytophilum* and *Babesia* species infection can result in aggravated disease manifestations in man.

As *I. ricinus* ticks may harbour and transmit many pathogens, co-infection with two or more pathogens is possible. Both animals and humans can be co-infected with various *Anaplasma*, *Ehrlichia*, *Borrelia*, *Bartonella*, *Rickettsia*, *Babesia* and arboviral species. Infection with any of these organisms causes a wide range of clinical and pathological abnormalities, ranging in severity from asymptomatic infection to death. The risk of acquiring one or more tick-borne infections may be dependent on the prevalence of multi-infected vectors. It has been shown that ticks dually infected with *A. phagocytophilum* and *Borrelia burgdorferi* transmit each pathogen to susceptible hosts as efficiently as ticks infected with only one pathogen. The presence of either agent in the tick does not affect acquisition of the other agent from an infected host. Since *Borrelia burgdorferi* and *A. phagocytophilum* to a large extent share both reservoir hosts and vectors, it is hardly surprising that the geographical areas where granulocytotropic anaplasmosis is endemic overlap areas where borreliosis is prevalent. The general capacity of one tick-borne infection to predispose to or aggravate another infection is not well understood.

CLINICAL SIGNS

The spectrum of clinical manifestations caused by *A. phagocytophilum* is wide, but disease presents most commonly as an acute febrile syndrome. The incubation period may vary from 4–14 days depending on the immune competence of the infected individual and the *Anaplasma* strain involved. Dogs with granulocytotropic anaplasmosis usually present with a history of lethargy and anorexia. Clinical examination commonly reveals fever, reluctance to move and, occasionally, lymphadenomegaly and splenomegaly. More localized presenting signs referable to the musculoskeletal system (e.g. lameness), respiratory system (e.g. coughing) and gastrointestinal system (e.g. diarrhoea) may be seen. Systemic manifestations may include haemorrhage, shock and multi-organ failure. However, seroepidemiological data suggest that mild and subclinical infections are common.

LABORATORY FINDINGS

The observation of *Anaplasma* inclusion bodies or morulae within neutrophils is the most helpful laboratory finding. During and after the period of bacteraemia, the disease is characterized by mild to severe thrombocytopenia and leucopenia **(Figure 12.13)**. Thrombocytopenia is one of the most consistent haematological abnormalities in infected dogs. It may persist for a few days before the platelet numbers return to normal. The leucopenia is a result of early lymphopenia later accompanied by neutropenia. The leucopenia may be followed by transient leucocytosis. Serum biochemical abnormalities include mildly elevated serum ALP activity and mild to moderate hypoalbuminaemia.

DIAGNOSIS

Granulocytotropic anaplasmosis should be considered when a patient presents with an acute febrile illness in a geographical area in which the disease is endemic, during a season when ticks are seeking hosts. There is no generally accepted case definition for granulcyto-tropic anaplasmosis in cats and dogs, but a case definition adapted from the Centers for Disease Control and Prevention (Atlanta, USA) definition for humans is given in **Table 12.3.**

As intracytoplasmic clusters of the bacteria (morulae) may be visible, a Wright's-stained blood smear should be examined. Morulae typically appear as dark blue, irregularly stained densities in the cytoplasm of neutrophils. The colour of the morulae is usually darker than that of the cell nucleus **(Figure 12.14)**. Morulae are often sparse and difficult to detect and a negative blood smear cannot rule out *A. phagocytophilum* infection.

PCR analysis using *A. phagocytophilum*-specific primers is a very sensitive and specific method for estab-

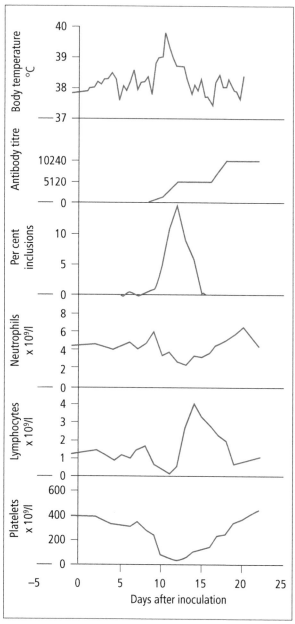

Fig. 12.13 Serial changes in a range of parameters in a dog infected experimentally with a European isolate of *Anaplasma phagocytophilum* and monitored for a 25-day period. The dramatic haematological changes during the acute stage of infection may be seen. (From *Veterinary Record* (1998) 143:412–417, with permission.)

lishing the cause of an infection. PCR is more sensitive than direct microscopy and *Anaplasma* are detected in the circulation for a longer time period by PCR com-

Table 12.3 **Case definition of acute canine or feline granulocytotropic anaplasmosis.**

Clinical description

- A tick-borne illness characterized by acute onset of fever and one or more of the following signs: myalgia, malaise, anaemia, leucopenia, thrombocytopenia or elevated hepatic transaminases.
- History of having been in a tick habitat in the 14 days prior to the onset of illness or a history of tick bite.

Laboratory criteria for diagnosis

Supportive:

- Serological evidence of elevated IgG antibody reactive with *A. phagocytophilum* antigen by indirect immunofluorescence antibody test (IFAT), enzyme-linked immunosorbent assay (ELISA), dot-ELISA or assays in other formats, **or**
- Identification of morulae in the cytoplasm of neutrophils or eosinophils by microscopic examination.

Confirmed:

- Serological evidence of a fourfold change in IgG antibody titre to *A. phagocytophilum* antigen by IFAT in paired serum samples (one taken in first week of illness and a second 2–4 weeks later), **or**
- Detection of *A. phagocytophilum* DNA in a clinical specimen via amplification of a specific target by polymerase chain reaction assay, **or**
- Demonstration of *Anaplasma* antigen in a biopsy/necropsy sample by immunohistochemical methods, **or**
- Isolation of *A. phagocytophilum* from a clinical specimen in cell culture.

Adapted from Centers for Disease Control and Prevention, 2009 Council of State and Territorial Epidemiologist's Position Statement 09-ID-15.

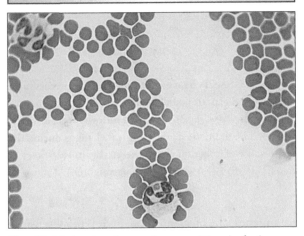

Fig. 12.14 An *Anaplasma phagocytophilum* inclusion (morulla) in a neutrophil.

pared with microscopy (**Figure 12.15**). In addition to blood, synovial fluid, cerebrospinal fluid and tissue samples may be analyzed by PCR.

Other useful diagnostic tests include anti-*A. phagocytophilum* IgG antibody evaluation by indirect IFAT, immunoblot analysis or ELISA. Some research laboratories also offer the service of *in-vitro* culture for *Anaplasma* (**Figure 12.16**). The most widely accepted diagnostic criterion is a fourfold change in titre by IFAT (**Figure 12.17**).

TREATMENT AND CONTROL

In vitro, *A. phagocytophilum* is susceptible to several intracellularly active antibiotics including tetracyclines. *A. phagocytophilum* is resistant to gentamicin and trimethoprim–sulphamethoxazole among others, and to all antibiotics that do not penetrate intracellularly including betalactam antibiotics. Doxycycline (5–10 mg/kg PO q24h for 10–21 days) appears to be the most effective regimen for treating granulocytotropic anaplasmosis in dogs and cats. In young animals, doxycycline is still considered the drug of first choice. The risks of enamel hypoplasia and discolouration are considered low when balanced against the risk of serious infection. The most common side-effects of doxycycline treatment are nausea and vomiting, which are avoided by administering the drug with food. Simultaneous feeding does not affect drug absorption.

A. phagocytophilum infection has been demonstrated to be persistent in experimentally infected, untreated dogs for up to 5.5 months after inoculation. Considering the high seroprevalence of *A. phagocytophilum* in some geographical areas, with only a small number of acute cases, self-limiting infections are likely not uncommon.

Particular caution should be taken when transfusing blood to critically ill patients. *A. phagocytophilum* PCR-positive blood donors can transmit the infection to a recipient with severe consequences. Routine screening of blood at every collection is recommended, as blood from apparently healthy blood donors may contain *A. phagocytophilum*.

No vaccines for protection or immunoglobulins for post-exposure prophylaxis are available. The most reliable, although not the most realistic way, to prevent infections is to avoid tick-infested areas. Careful daily

Fig. 12.15 Comparison of (a) microscopy,
(b) PCR and (c) serology in an experimental
infection of a dog with a European isolate of
Anaplasma phagocytophilum. The dog was given
prednisolone on days 55 and 153 (red arrows) and
was monitored for a 180-day period. It can be
seen that persistent infection results in prolonged
seropositivity that does not discriminate the
cyclical infection demonstrated by PCR. (From
Veterinary Record (2000) 146:186–190, with
permission.)

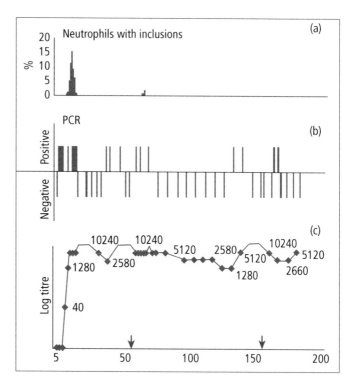

inspection for and removal of ticks is recommended in
combination with the application of residual acaricidal
products. Spray, spot-on liquid or collar formulations
are available with residual efficacy of 1 month or more
depending on the product.

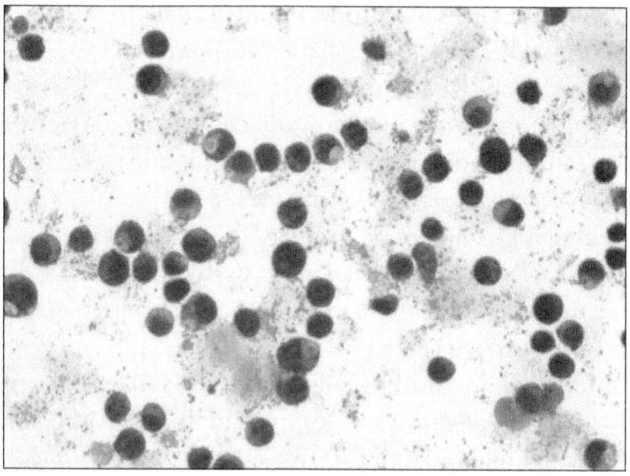

ZOONOTIC POTENTIAL/PUBLIC HEALTH SIGNIFICANCE

The catholic feeding behaviour of the *Ixodes* species
tick vectors permits transmission of *A. phagocytophilum*

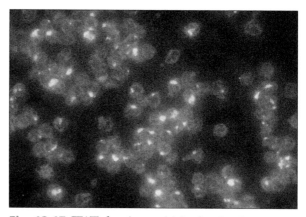

Fig. 12.16 *Anaplasma phagocytophilum*-infected HL-60
cells.

Fig. 12.17 IFAT showing positivity for *Anaplasma
phagocytophilum*. A whole cell *A. phagocytophilum* antigen
is often used in the diagnostic IFAT. The primary
antibody–antigen reaction is demonstrated by the use
of a secondary fluorescein-labelled antibody. If the
serum sample contains antibodies to the antigen, strong
fluorescence is seen.

to a wide range of vertebrate species including man; however, few cases of human infection have been reported from Europe. Seroprevalence data suggest that the infection is mild and self-resolving. The majority of cases of human granulocytotropic anaplasmosis have been reported from the USA. The most common clinical manifestations of human granulocytotropic anaplasmosis are fever and headache. The clinical disease is often accompanied by non-specific symptoms such as myalgia, stiffness, malaise and arthralgia. Symptoms implicating involvement of other organ systems are also present and include gastrointestinal (e.g. nausea, vomiting and diarrhoea), respiratory (e.g. non-productive cough) and central nervous system signs (e.g. confusion). Skin rashes are reported uncommonly and involvement of concurrent infectious agents has been suggested in these cases. However, such rashes may well be part of the host inflammatory response to infection. Laboratory data frequently demonstrate thrombocytopenia, leucopenia and elevated levels of hepatic transaminases. Severe complications include prolonged fever, shock, seizures, pneumonitis, acute kidney injury, rhabdomyolysis, opportunistic infections, adult respiratory distress syndrome and death. Pre-existing immune dysfunction predisposes to poor prognosis and the risk of serious illness or death increases with advanced age and delayed onset of therapy.

FURTHER READING

Ayllón T, Villaescusa A, Tesouro MA *et al.* (2009) Serology, PCR and culture of *Ehrlichia/Anaplasma* species in asymptomatic and symptomatic cats from central Spain. *Clinical Microbiology and Infection* **15**:4–5.

Billeter SA, Spencer JA, Griffin B *et al.* (2007) Prevalence of *Anaplasma phagocytophilum* in domestic felines in the United States. *Veterinary Parasitology* **147**:194-198.

Birkner K, Steiner B, Rinkler C *et al.* (2008) The elimination of *Anaplasma phagocytophilum* requires CD4+ T cells, but is independent of Th1 cytokines and has a wide spectrum of effector mechanisms. *European Journal of Immunology* **38**:3395–3410.

Egenvall A, Björersdorff A, Lilliehöök I *et al.* (1998) Early manifestations of granulocytic ehrlichiosis in dogs inoculated experimentally with a Swedish *Ehrlichia* species isolate. *Veterinary Record* **143**:412–417.

Egenvall A, Lilliehöök I, Björersdorff A *et al.* (2000) Detection of granulocytic *Ehrlichia* species DNA by PCR in persistently infected dogs. *Veterinary Record* **146**:186–190.

Kohn B, Galke D, Beelitz P *et al.* (2008) Clinical features of canine granulocytic anaplasmosis in 18 naturally infected dogs. *Journal of Veterinary Internal Medicine* **22**:1289–1295.

Maggi RG, Birkenheuer AJ, Hegarty BC *et al.* (2014) Comparison of serological and molecular panels for diagnosis of vector-borne diseases in dogs. *Parasites and Vectors* **7**:127.

Ravnik U, Bajuk BP, Lusa L *et al.* (2014) Serum protein profiles, circulating immune complexes and proteinuria in dogs naturally infected with *Anaplasma phagocytophilum*. *Veterinary Microbiology* **173**:160–165.

Ravnik U, Tozon N, Smrdel KS *et al.* (2011) Anaplasmosis in dogs: the relation of haematological, biochemical and clinical alterations to antibody titre and PCR confirmed infection. *Veterinary Microbiology* **149**:172–176.

Sainz Á, Roura X, Miró G *et al.* (2015) Guideline for veterinary practitioners on canine ehrlichiosis and anaplasmosis in Europe. *Parasites and Vectors* **8**:75.

Scorpio DG, Dumler JS, Barat NC *et al.* (2011) Comparative strain analysis of *Anaplasma phagocytophilum* infection and clinical outcomes in a canine model of granulocytic anaplasmosis. *Vector-Borne and Zoonotic Diseases* **11**:223.

Seidman D, Ojogun N, Walker NJ *et al.* (2014) *Anaplasma phagocytophilum* surface protein AipA mediates invasion of mammalian host cells. *Cellular Microbiology* **16**:1133–1145.

Stuen S, Granquist EG, Silaghi C (2013) *Anaplasma phagocytophilum* – a widespread multihost pathogen with highly adaptive strategies. *Frontiers in Cellular and Infection Microbiology* **3**:31.

Woldehiwet Z (2009) The natural history of *Anaplasma phagocytophilum*. *Veterinary Parasitology* **167**:108–122.

Part 4: Infectious Canine Cyclic Thrombocytopenia (*Anaplasma platys*)

Trevor Waner and Shimon Harrus

BACKGROUND, AETIOLOGY AND EPIDEMIOLOGY

Infectious canine cyclic thrombocytopenia, caused by *Anaplasma platys*, was first described in the USA in 1978 and since then it has been found worldwide. It has been reported from Africa, southern Europe, the Mediterranean basin, Southeastern and Eastern Asia, South America and Australia. The aetiologial agent is an obligate intracellular rickettsial organism with tropism for platelets. Although originally referred to as *Ehrlichia platys*, based on phenotypic similarities to other organisms of this genus, it was formally classified in 2001 according to its 16S rRNA gene sequence as a member of the genus *Anaplasma*. Although *A. platys* is reported predominantly from domesticated dogs, the extent of its host spectrum has not been determined fully. Similar organisms have been reported from North American deer and from sheep species in South Africa. Two reports of infections of cats from Brazil and North America, respectively, have been documented. In the former, the finding was accidental without any significant clinical or haematological changes. In the latter, the cat had splenic plasmacytosis and multiple myeloma and was concurrently infected with *A. platys*, two *Bartonella* species and a *Mycoplasma* species. In both cases, *A. platys* was identified by PCR analysis.

A. platys organisms are round to oval in shape, 0.3–1.2 μm in diameter are enclosed by a double membrane. The mechanism by which the organisms attach and penetrate platelet membranes is unknown. *A. platys* bacteria aggregate and divide within the platelet cytoplasm, producing morulae identified on light microscopy. Further bacteriological characterization is limited, as the organism remains unculturable.

A. platys is presumed to be transmitted by the tick *Rhipicephalus sanguineus*, and its widespread geographical distribution supports this mode of transmission. In particular, *R. sanguineus* is the only tick species that has been identified in isolated areas of central Australia where *A. platys* infection has been reported. In addition, co-infection with *Ehrlichia canis*, which is transmitted by the same tick species, is reported from several areas of the world. *A. platys* DNA has been identified in *R. sanguineus* ticks collected from dogs from different parts of the world, but definitive evidence of natural transmission by this tick is still lacking and experimental transmission by *R. sanguineus* has not been successful.

There is limited information available on other epidemiological aspects of *A. platys* infection, although studies would suggest that the prevalence is relatively high in some dog populations. Using the IFAT, seropositivity in two southern states of the USA was widespread. Thirty-three percent of thrombocytopenic dogs in endemic areas were positive. In addition, 13/28 apparently healthy dogs sampled from one study site in northern Australia were positive for *A. platys* DNA by PCR. Although puppies may be more susceptible to clinical *A. platys* infection in northern Australia, there are no reported breed, gender, individual predispositions or risk factors for infection. However, as mentioned above, concurrent infection with other arthropod-borne pathogens is a considerable risk factor for the clinical expression of infection. Up to 50% of dogs seropositive for *A. platys* in one study from the USA were concurrently seropositive for *E. canis*.

PATHOGENESIS

In dogs, the period of time from experimental inoculation of *A. platys*-infected blood to the appearance of circulating parasitized platelets ranges from 8–15 days. The period of maximum parasitaemia is followed by severe thrombocytopenia, possibly due to direct platelet injury. The number of circulating organisms decreases and recovery in the platelet count occurs in 3–4 days. Repeated episodes of parasitaemia and thrombocytopenia occur at intervals of 1–2-weeks. Although the degree of parasitaemia is much reduced (1% of platelets affected) in recurrent episodes, the thrombocytopenia remains severe. Immune-mediated platelet destruction is a more likely mechanism for thrombocytopenia occurring during this phase. Chronic infection is associated with cyclic low-level parasitaemia, which may reflect host–*A. platys* adaptation. Antibody titres may persist for 4 months up to several years.

CLINICAL SIGNS

A. platys strains in the USA are considered to cause minimal clinical disease. Infection with *A. platys* is commonly asymptomatic unless the dog undergoes surgery or has a concurrent bleeding disorder such as that produced by co-infection with *E. canis*. However, there are reports from Greece and Israel of more severe disease associated with cyclical epistaxis and bleeding from venipuncture sites in adult dogs, and severe thrombocytopenia with anaemia and increased mortality rate in puppies in northern Australian. Bilateral uveitis has been reported in a dog with *A. platys* infection.

The spectrum of clinical signs is suggestive of geographical strain variation and minor sequence differences have been detected in *A. platys* samples from the USA and Australia. It is widely accepted that clinical signs associated with *A. platys* infection may be precipitated through co-infection with other arthropod-borne pathogens such as *Babesia* species and *Ehrlichia canis*.

LABORATORY FINDINGS

Thrombocytopenia is the major haematological finding, although leucopenia has been reported in rare cases. Cyclic thrombocytopenia of 3–4 days' duration, followed by asymptomatic periods of 7–21 days, are characteristics of *A. platys* infection. Moderate non-regenerative anaemia may occur and is probably a result of inflammation. However, in cases that experience severe bleeding, a regenerative anaemia may be expected. Moderate hypergammaglobulinaemia, occasional hypoalbuminaemia and hypocalcaemia have also been reported.

Bone marrow examination of *A. platys*-infected dogs may reveal hyperplasia of lymphocyte, monocyte or plasma cell populations, dysmyelopoiesis, megakaryocyte hyperplasia and dysplasia, emperipoiesis (engulfing of various bone marrow cells by megakaryocytes), eyrthrophagocytosis and platelet phagocytosis.

DIAGNOSIS

The microscopic identification of morulae in platelets with morphology characteristic of *A. platys* in blood smears is diagnostic for infection. However, the sensitivity of this technique is limited by the low levels of parasitaemia seen during severe thrombocytopenic episodes and in chronic infections. Attempts to culture *A. platys* have been uniformly unsuccessful.

Historically, serology has been the major technique used for *A. platys* diagnosis. An IFAT for *A. platys* has been developed, but its availability is limited by lack of antigen substrate. Cross-reactions with *E. canis* reportedly do not occur, but cross-reactivity with *A. phagocytophilum* has been demonstrated. Because of the serological cross-reactivity between *A. platys* and *A. phagocytophilum*, differentiation between these two species can be made on the basis of the target cell when morulae are detected, and confirmed by molecular characterization.

Several methods of species-specific PCR testing are available and, considering the limitations of serology and microscopy in the diagnosis of this infection, they are considered sensitive and specific adjuncts to diagnosis. A LAMP method has been recently developed for the diagnosis of *A. platys*. No cross-reactivity was shown for this LAMP-based assay with other *Anaplasma* or *Ehrlichia* species.

TREATMENT AND CONTROL

A. platys infection should be treated with tetracylines using protocols discussed for other members of the genera *Ehrlichia* and *Anaplasma*. Prevention is dependent on vector control using effective acaricides with long duration.

ZOONOTIC POTENTIAL/PUBLIC HEALTH SIGNIFICANCE

There is some preliminary evidence that *A. platys* has zoonotic potential and two reports of human *A. platys* infection have been documented in Venezuela. In the first, *A. platys* was identified ultrastructurally and in the second *A. platys* DNA was amplified and sequenced from blood drawn from two women. In another case, a veterinarian was diagnosed with a co-infection of *A. platys*, *Bartonella henselae* and a *Mycoplasma* species. In the USA, two people were found to be PCR positive for *A. platys*, *Ehrlichia chaffeensis* and *Ehrlichia ewingii*.

FURTHER READING

Breitschwerdt EB, Hegarty BC, Qurollo BA *et al.* (2014) Intravascular persistence of *Anaplasma platys*, *Ehrlichia chaffeensis*, and *Ehrlichia ewingii* DNA in the blood of a dog and two family members. *Parasites and Vectors* **7:**298.

De Tommasi AS, Otranto D, Furlanello T *et al.* (2014) Evaluation of blood and bone marrow in selected canine vector-borne diseases. *Parasites and Vectors* **7:**534.

Lanza-Perea M, Zieger U, Qurollo BA *et al.* (2014) Intraoperative bleeding in dogs from Grenada seroreactive to *Anaplasma platys* and *Ehrlichia canis*. *Journal of Veterinary Internal Medicine* **28:**1702–1707.

Latrofa MS, Dantas-Torres F, Giannelli A *et al.* (2014) Molecular detection of tick-borne pathogens in *Rhipicephalus sanguineus* group ticks. *Tick Borne Diseases* **5:**943–946.

Li HT, Sun LS, Chen ZM *et al.* (2014) Detection of *Anaplasma platys* in dogs using real-time loop-mediated isothermal amplification. *Veterinary Journal* **199:**468–470.

Lima ML, Soares PT, Ramos CA *et al.* (2010) Molecular detection of *Anaplasma platys* in a naturally-infected cat in Brazil. *Brazilian Journal of Microbiology* **41:**381–385.

Qurollo BA, Balakrishnan N, Cannon CZ *et al.* (2014) Co-infection with *Anaplasma platys*, *Bartonella henselae*, *Bartonella koehlerae* and 'Candidatus Mycoplasma haemominutum' in a cat diagnosed with splenic plasmacytosis and multiple myeloma. *Journal of Feline Medicine and Surgery* **16:**713–720.

Stillman BA, Monn M, Liu J *et al.* (2014) Performance of a commercially available in-clinic ELISA for detexion of antibodies against *Anaplasma phagocytophilum*, *Anaplasma platys*, *Borrelia burgdorferi*, *Ehrlichia canis*, *Ehrlichia ewingii* and *Dirofilaria immitis* antigen in dogs. *Journal of the American Veterinary Medical Association* **245:**80–86.

CASE STUDY 1: CANINE MONOCYTIC EHRLICHIOSIS

History

Kika, a 6-year-old, neutered female Siberian Husky, was admitted to the Veterinary Teaching Hospital, Koret School of Veterinary Medicine, Hebrew University, Israel, with a chief complaint of intermittent epistaxis for the last 2 days. The owner also reported that the dog had been anorexic and lethargic for 6 days.

Clinical examination

The dog had pyrexia (body temperature 39.8°C); tachycardia (pulse 104 beats/minute) and tachypnoea (35 breaths/minute). On physical examination, the dog was depressed, lethargic and had pale mucous membranes. Bilateral epistaxis as well as mucosal petechiae and ecchymoses were present (**Figure 12.18**). Palpation revealed generalized lymphadenomegaly and splenomegaly.

Laboratory diagnostics
Haematology
Abnormal haematological findings included anaemia (RBC count 4.28×10^{12}/l, reference range 5.4–7.8×10^{12}/l; haemoglobin 102 g/l, reference range 130–190 g/l; PCV 0.3 l/l, reference range 0.35–0.54 l/l) and thrombocytopenia (platelets 145×10^9/l, reference range 160–450×10^9/l). Blood smear evaluation revealed thrombocytopenia and reactive monocytes.

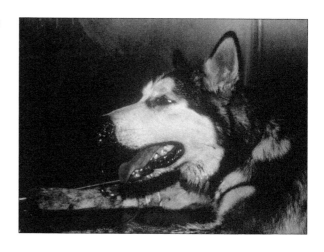

Fig. 12.18 Bilateral epistaxis in this Siberian Husky. (Courtesy Prof. G. Baneth)

Serum biochemistry

Abnormal serum biochemical findings included hypoalbuminaemia (26 g/l, reference range 28.3–38.3 g/l), hyperglobulinaemia (51 g/l, reference range 24–44 g/l), reduced albumin to globulin ratio (0.6, reference range >0.7) and increased alkaline phosphatase activity (188 U/l, reference range 4–140 U/l).

Urinalysis

No abnormal findings.

Buccal mucosal bleeding time

Prolonged (8 minutes, reference range 2–4 minutes).

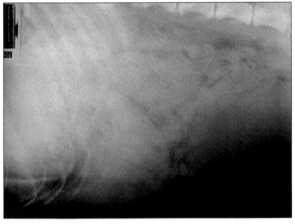

Fig. 12.19 Radiograph (lateral projection) showing an abdominal mass (enlarged spleen) in the cranial ventral abdomen.

Coagulation assays

Prothrombin time, partial thromboplastin time and capillary clotting time were all within the reference ranges.

Radiography

Abdominal radiography revealed an abdominal mass (diagnosed as an enlarged spleen) in the cranial ventral abdomen (**Figure 12.19**).

Serology for *E. canis*

Positive for *E. canis* antibodies using a dot-ELISA kit (Immunocomb, Biogal, Galed Laboratories) (**Figure 12.20**). The 'S score' was 5/6 (roughly equivalent to an IFAT titre of 320 to 640).

PCR

PCR targeting the *E. canis* 16S rRNA gene was positive.

Treatment

Kika was hospitalized and received intravenous fluids and doxycycline (10mg/kg PO q24h). There was clinical improvement within 48 hours; the dog started eating and was sent home with instructions to continue the doxycycline treatment for an additional 3 weeks. The owners were instructed to visit the Veterinary Teaching Hospital for a recheck in 14 days.

Outcome

After 14 days, the owners reported that Kika has completely recovered. The dog was bright, alert and responsive during the return visit. Temperature, pulse and respiratory rate, haematology and biochemistry parameters were all within reference ranges.

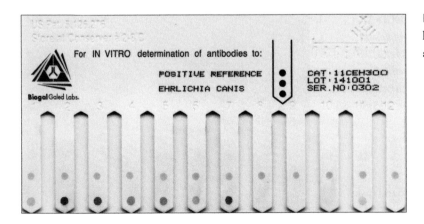

Fig. 12.20 Lane 3 (from the left; lower dot) indicates the presence of anti-*E. canis* antibodies in this dog.

CASE STUDY 2: GRANULOCYTOTROPIC ANAPLASMOSIS

History

A 5-year-old Basset Griffon Vendeen was presented with a 2-day history of depression, fever, anorexia and a mild cough (**Figure 12.21**). The dog had been out hunting several times during recent weeks without any problems. For the past 2 days it had been reluctant to stand or take walks and had mostly been sleeping.

Physical and laboratory examinations

Initial physical examination revealed pale mucous membranes, pronounced lethargy, mildly increased lung sounds and a body temperature of 39.7°C. Haematological examination revealed marked thrombocytopenia (76.8 × 10^9/l, reference range 150–500 × 10^9/l), a slight decrease in haemoglobin concentration (119 g/l, reference range 125–190 g/l) and a moderately decreased total white blood cell count (4.4 × 10^9/l, reference range 5.5–14.5 × 10^9/l) with the most pronounced changes in the neutrophil (2.5 × 10^9/l, reference range 3.2–11.5 × 10^9/l) and lymphocyte (0.6 × 10^9/l, reference range 1.0–5.0 × 10^9/l) counts. Fifteen percent of the neutrophils contained basophilic inclusions (morulae).

The serum biochemistry profile showed moderate hypoalbuminaemia (18 g/l, reference range 27–40 g/l) and mildly elevated serum alkaline phosphatase activity (230 U/l, reference range 22–200 U/l). A nested PCR test performed on an EDTA blood sample was positive for *Anaplasma phagocytophilum* and confirmed the diagnosis of granulocytotropic anaplasmosis.

Treatment

Treatment with doxycycline (10 mg/kg PO q24h) was initiated. The dog was hospitalized and monitored for the rest of the day and for that night. After 12 hours the body temperature had started to decline and after 18 hours the temperature had returned to normal (38.1°C). The dog also showed interest in food and ate with good appetite when fed after 18 hours. The dog was sent home on doxycycline (10 mg/kg PO q24h) for another week. Follow up physical and blood examinations after one week showed no abnormalities. No *Anaplasma* morulae were detected on the blood smear at this time. The owner reported that the dog had a normal appetite, but was not yet completely returned to normal activity. However, on telephone consultation 25 days after the initial visit, the owner reported that the dog was now completely normal.

Fig. 12.21 The 5-year-old Basset Griffon Vendeen in case study 2.

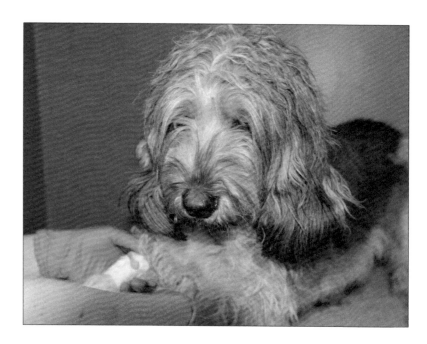

Chapter 13

Rickettsial Infections

Casey Barton Behravesh
Robert Massung

INTRODUCTION

Rickettsia species are gram-negative, obligate intracellular microorganisms with a global distribution. Serologically and pathogenically distinct members of the genus *Rickettsia* exist throughout the world and cause febrile exanthems in people. Rickettsial infections are transmitted by ticks, fleas or mites.

TICK-TRANSMITTED RICKETTSIAL INFECTIONS

In the western hemisphere, *Rickettsia rickettsii*, the most important and most pathogenic organism and a member of the spotted fever group (SFG) of *Rickettsia*, causes Rocky Mountain spotted fever (RMSF). This disease is important as a potentially fatal illness in people, and dogs are known to be similarly affected. Naturally occurring disease has not been reported in cats. *Dermacentor andersoni* and *D. variabilis* ticks have been defined traditionally as the vectors for transmission of *R. rickettsii* in North America. More recently, *Rhipicephalus sanguineus*, the brown dog tick, was found to be important for transmission in parts of the state of Arizona and along the USA–Mexico border. *R. sanguineus* is also known to be involved in transmission of RMSF in Mexico and South America. Additionally, several other tick species of the genus *Amblyomma* are recognized as vectors of *R. rickettsii* from Mexico to Argentina, including *A. cajennense*, *A. aureolatum* and *A. imitator*. Other closely related members of the SFG in North America include *R. montanensis*, *R. rhipicephali*, *R. bellii* and *R. canada*. Of these, only *R. montanensis* has been linked to human disease. However, these have been suggested to produce subclinical infections in dogs and *R. canada* may have some virulence.

In other parts of the world, similar SFG *Rickettsia* and tick–reservoir cycles exist. *R. conorii*, which causes Boutonneuse or Mediterranean spotted fever, is an analogous organism to *R. rickettsii* and is found in parts of Europe, Asia and Africa. It is primarily transmitted by dog ticks of the genus *Rhipicephalus*, and dogs and rodents are the chief animal reservoirs. Dogs appear to have subclinical infection, but they may facilitate transport of ticks and serve as reservoir hosts for infection of humans. Although infection of dogs by *R. massiliae* has been suggested based on serological results, the agent has yet to be detected by polymerase chain reaction (PCR) or isolated from dogs. African tick bite fever (*R. africae*), *R. parkeri* rickettsiosis, Queensland tick typhus (*R. australis*), Flinder's Island spotted fever (*R. honei*), Astrakhan fever (Astrakhan fever rickettsia), Japanese spotted fever (*R. japonica*), North Asian tick typhus (*R. sibirica*) and unnamed European rickettsioses (*R. helvetica*, *R. mongolotimonae* and *R. slovaca*) are diseases of humans caused by other SFG rickettsiae and transmitted by arthropods in geographically distinct regions. The clinical significance in, or reservoir status of, dogs or cats for these infections has not been determined.

In this section, RMSF is emphasized as the model disease for tick-transmitted rickettsioses because it is the most severe infection caused by tick-borne rickettsiae in dogs. It is important for human and animal health care providers to be aware of tick vectors present in their areas as well as those in areas where their patients may have travelled.

TICK INFECTION AND TRANSMISSION

Ticks may acquire infection with *R. rickettsii* by the transovarial route or by feeding on dogs or other animals that have sufficient rickettsaemia to allow transmission. Infected ticks maintain the infection transstadially and can pass *R. rickettsii* to progeny transovarially. Therefore, the disease becomes established in a given geographical region. Despite the presence of adequate hosts and ticks, *R. rickettsii*-infected ticks are limited to a small proportion of ticks in the overall population within an area. This is caused by the deleterious effects that the organism has on tick metabolism and antagonism or immunity from co-infecting non-pathogenic rickettsiae. In addition to the low prevalence of infection, *R. rickettsii* organisms in infected ticks are not immediately infectious, but reactivate their virulence following tick attachment and uptake of a blood meal. Generally, attachment periods of 5–20 hours are required for successful transmission.

PATHOGENESIS

Once *R. rickettsii* are inoculated into the body, they enter the bloodstream and infect and replicate in endothelial cells. A widespread vasculitis occurs, as the organisms cause endothelial necrosis and spread to infect new endothelial cells. Vascular injury leads to activation of the coagulation and fibrinolytic pathways. Platelet consumption and destruction can be caused by coagulatory and immune-mediated mechanisms, respectively. In serious or long-standing untreated cases, organ systems with end-arterial circulation (e.g. the skin, brain, heart and kidneys) may develop multiple foci of necrosis. Severe organ failure occurs less commonly in dogs than in people. Vascular injury leads to leakage of intravascular fluids into extracellular fluid spaces and resultant oedema formation. Fluid accumulation in tissues such as the central nervous system (CNS) can cause significant brain oedema, resulting in a progressive mental and cardiorespiratory depression.

CLINICAL SIGNS

In dogs, RMSF manifests with fever, lethargy, decreased appetite, tremors, scleral injection, maculopapular rash on ears and exposed skin and petechial lesions on mucous membranes. Most dogs develop illness during the warmer months of the year when the tick vectors are most active; however, this seasonality is less noticeable at lower latitudes. Fever is one of the most consistent signs of illness. It may develop within several days after tick exposure and is associated with lethargy, mental dullness and inappetence (**Figure 13.1**). Animals develop a stiff gait and show arthralgia and myalgia, as demonstrated by difficulty in rising and eventual reluctance to walk. Lymphadenomegaly of all peripheral lymph nodes is apparent (**Figure 13.2**). Hyperaemia of mucosal surfaces and subcutaneous oedema develop (**Figures 13.3, 13.4**) and in severely affected animals, dermal necrosis ensues (**Figure 13.5**). Scrotal oedema may occur in male dogs (**Figure 13.4**).

Macropapular skin rash can occur in exposed areas of skin starting with the ears and spreading to the trunk and limbs (**Figure 13.6A**). In contrast to the disease in people, dogs develop petechial haemorrhages infrequently, and when they do the distribution is generally on the mucous membranes including the gums and buccal mucosa (**Figure 13.6B**). Fine petechiae on the

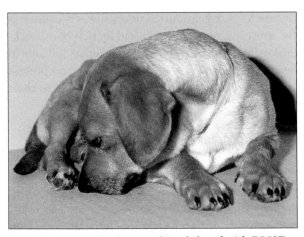

Fig. 13.1 Mentally depressed Dachshund with RMSF. (Courtesy C.E. Greene)

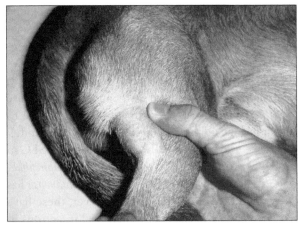

Fig. 13.2 Enlarged popliteal lymph node of a Dachshund with systemic manifestations of RMSF. (Courtesy C.E. Greene)

Fig. 13.3 Subcutaneous oedema of the limb of a mixed breed dog with RMSF. (Courtesy C.E. Greene)

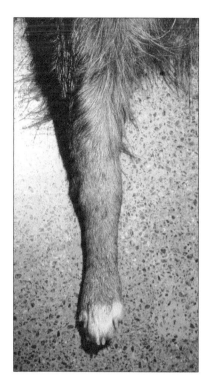

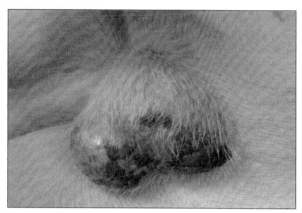

Fig. 13.4 Scrotal oedema in a dog with RMSF (Courtesy M.L. Levin)

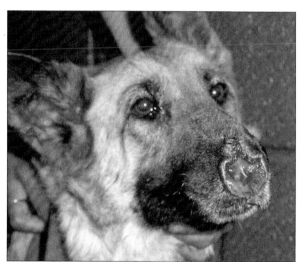

Fig. 13.5 Necrosis of the planum nasale in a German Shepherd Dog with RMSF. (Courtesy C.E. Greene)

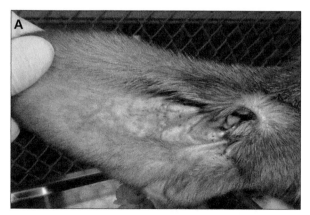

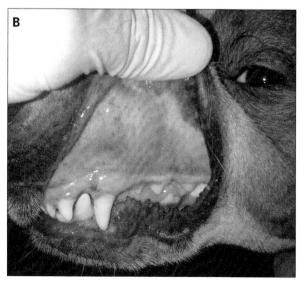

Figs. 13.6A, B (A) Maculopapular rash on the ear of a dog with RMSF. (B) Fine petechiae on the lip mucosa of a dog with RMSF. (Courtesy M.L. Levin)

penile mucosa of male dogs may be present (**Figure 13.7**). Vascular injection of the sclera (**Figure 13.8**) with petechiae in the conjunctiva can occur. Haemorrhages are also found more consistently in the ocular fundus. Overt haemorrhage is rare and found only in the most severely affected animals. Neurological complications often result in animals that suffer a delay in diagnosis and treatment. These are caused by meningitis and can include hyperaesthesia, seizures, vestibular dysfunction and a variety of manifestations depending on the lesion localization. Necrosis of the extremities (acryl gangrene) or disseminated intravascular coagulation (DIC) can develop in severely affected dogs. Recovery is rapid and complete in those animals receiving treatment with appropriate antibiotics early, before the onset of organ damage or neurological complications. Once the neurological signs have developed, recovery is delayed or deficits may be permanent.

DIAGNOSIS

Clinical laboratory findings are non-specific for a generalized acute-phase inflammatory reaction. Leucopenia in the acute stages is followed by a moderate leucocytosis and stress leucogram. A left shift and toxic granulation of neutrophils may be observed in animals with the most severe tissue necrosis. Thrombocytopenia is one of the most consistent laboratory findings.

Coagulation times are usually within normal limits unless dogs develop overt DIC. Serum biochemical abnormalities include hypoalbuminaemia, elevated serum ALP activity and variable hyponatraemia and hyperbilirubinaemia. Analysis of cerebrospinal fluid may reveal a mild increase in protein and a neutrophil pleocytosis. Cell counts are increased in joint fluid, with a predominance of neutrophils. Results of tests for autoimmunity are usually negative, with the exception of platelet autoantibody. Electrocardiographic testing may show conduction disturbances related to myocarditis. Thoracic radiography may show a diffuse increase in pulmonary interstitial density.

The indirect immunofluorescence antibody test (IFAT) is used by most laboratories to determine specific IgG and IgM serum antibodies. When IgM levels are not increased in the initial sample, the most definitive results are obtained by measuring convalescent IgG in sera, collected after a 2–3 week interval. Seronegative results on the first sample do not eliminate the possibility of infection, and a subsequent serum sample should be taken under these conditions. Although inter-laboratory variation exists in measured antibody titres, high IgG levels (e.g. a titre of ≥1,024) generally indicate exposure within the last year and may be presumed to indicate recent infection if clinical signs are compatible. A fourfold or greater increase in IgG level in the convalescent sample relative to the acute sample

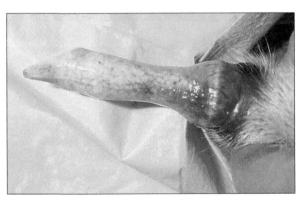

Fig. 13.7 Fine petechiae on the penile mucosa of a dog with RMSF. (Courtesy C.E. Greene)

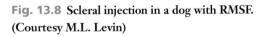

Fig. 13.8 Scleral injection in a dog with RMSF. (Courtesy M.L. Levin)

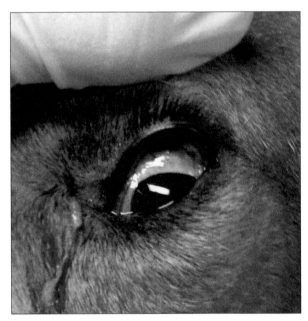

Table 13.1 Drug therapy for treatment of spotted fever group rickettsial infections.

DRUG	DOSE (MG/KG)	ROUTE	FREQUENCY (HOURS)	DURATION (DAYS)
Doxycycline	5–10	PO, IV	12	10–21
Tetracycline	22	PO	8	14
Chloramphenicol	15–30	PO, IV	8	7

confirms an infection. Both IgM and IgG levels may remain elevated for months or longer after the disease has resolved. Additionally, elevated IgM or IgG levels may be detected in dogs that were previously exposed to antigenically related organisms.

Direct immunolabelling of tissues has been used for clinical or postmortem diagnosis of RMSF. Full-thickness skin biopsy samples have been submitted to detect the presence of the rickettsiae in dermal blood vessels. This method allows for rapid confirmation of infection; however, it is not widely available. Molecular detection methods (e.g. PCR) have been used to identify rickettsiae in blood or tissue specimens, and are increasing in availability and sensitivity. Rickettsial isolation is technically difficult and involves a significant risk for infection, and should only be done in high biocontainment (≥biosafety level 3) facilities. At necropsy examination, pathological lesions include petechial and ecchymotic haemorrhages throughout all body tissues, lymphadenomegaly and splenomegaly. Microscopically, widespread necrotizing vasculitis occurs in many organs.

TREATMENT

Untreated RMSF is a highly fatal disease in both people and dogs. Because of the delay in obtaining antibody titres for laboratory confirmation, empirical treatment should be instituted whenever the disease is suspected. Tetracyclines are the antibiotics of choice and treatment should be for 1–3 weeks depending on the dosage (**Table 13.1**). Doxycycline is the recommended treatment for RMSF in people and in dogs of all ages. Appropriate antibiotic therapy with doxycycline of a sufficient dose and duration is crucial for the prevention of RMSF relapses in dogs.

If doxycycline is not readily available, other options for antibiotics to treat dogs with suspected RMSF include tetracycline or chloramphenicol. Tetracycline is reported to be as effective as the more lipid-soluble doxycycline, because intracellular penetration is not essential to eliminate the organism. Chloramphenicol should only be used as a last resort since use of this antimicrobial can be associated with higher rates of fatal outcome in human patients. Adequate supportive care must be provided if the dog has evidence of dehydration, kidney failure, shock or a haemorrhagic diathesis. Negative samples from initial serological testing should not be considered as a reason to stop antimicrobial therapy, since antibodies may take more than a week to develop in acute cases. Additionally, early therapy may delay or suppress the rise in antibody titre of convalescent samples. Fluid therapy must be restricted because of the danger of causing more oedema in the CNS. Appropriate antibiotics should be administered as soon as disease is suspected, and antibiotics are only effective if they are instituted prior to the onset of tissue necrosis or organ failure. The response to treatment, as noted by a reduction in body temperature and improvement in clinical illness, is apparent typically within 24–48 hours if the diagnosis is correct. Supportive care is needed in dogs with hypotension, coagulopathy or evidence of organ dysfunction. Based on experimental studies where dogs were infected with RMSF via tick bites, the best indicator to mark the beginning of a dog's recovery and to predict a favourable outcome is the apex and subsequent subsidence of neutrophilia, even despite the continuing persistence of mucosal petechiae and rash. Therefore, differential blood cell counts should be monitored continuously in dogs during RMSF treatment because it is recommended that treatment continue at least until the total white blood cell, neutrophil, lymphocyte and monocyte counts return to their normal range.

Recovery from infection is associated with protective immunity against infection with the same rickettsial species. Vaccines are not available commercially, although experimental vaccines have been shown to be protective against severe or prolonged infection.

Vaccines containing outer membrane proteins have produced protection against challenge infection in experimental animals. However, no vaccine is currently licensed for the prevention of tick-borne rickettsial diseases in dogs.

A single human case of RMSF transmission was documented through a blood transfusion; this should be considered when selecting canine blood donors. Direct transmission of *R. rickettsii* from dogs to people has not been reported and transmission typically requires a tick bite. One exception, though uncommon, is that human infection may occur after contact of abraded skin or conjunctiva with tick haemolymph or excreta during removal of infected engorged ticks from pets. Gloves should be worn when removing ticks from potentially infectious dogs as the ticks may contain live rickettsial agents. Removed ticks should not be crushed between the fingers to prevent contamination and potential infection through skin abrasions. When possible, the tick bite site should be cleansed with soap and water following tick removal.

ZOONOTIC POTENTIAL AND PUBLIC HEALTH SIGNIFICANCE

RMSF is an important zoonotic disease because of the potential for fatal outcome in humans if effective treatment is absent or delayed. Dogs may serve as sentinels for RMSF in human populations. Additionally, dogs may serve as transport hosts by carrying infected ticks into closer proximity with humans in household settings; this can lead to establishment of a focus of infection at or near the home environment. RMSF is a significant public health concern because of the potential for household clustering and large urban outbreaks, particularly in areas with transmission by brown dog ticks.

Infection rate and seasonality in the dog parallels these parameters in people, as both species are exposed to the same ticks in the environment. Dogs and their owners may be infected with RMSF simultaneously by a common exposure in areas where *Rickettsia*-infected ticks are present. Canine RMSF infections have been repeatedly associated with an increased risk of the disease in pet owners in the same household environment. One example of household clustering occurred when two dogs died, followed by their owner dying, all within a 3-week period. The two dogs had tick infesta-

tions and clinical signs consistent with RMSF before their death, but were not tested for the disease due to economic reasons. The owner became ill 2 weeks after the second dog died, was hospitalized and subsequently died with the presumed cause of death as cerebral oedema secondary to RMSF; the owner was confirmed to have RMSF through postmortem diagnostic testing. Four days after the owner died, two additional dogs from the household became ill, were hospitalized and were treated with doxycycline. These two dogs, both of which had tick infestations, were confirmed as having RMSF by their veterinarian; they survived after appropriate treatment with doxycycline. Documentation of a tick-borne rickettsial disease in a dog should prompt veterinary professionals to warn pet owners about the risk of tick-borne disease in household members and to seek consultation with a physician when potential human illnesses are suspected in order to guide prompt treatment and facilitate confirming a diagnosis.

Although clinical disease can occur in both dogs and humans, the involvement of a required intermediate tick vector for transmission means that dogs do not pose a direct transmission risk to people in normal circumstances. Serological studies of dogs in emerging areas may help predict human risk of infection because dogs generally have greater exposure to ticks than humans, and infection in dogs indicates a heightened risk of human infections related to tick exposures in shared environments. Particularly in areas with transmission by the brown dog tick, close cooperation using a One Health approach between animal, human and environmental health officials is critical to the prevention and control of RMSF.

PREVENTION AND CONTROL

Avoiding tick bites and promptly removing attached ticks on people and pets remain the best disease prevention strategies. Tick checks should be performed on people and pets after being outdoors and especially in known tick areas. Pets should be checked routinely for ticks because they have the potential to carry ticks back to their home environment, which increases the risk of human exposure to ticks. Veterinary professionals should advise pet owners to check dogs, other pets and household members routinely for ticks. Several hours elapse before ticks attach and transmit pathogens; therefore, frequent tick checks on people and pets are important to increase the likelihood of finding and removing ticks before they transmit a pathogen. Attached ticks should be removed immediately, preferably by grasping the tick with tweezers or fine-tipped forceps close to the skin and gently pulling with constant pressure. Additionally, people should apply tick repellents when spending time in tick-infested areas. Regular use of pet ectoparasite control products, such as topical acaricides, tick collars and acaricidal shampoos, can help reduce the risk for human exposure to ticks. Additionally, prevention is enhanced by the strict control of tick vectors on dogs and properly timed treatment of the environment with acaricides.

FLEA-TRANSMITTED RICKETTSIAL INFECTIONS

Two causes of flea-transmitted human typhus are now recognized: *Rickettsia typhi*, which is transmitted by rodent fleas and has a worldwide distribution; and *R. felis*, which has been identified in cats, dogs and in cat fleas (*Ctenocephalides felis*) and is found in the Americas, Africa, Asia, Australia and Europe. In endemic areas of the USA, peri-urban opossums are major reservoir hosts for *R. felis*, but the reservoir potential of cats and dogs has not yet been determined. In North America, *R. typhi* infections have been found in fleas and people in the same geographical areas where *R. felis* exists, although co-infection is not common.

Experimental infection of cats with *R. felis* has been demonstrated, as has seropositivity to *R. typhi*. Cats infected with *R. felis* by repeat exposure to feeding fleas develop a subclinical illness with an incubation period of 2–4 months. However, the pathogenic potential of natural infection with either rickettsial species in dogs and cats is unknown. What is known is that cats and dogs will transport *Ct. felis* into domestic surroundings and, as transovarial and transstadial transmission of *R. felis* has been demonstrated, a domestic focus of infection for humans could be established.

MITE-TRANSMITTED RICKETTSIAL INFECTION

Rickettsia akari is the agent of rickettsialpox, a febrile and vesicular disease in humans. It is a self-limiting zoonotic disease, which may occur worldwide. Limited information is available on *Rickettsia akari* in companion animals. One severe canine case of *Rickettsia akari* infection has been documented in Mexico. Additionally, seroprevalence studies of dogs in New York, and dogs and cats in Japan, identified antibodies for *Rickettsia akari*. The clinical significance in, or reservoir status of, dogs or cats for *Rickettsia akari* has not yet been determined.

FURTHER READING

Drexler N, Miller M, Gerding J *et al.* (2014) Community-based control of the brown dog tick in a region with high rates of Rocky Mountain spotted fever, 2012–2013. *PLoS One* **9**:e112368.

Elchos BN, Goddard J (2003) Implications of presumptive fatal Rocky Mountain spotted fever in two dogs and their owner. *Journal of the American Veterinary Medical Association* **223**:1450–1452.

Levin ML, Killmaster LF, Zemtsova GE *et al.* (2014) Clinical presentation, convalescence, and relapse of Rocky Mountain spotted fever in dogs experimentally infected via tick bite. *PLoS One* **9**:e115105.

Paddock CD, Brenner O, Vaid C *et al.* (2002) Short report: concurrent Rocky Mountain spotted fever in a dog and its owner. *American Journal of Tropical Medicine and Hygiene* **66**:197–199.

Parola P, Paddock CD, Socolovschi C *et al.* (2013) Update on tick-borne rickettsioses around the world: a geographic approach. *Clinical Microbiology Reviews* **26**:657–702. Erratum in: *Clinical Microbiology Reviews* **27**:166.

Martin Pfeffer
Michael Leschnik
Gerhard Dobler

RARE BACTERIAL INFECTIONS IN DOGS AND CATS

TULARAEMIA

Background, aetiology and epidemiology

Tularaemia is a zoonotic disease caused by the bacterium *Francisella tularensis*. There are several subtypes of the bacterium; however, the most important subtypes causing human disease are *Francisella tularensis tularensis*, occurring exclusively in North America, and *Francisella tularensis holarctica*, which occurs in the Eurasian northern hemisphere. The natural transmission cycle involves mainly small rodents (e.g. voles, mice and lemmings); however, other rodents and lagomorphs may be infected and may develop a fatal infection.

Pathogenesis, clinical signs and diagnosis

Dogs appear to be relatively resistant to infection with *F. tularensis* senso lato. Occasional reports of natural infection of dogs with the subtype *F. tularensis tularensis* exist and infections of hunting dogs with *F. tularensis holarctica* are documented. In Norway, a 1.5-year-old Hamilton Hound developed non-specific lethargy, pyrexia (>39.5°C), loss of appetite, vomiting and abdominal pain 2 days after contact with an infected mountain hare. Physical examination of this dog revealed enlargement of the pharyngeal, prescapular and popliteal lymph nodes. There were no abnormalities on haematological or serum biochemical screening. The mild clinical signs lasted for a few days and the dog recovered spontaneously.

Tularaemia is also rare in cats. Symptomatic feline tularaemia is most often detected after contact with humans and human infection is reported to occur after cat bites. Seroprevalence rates of 12–24% in some endemic areas of the USA imply a high rate of subclinical or mild clinical forms, which might not be recognized as tularaemia. The clinical signs may range from a mild localized infection (ulceroglandular form) to acute fatal disease (typhoidal form). Kittens usually present with more severe signs than adult cats. The ulceroglandular form is characterized by chronically draining subcutaneous abscesses or ulceration of the oral cavity. The systemic (typhoidal) form presents with pyrexia, marked depression, enlargement of lymph nodes, splenomegaly and hepatomegaly and jaundice. Haematological abnormalities include leucocytosis, panleukopenia or thrombocytopenia. Serum biochemistry may reveal increased serum ALT and ALP activities and hyperbilirubinaemia.

Diagnosis can be made in the acute stage of infection by cultivation of bacteria or by molecular detection of organisms in biopsy samples of lymph node or ulcerated oral mucosa. Antibodies against *F. tularensis* may be detected by an indirect immunofluorescent antibody test (IFAT) or by haemagglutination testing. A fourfold increase in titre may be indicative of an acute infection; however, antibodies may only occur up to 3 weeks after acute infection. In antibody-positive animals culture and molecular detection is no longer possible, because by this time the organism will have been eliminated from the animal.

Treatment and control

Treatment of tularaemia in dogs and cats is similar to treatment for human patients. Aminoglycosides (e.g. gentamicin) are the antibiotics of choice. According to limited information, doxycycline or fluoroquinolones may also be used in cases where there are contraindications for administration of gentamicin. Application of acaricides will help to prevent tick- and flea-transmitted tularaemia in companion animals.

Zoonotic potential/public health significance

Humans can be infected by direct contact with infected rodents and hares (e.g. during skinning), by eating or drinking contaminated or uncooked meat from hares and by inhaling contaminated dust. Arthropods (e.g. mosquitoes, ticks and horse flies) may transmit the bacteria to humans while taking a blood meal. A recent study found that almost half of human cases of tularaemia in Nebraska, USA, recorded between 1998 and 2012, were cat-associated. The North American subtype is highly infectious and pathogenic for humans and was tested as a potential bioweapon. The European/Asian subtype shows lower pathogenicity for humans and fatal cases are unusual.

PLAGUE

Background, aetiology and epidemiology

Plague is a zoonotic bacterial disease caused by *Yersinia pestis*. It is maintained in nature principally by transmission among rodent populations by fleas. Fleas also play a major role in the transmission of plague to humans. Because of their hunting behaviour, dogs and cats may become infected with *Yersinia pestis* and play a role in the transmission of plague bacteria to humans. The significance of this route of transmission may have been underestimated in the past.

Pathogenesis and clinical signs

Cats may develop clinical forms of plague similar to the human disease (i.e. bubonic and pneumonic forms). After the bite of an infected flea, *Y. pestis* infects macrophages, which accumulate in the closest draining lymph node, leading to visible and painful lymphadenitis (a 'bubo'). Bacteria may be released from here to cause a bacteraemia, which in turn leads to pneumonic plague or dissemination to other organs. The pneumonic form of plague may also develop directly after ingestion or, more frequently, inhalation of the bacterium. The latter cases develop more rapidly and have a more severe clinical presentation. The window of time in which to successfully treat these patients is shorter than that for bubonic plague. In a description of 119 cases of plague in cats in California, more than half of the naturally infected cats developed bubonic plague with high fever and purulent lymphadenitis and 10% developed the pneumonic form

of the disease. Even more important was the observation that 20% of the cats had a subclinical form of disease. In 75% of these infected cats, *Y. pestis* could be isolated from pharyngeal swabs and some of these culture-positive cats were asymptomatic. In a study of 16 experimentally infected cats, the outcomes were fatal disease (38%), transient illness and recovery (44%) or subclinical infection (19%).

Dogs appear to be less susceptible to plague than cats; however, there are a number of descriptions of clinical plague in dogs. In a study describing 62 canine cases of plague in New Mexico, all of the sick dogs were pyrexic and most of them (97%) showed lethargy, but lymphadenomegaly (23%), vomiting (13%), diarrhoea (2%) or abscesses (2%) were observed rarely. Fatality appears to be uncommon. A number of infections with *Y. pestis* in dogs may be subclinical, as a study from China showed antibodies against the specific F1-antigen in 22% of dogs tested in known endemic areas.

Diagnosis

Suspected cases with bubos can be diagnosed when the bacteria are identified in lymph node aspirates by culture, Gram stain or polymerase chain reaction (PCR) testing. Pulmonary lesions may be detected by thoracic radiology, but caution should be taken in any suspected plague case while handling and treating the animal. The bacteria are highly contagious and safety measures should be implemented at each stage, including the shipment of diagnostic samples to the laboratory and notification of health officials (see below).

Treatment and control

Y. pestis is sensitive to most antibiotics, but the most commonly used is doxycyline, which should be given for at least 3 weeks. Doxycycline may also be used preventively in free-roaming cats when plague cases are noticed in the area. The decision as to whether to treat an infected cat depends on how the cat is kept in the household and the risk of transmission of the infection to the owner. As no vaccines are available for cats or dogs, ectoparasitic control is the key in preventing plague in companion animals.

Zoonotic potential/public health significance

Cats are a direct source of infection for humans and may transmit the pathogens by the aerosol route, shedding the bacteria in nasal fluid. Cats may also transport infected rodent fleas from ill or dead rodents to humans and therefore may serve as vehicles for the vector and reservoir of plague bacteria, the rodent fleas. About 8% of all registered human cases of plague were associated with cats in one study. Dogs are probably less likely than cats to be involved in transmission to humans, but one study showed that plague patients were significantly more likely to sleep with dogs in their beds. However it is unclear whether there is direct transmission of the bacterium from dogs to humans via aerosol transmission or if transmission involves direct contact, which may facilitate the transition of infected fleas to humans. In humans the infection may be bubonic or, more rarely, pneumonic or presenting as meningitis. Patients with pneumonic plague may transmit the pathogen by aerosol infection to other patients who will again develop the pneumonic form of disease. Pneumonic and meningitic plague follows bacteraemia when localized bubos release the bacteria into blood or lymphatic vessels. While treatment of bubonic plague may be successful, these cases can have fatality rates as high as 80%. Plague is a notifiable disease in most countries in the world.

COXIELLOSIS/Q FEVER

Background, aetiology, epidemiology and zoonotic significance

Coxiella burnetii is an obligate intracellular, gram-negative bacterium. In cats and dogs the bacterium produces subclinical infection, but in humans it causes Q fever, a disease associated with fever, arthralgia, myalgia, hepatitis and respiratory signs. A wide range of wild and domesticated animals can be infected, but only domestic ruminants are considered to be common reservoirs for human infection. In wildlife reservoir cycles, *C. burnetii* is arthropod-transmitted, mostly by ticks. In addition, the sporulated form of *C. burnetii* is highly resistant to environmental extremes and can be spread between hosts by ingestion or aerosol dissemination of infected fluids (e.g. milk, urine or vaginal/uterine secretions) or by ingestion of infected tissues (e.g. placental material). Infected cats are considered to be important reservoirs for human coxiellosis. *C. burnetii* appears to be carried frequently in the vagina of healthy cats in endemic areas and contact with infected parturient cats is a risk factor for human infection.

Seropositivity to *C. burnetii* is reported at 16–20% of populations of stray and companion cats in the USA, Canada and Japan, while lower seroprevalences are reported from Africa. A seropositivity rate of 21.8% was recently reported from Australia. Cross-reactivity between *C. burnetii* and *Bartonella henselae* has been reported in human studies and although this has not been investigated in cats, it may inflate seroprevalence figures for *Coxiella*.

Reports of *Coxiella* infections in dogs are very scarce, but dogs may be involved temporarily during outbreak situations. In one report, a dog was responsible for a family cluster of Q fever cases in Canada and in two other studies dogs were found to be PCR positive or culture positive during Q fever endemics in Brazil and the Netherlands.

Diagnosis

Diagnosis of active infection with *Coxiella* is made by demonstration of a rising antibody titre, PCR or immunohistochemical techniques on tissue biopsy samples.

Treatment and control

Treatment of cats may be required in households where there is increased risk of human infection. *Coxiella* infections are variably susceptible to single agent therapy for 2–4 weeks with macrolides (e.g. erythromycin, azithromycin), potentiated sulphonamides or fluoroquinolones. Combination therapy of doxycycline and fluoroquinolones with rifampicin may be more effective. Clinical infections in cats should be treated with tetracyclines and chloramphenicol. *C. burnetii* is shed in extremely high doses when infected ruminants give birth or abort, as the bacterium has a tropism for the uterus and the placenta. Therefore, gloves and masks should be worn and the development of a spore-containing aerosol should be prevented. There are no vaccines licensed for cats or dogs.

'CANDIDATUS NEOEHRLICHIA MIKURENSIS'

'*Candidatus* Neoehrlichia mikurensis' (Rickettsiales, 'Anaplasmataceae') is a tick-borne pathogen that should be mentioned briefly, although there is only a single case report of canine infection. This 8-year-old dog displayed lethargy, mild anaemia, thrombocytopenia and profuse subcutaneous haemorrhage after ovariohysterectomy and removal of the mammary glands. Treatment with high-dose doxycycline for 4 weeks resulted in a full recovery. 'Candidatus N. mikurensis' has been described only recently, but has not yet been cultured *in vitro*, although PCR can readily detect DNA from the organism. It is a zoonotic bacterium, causing sometimes fatal infections in people with underlying diseases and/ or immunosuppression. Only ticks of the genus *Ixodes* have thus far been found to harbour this pathogen, with prevalences of 1.7% reported in France and 26.6% in Germany. Many small mammal species, mainly rodents, tested positive for this bacterium suggesting that they may function not only as a blood source for the blood-feeding ticks, but also as a reservoir host for the bacterium. Recently, transplacental infection of rodent fetuses was demonstrated, further substantiating the reservoir role of rodents for the organism.

RARE VIRAL INFECTIONS IN DOGS AND CATS

ALPHAVIRUS INFECTIONS

Alphaviruses comprise a genus in the family Togaviridae. The genus contains some 30 different recognized viruses. Alphaviruses are enveloped viruses with a size of about 70 nm. The viral nucleocapsid is formed in an icosahedral structure and contains positive-strand RNA of about 11,000 nucleotides in length.

Most alphaviruses are transmitted in a natural transmission cycle between arthropods (e.g. mosquitoes or bugs) and vertebrates (e.g. rodents, birds, ungulates or humans). Many of the known alphaviruses cause mild (febrile) to severe (encephalitis) disease in humans and animals and are of medical and veterinary importance. Only a few alphaviruses are known to infect dogs or cats, namely eastern equine encephalitis (EEE) virus and Venezuelan equine encephalitis (VEE) virus.

EASTERN EQUINE ENCEPHALITIS
There are anecdotal reports of infections of EEE virus infection in dogs. In a study of causes of encephalitis in dogs in southern Georgia, USA, 12 out of 101 dogs with neurological diseases showed infection with EEE virus. The virus was detected by molecular methods and/or by virus isolation from the brain. All of the dogs were puppies aged 10 days to 6 months and were of

different breeds. Clinically, the dogs presented with fever, anorexia and diarrhoea and a range of neurological signs including recumbency, nystagmus, depression and seizures. Histologically, inflammation was found in the cerebral cortices and midbrains of all affected dogs. No information on haematological changes was given. There is no information about EEE infection of cats.

VENEZUELAN EQUINE ENCEPHALITIS
Infections with VEE virus in dogs are described rarely. One study showed that Beagle dogs (aged 12–18 months) infected experimentally with two different strains of VEE virus (attenuated and unmodified Trinidad donkey strain, subtype IA) developed viraemia high enough to re-infect blood-sucking mosquitoes. All of these dogs developed a leucopenia. Some dogs infected with the original Trinidad donkey virus strain exhibited fever and showed aggression at the time of peak viraemia. No other clinical signs were observed. However, two dogs succumbed at 58 and 70 days post infection, respectively, and VEE virus was isolated from their brains. Beagle dogs infected experimentally by mosquitoes (*Aedes triseriatus*) all showed pyrexia (1–5 days post infection), leucopenia and lymphopenia (2–4 days post infection) and decreased haematocrit (4–5 days post infection). No clinical disease or fatal cases were observed in that study. Experimental studies have not yet investigated whether VEE virus can infect dogs of other breeds or ages; however, there is some evidence of subclinical infection of military and domestic dogs with Everglades virus (formerly VEE virus subtype II), which showed that the dogs developed antibodies against Everglades virus, but did not develop any clinical signs. There is no evidence of subclinical or clinical infection of VEE virus in cats.

FLAVIVIRUS INFECTIONS

Flaviviruses comprise a genus in the family Flaviviridae that contains more than 70 different viruses and virus subtypes. Flaviviruses are enveloped viruses with a virion measuring approximately 70 nm. The viral nucleocapsid is formed in an icosahedral structure and contains a single positive-strand RNA of about 11,000 nucleotides.

Flaviviruses are transmitted in a natural transmission cycle between arthropods (e.g. mosquitoes or ticks) and vertebrates (e.g. rodents, birds, ungulates or humans) or by rodents or bats. Recently, a group of flaviviruses was detected that seem to occur only in mosquitoes. Their role in pathogenesis is unclear. Many of the known flaviviruses cause severe diseases (e.g. haemorrhagic fever, encephalitis) in humans and animals and are of global medical and veterinary importance. Some flaviviruses are known to infect dogs or cats and may occasionally lead to severe and fatal disease (e.g. tick-borne encephalitis [TBE] virus).

TICK-BORNE ENCEPHALITIS
Background, aetiology and epidemiology
TBE is the most important viral tick-borne disease in humans in Europe and Asia, with up to 10,000 human cases per year. The disease is caused by TBE virus (TBEV), which is a member of the tick-borne group in the family Flaviviridae. There are three subtypes of TBEV: the European type, the Siberian type and the Far

Eastern type, which are prevalent in different but partially overlapping geographical areas (**Figure 14.1**) and cause neurological syndromes of different severity and with different rates of chronic neurological sequelae.

TBEV is transmitted in a natural transmission cycle, consisting of ticks, the vectors of TBEV, and rodents, which act as reservoir hosts for the virus. *Ixodes ricinus* (European subtype) and *Ixodes persulcatus* (Siberian and Far Eastern subtypes) are the main vectors of the three TBEV subtypes. Infected ticks may have lifelong infection and transmit the TBEV to the next developmental stage (i.e. transstadial persistence), while only minor transovarial transmission is recognized. Other tick species (e.g. *Dermacentor reticulatus*) may play a role in transmitting TBEV in some localized areas. TBEV is distributed over large areas of Central Europe, Northern Europe (i.e. Scandinavia and Russia), Eastern Europe, Southeastern Europe, in Asia along the so-

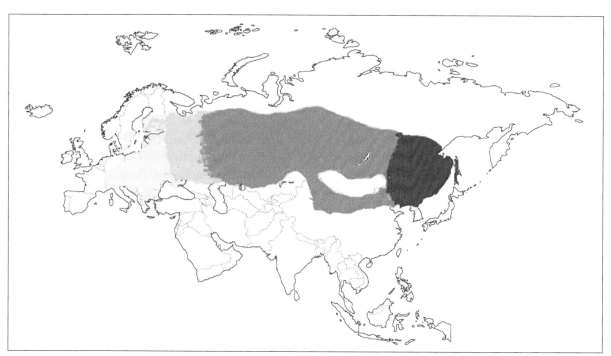

Fig. 14.1 Geographical distribution of the three different tick-borne encephalitis (TBE) virus subtypes in Eurasia. In Western Europe, only the European subtype TBE virus (yellow), transmitted by *Ixodes ricinus*, is found. Moving east, there is a mixed zone where the European and Siberian subtype TBE virus (ochre) is present. In central Asia, the Siberian subtype TBE virus (orange), transmitted by the Taiga tick *Ixodes persulcatus*, predominates but is not the exclusive TBE virus subtype. As suggested, the Far Eastern subtype TBE virus (red) follows eastwards to the Pacific coast and Japan. This map gives an approximate picture of the so-called TBE belt, but the European TBE virus subtype has, for example, also been documented in Japan.

called 'Taiga Belt' up to China and the Northern Japanese islands (**Figure 14.1**).

Both tick species involved in the transmission cycle in nature, *I. ricinus* and *I. persulcatus*, are found as ectoparasites on dogs. Despite the high frequency of tick infestation, dogs appear to be very resistant to clinical illness after TBEV infection, although the virus can infect dogs and also cause neurological disease. There are a number of canine cases of TBEV infection described.

Pathogenesis and clinical signs

No studies on the pathogenesis of TBEV in dogs are available. In humans it is thought that after a tick bite the TBEV replicates locally in dendritic cells and possibly in lymphocytes. The TBEV will then spread in the body and may infect the reticuloendothelial cells of the liver, spleen and lymph nodes. There, a first virus replication takes place, causing a viraemia. This phase in humans is often accompanied by febrile and systemic symptoms ('summer flu'). After this primary virus replication, the virus, in a low percentage (10–20%) of patients, enters the brain and causes neurological disorders (i.e. meningitis, encephalitis or myelitis) with minor or major neurological symptoms that reflect the chronic sequelae of infection.

The clinical signs in dogs usually start with an elevated body temperature. Ill dogs show signs of paralysis (tetraparalysis) and changes in behaviour (e.g. denying food, aggressiveness, skittishness or lethargy). In addition to these non-specific changes, dogs may show vestibular signs (e.g. nystagmus), facial nerve paralysis, anisocoria, strabismus, myosis and loss of the palpebral reflex. Experimentally infected puppies of wolves and foxes showed fever, paresis, convulsions and signs of meningoencephalitis. Experimental infection of dog puppies with subcutaneous administration of TBEV did not lead to any clinical signs.

Diagnosis

Haematological findings during neurological infections may include monocytosis, leucopenia and lymphopenia. Analysis of cerebrospinal fluid (CSF) may show monocytosis and lymphocytosis and high protein content, which are typical features of viral encephalitis.

Specific diagnostic procedures are necessary to exclude or confirm TBEV infection. In most cases specific diagnosis is based on serology using a range of techniques including enzyme-linked immunosorbent assay, indirect IFAT or complement fixation and the haemagglutination inhibition test. All of these tests show varying degrees of cross-reactivity with other flaviviruses. The detection of IgM antibody allows classification of the infection as a possible TBEV infection, because cross-reactions of IgM antibodies are not very common. For diagnosing an acute TBEV infection, a significant (fourfold) increase in IgG antibodies must be demonstrated in paired sera taken at least 2 weeks apart. Detection of TBEV antibodies on a single occasion does not indicate an acute infection. The detection of TBEV in CSF or blood during the encephalitic phase of disease is usually not very successful and a negative result does not exclude TBEV infection. For detection and isolation in cell culture or animals, brain material is the clinical material of choice. Viral infection can also be detected in the brain by immunohistochemistry. There is no evidence of clinical disease after TBEV infection in cats.

Treatment and control

No treatment for TBEV infection is available currently. TBE in dogs and humans is treated symptomatically. An important issue is the prevention of secondary harm by the patient itself during convulsions or episodes of aggressive behaviour. The dog owner may also become injured during the encephalitic phase of disease. The use of glucocorticoids is controversial and nonsteroidal anti-inflammatory drugs are most often used to treat the fever. Antibiotics are often given to prevent secondary bacteraemia. The fatality rate of TBE in dogs is high and surviving dogs may take 6–12 months to recover.

Preventive measures include the use of acaricides in endemic areas. There is no licensed vaccine against TBEV for dogs; however, human vaccines have been used successfully in dogs. Vaccination may be considered when dogs live in highly endemic areas and when they attract high numbers of ticks.

LOUPING-ILL

Louping-ill is a disease of sheep and humans caused by louping-ill virus. The virus is also a member of the tick-borne group of the family Flaviviridae. The virus is closely related to, but distinct from, TBEV. The disease is prevalent in parts of the UK, mainly in Scotland, where it has been known for more than 200 years. It is transmitted by *I. ricinus* and the natural transmission cycle appears to involve sheep and possibly red grouse. In humans it causes a severe form of encephalitis.

Louping-ill virus infections are reported to cause clinical signs in the dog. Descriptions of the canine disease have been made since the 1970s and involve primarily shepherding dogs such as Labrador Retrievers and Collies. Affected dogs show signs of central nervous system (CNS) infection including ataxia, trembling of the forelimbs and clonic spasms. The dogs show also dyspnoea and coughing and loss of appetite. Sometimes, neurological sequelae, such as radial paralysis or altered temperament, occur up to 18 months after the acute disease.

There is no cure for louping-ill encephalitis and only symptomatic treatment is used. In man, TBE vaccines may also protect against infection by louping-ill virus, but there are no data for dogs. There is no evidence that louping-ill virus causes any clinical disease in cats.

POWASSAN ENCEPHALITIS

Powassan virus is the only known flavivirus of the tick-borne group to occur on the American continent. The virus is not closely related to TBEV. Powassan virus and a closely related variant of Powassan virus, deer tick virus, has been identified in Canada (Ontario) and the USA (East Coast states, Colorado). Powassan virus has also been isolated in the Primor'ye District in Far Eastern Russia. Powassan virus has been detected and isolated from ticks of the genera *Ixodes*, *Dermacentor* and *Haemaphysalis*. The most important vector appears to be the groundhog tick *Ixodes cookei*. The transmission cycle in nature appears to be similar to the transmission cycle of TBEV; however, many aspects are unclear, such as the importance of mosquitoes as vectors and of birds as hosts of the virus. Human cases have been seen in Canada and in the USA and in the few human cases observed the disease takes a more severe clinical course than that of TBE.

Experimental infection of dogs with high levels of virus may lead to febrile illness, but after natural infection (as determined by seroconversion), no clinical signs have been described. Infections in dogs may be identified by antibody testing or by the detection of virus in the brain of ill or dead animals. There are no recommended preventive measures except the use of acaricides. The use of TBEV vaccine may not prevent disease as the viruses are quite different from each other. Cats do not show any clinical signs after experimental infection with Powassan virus.

WEST NILE VIRUS INFECTION

West Nile virus (WNV) is a member of the Japanese encephalitis (JE) serogroup in the family Flaviviridae. WNV was first detected in 1937 in Uganda during a yellow fever epidemic. Until 1999, WNV was restricted geographically to Europe, Asia, Africa and Australia. In 1999, WNV invaded the North American continent and, within only 4 years, spread throughout the entire USA and parts of southern Canada, Central America and South America.

The main vectors are mosquitoes of the genus *Culex*. The virus can also be found in ticks, but their epidemiological relevance is questionable. The natural hosts are wetland and terrestrial birds of various species, but the virus can be found in a number of other birds, some of which become ill and may die from the infection. The virus has been detected rarely in rodents, camels, horses, cattle and dogs. Horses and lemurs may develop moderate viraemia, but other mammals do not appear to play a role in the transmission cycle of the virus as they do not develop viraemia sufficient enough to infect sucking mosquitoes.

Although thousands of human WNV infections are reported from Europe, Asia, Africa and America, reports of illness in dogs are rare. However, seroprevalence rates of up to 26% in dogs and 9% in cats imply a high rate of subclinical infection in these species. There are several case reports of WNV infections in dogs and one in a wolf. The infected dogs developed signs of encephalitis with fever, stupor or paralysis of the limbs. Several dogs showed tremors, uncontrolled involuntary erratic movements, lethargy and depression. In the later stages of disease, dyspnoea, diarrhoea with melena, anorexia, pulmonary oedema or arrhythmias are reported. A moderate to severe thrombocytopenia and moderate leucocytosis with a left shift are detected. Hypokalaemia, hypoglycaemia and hypoproteinaemia are reported in hospitalized dogs with WNV encephalitis.

There is no cure for WNV infection. The only available option is symptomatic treatment using modern intensive care medicine. Commercial vaccines have been developed and licensed for horses in the USA and in Europe. They are based on the genetic lineage 1 of the virus; however, cross-protection for WNV lineage 2 strains was demonstrated. They can also be used for the vaccination of pets and endangered bird species.

MURRAY VALLEY ENCEPHALITIS

Murray Valley encephalitis is a flavivirus infection transmitted by mosquitoes. The virus is closely related to JE virus and WNV and is grouped in the JE serogroup of flaviviruses. It is mainly distributed on the Australian continent, with some evidence that it is also prevalent in New Guinea. The virus causes sporadic cases and epidemic outbreaks of severe and sometimes fatal encephalitis in Australia. The virus is transmitted in Australia by mosquitoes (*Culex annulirostris*). The virus circulates in nature between mosquitoes and egrets and herons near watercourses. Dogs are a known host for the main vector of Murray Valley encephalitis, *C. annulirostris*, and there is evidence that Murray Valley encephalitis virus also infects dogs. Reports from Australia indicate that during epidemics dogs often die from severe neurological disease, but Murray Valley encephalitis virus has never been isolated from ill or dead dogs.

BUNYAVIRUS INFECTIONS

LA CROSSE ENCEPHALITIS

La Crosse virus is a member of the California serogroup, genus *Orthobunyavirus* of the family Bunyaviridae. It is an important cause of CNS infections in the mid-western and southern states of the USA. It is transmitted by tree hole-breeding mosquitoes (e.g. *Aedes triseriatus* and *Aedes canadensis*). The natural hosts include squirrels and chipmunks, but woodchucks and foxes may also contribute to the natural circulation of the virus.

Few natural infections in dogs are reported. A 4-year-old mixed breed dog was presented with depression, lethargy, anorexia, left head tilt and ataxia, mild fever, difficulty in standing, body twisting and repeated falling. The dog died after a series of seizures, each of which lasted seconds to minutes. La Crosse virus was detected in the brain of the dog by immuno-histochemistry; however, there were no serum antibodies, possibly due to sequestration of the antibodies in the CNS. In another case report, 1–2-week-old puppies (mixed breed or Brittany) developed gener-

ally fatal necrotizing encephalitis after natural infection with La Crosse virus. The puppies were either found dead or suffered from breathing difficulties and seizures before dying. The puppies were reportedly healthy only 5 days before. Histologically, there was panencephalitis and La Crosse virus was isolated from the brain.

Experimental infection of puppies with high-titred virus leads to CNS signs with tremors, disorientation and arching of the back. Three of four such infected puppies died, but none of them developed detectable viraemia. In another experiment, dogs inoculated with La Crosse virus were not able to infect blood-sucking non-infected mosquitoes (*A. triseriatus*).

Experimental infection of cats by feeding them with La Crosse virus-infected suckling mice resulted in the detection of low titres of the virus in the oral cavity of the cats, but the cats did not develop viraemia. Inoculation of cats with La Crosse virus did not result in the detection of the virus in any body fluid tested. After the infection most, but not all, of the inoculated cats developed serum antibodies against La Crosse virus.

RIFT VALLEY FEVER

Rift Valley fever is a febrile disease of ungulates and humans caused by Rift Valley fever virus (RVFV), a virus in the genus *Phlebovirus* of the family Bunyaviridae. The virus is prevalent in large parts of sub-Saharan Africa. Epidemics have been described repeatedly in Egypt and recently also in parts of the Arabian Peninsula. RVFV is transmitted in nature by mosquitoes of at least 30 different species, mainly of the genera *Aedes* and *Culex*. Natural hosts of the virus are mostly wild ungulates. In nature, the virus appears to be maintained mainly by transovarial transmission from female mosquitoes to their offspring. In humans, RVFV causes a febrile disease, which in some patients may cause haemorrhagic manifestations or encephalitis, with high fatality rates and optical neuritis, which may cause blindness. Domestic ungulates (i.e. sheep, goats and cattle) may develop severe clinical signs with fatal outcome, especially in young animals. RVFV is also an important cause of stillbirth and fetal malformation of domestic animals, especially during epidemics ('abortion storms').

No reports on natural infections of RVFV in dogs or cats exist; however, in the 1970s a number of experimental studies were conducted to test the susceptibility and potential role of these species as sustaining hosts for the natural transmission. These studies showed that RVFV can infect dogs and cats and cause a fatal disease, especially in puppies and kittens. In puppies aged 1–7 days a fatal disease developed after inoculation with low to medium titres of virus. The dogs died from a generalized infection with gross lesions in the liver, spleen, heart and brain. Petechiae and ecchymoses were present on the epicardial surfaces of the heart, within the abdominal lymph nodes and on the mucosal surfaces of the gastrointestinal tract, a similar pathology to that in human haemorrhagic fever. A few hours to 1 day before death the moribund puppies exhibited signs of CNS involvement (e.g. ataxia, paddling and opisthotonos). The severity of clinical signs diminished rapidly with increasing age and puppies 21 days and older did not succumb to the infection. All infected dogs (1–84 days of age) developed viraemia high enough to infect blood-feeding mosquitoes and they may therefore be able to serve as sustaining hosts for the virus. When 70-day-old puppies were given an aerosol infection they developed no clinical signs, but viraemia was detected in 75% of the animals. Oral infection by milk containing high virus titres did not cause any signs or markers of infection.

Experimental infection of 1–21-day-old kittens resulted in anomalies in body temperature (either hypothermia or fever) and CNS signs (e.g. ataxia, loss of reflexes, paddling) and eventual death. Histologically, there was necrosis and inflammation in the liver, spleen, myocardium and brain. Cats 84 days and older did not show any clinical signs, but developed antibodies against RVFV.

REOVIRUS INFECTIONS

AFRICAN HORSE SICKNESS

African horse sickness is caused by the African horse sickness virus. The virus is a member of the genus *Orbivirus* of the family Reoviridae. There are nine serotypes of the virus and due to the segmented virus genome using fragment re-assortment, new variants may occur. The virus is mainly transmitted by midges (*Culicoides* species). Occasionally, the virus may also be transmitted by mosquitoes (i.e. *Aedes* species, *Culex* species). The virus circulates between midges and equids (i.e. horses, donkeys, mules and zebras). There seems to be a particular organotropism with particular genotypes being especially neurotropic.

In dogs, fatal febrile encephalitis was produced when dogs were fed with meat from infected horses. There are no data on infection of cats with African horse sickness virus.

YUNNAN VIRUS INFECTION

Yunnan virus is a virus of the genus *Orbivirus*. It was originally isolated in China, but closely related viruses were detected in Peru (Rioja virus) and northern Australia (Middle Point virus). The virus is transmitted by mosquitoes (*Culex* species). Apart from fever and neurological disorders in donkeys, fever and encephalitis with fatalities were also described in dogs from China. No detailed clinical descriptions of the encephalitis in dogs are available. There are no data available on Yunnan virus infection in cats.

CASE STUDY: TICK-BORNE ENCEPHALITIS

History
Simba, a 12-year-old female mixed breed dog, was referred to the emergency service of the Veterinary University, Vienna, with a tentative diagnosis of acute intoxication. The owner reported pica, circling and unusual vocalization for 12 hours. The dog had been vaccinated regularly against canine distemper and rabies and was dewormed 3 months prior to presentation, but no prophylactic measures had been taken to prevent tick or flea infestation.

Clinical examination
The dog was depressed and showed continual vocalization. Gait was ataxic and Simba was stumbling and circling to the left. The body temperature was slightly elevated (39.3°C) and mucosae were reddened and mildly cyanotic.

Laboratory diagnostics
Haematological findings were unremarkable and serum biochemistry was within normal limits. CSF analysis revealed 149 cells/µl (reference <5 cells/µl) and elevated protein (35 mg/dl; reference <25 mg/dl). The cellular population consisted of 85% small lympho-

cytes, 10% neutrophils and 5% monocytes. Serology for TBE virus (serum and CSF) was negative.

Treatment

Simba was hospitalized and put under quarantine. She received intravenous fluids and was fed by a nasal tube. Epileptic seizures started 6 hours after initial examination and were treated successfully with a single bolus of midazolam (0.5 mg/kg) given intravenously.

Outcome

The dog deteriorated progressively over 24 hours and eventually became comatose, although no further sedation was given. The dog showed marked salivation, as she was unable to swallow (**Figure 14.2**). The eye position was asymmetrical and the pupils were miotic (**Figure 14.3**). In lateral recumbency, truncal rigidity was obvious and the dog did not respond to stimulation of the digits. Simba was euthanized because of the poor prognosis.

Necropsy examination

Histological examination of the brain revealed severe non-purulent panencephalitis, especially involving the brainstem, and mild non-purulent leptomeningitis. Immunohistochemical analyses were positive for TBE virus and negative for rabies, Aujeszky and Borna viruses and for *Listeria* species.

FURTHER READING

Attoui H, Mendez-Lopez MR, Rao S *et al.* (2009) Peruvian horse sickness virus and Yunnan orbivirus, isolated from vertebrates and mosquitoes in Peru and Australia. *Virology* **394**:298–319.

Baldwin CJ, Panciera RJ, Morton RJ *et al.* (1991) Acute tularemia in three domestic cats. *Journal of the American Veterinary Medical Association* **199**:1602–1605.

Bivin WS, Barry C, Hogge AL *et al.* (1967) Mosquito-induced infection with equine encephalomyelitis virus in dogs. *American Journal of Tropical Medicine and Hygiene* **16**:544–547.

Black SS, Harrison LR, Pursell AR *et al.* (1994) Necrotizing panencephalitis in puppies infected with La Crosse virus. *Journal of Veterinary Diagnostic Investigation* **6**:250–254.

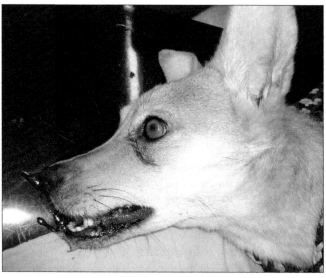
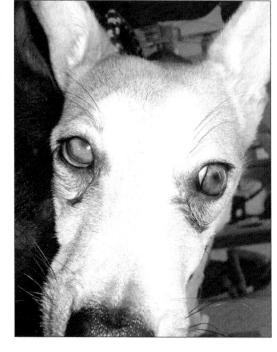

Figs. 14.2, 14.3 Clinical presentation of Simba. **(14.2) Note the rigid posture, miotic pupils and accumulation of saliva. (14.3) Note the asymmetrical positioning of the eyes and the miotic pupils.**

Boyce WM, Vickers W, Morrison SA *et al.* (2011) Surveillance for West Nile virus and vaccination of free-ranging Island scrub-jays (*Aphelocoma insularis*) on Santa Cruz Island, California. *Vector-Borne Zoonotic Diseases* **11**:1063–1068.

Buckweitz S, Kleiboeker S, Marioni K *et al.* (2003) Serological, reverse transcriptase-polymerase chain reaction, and histochemical detection of West Nile virus in a clinically affected dog. *Journal of Veterinary Diagnostic Investigation* **15**:324–329.

Buhariwalla F, Cann B, Marrie TJ (1996) A dog-related outbreak of Q fever. *Clinics in Infectious Disease* **23**:753–755.

Coffey LL, Crawford C, Dee J *et al.* (2006) Serologic evidence of widespread Everglades virus activity in dogs, Florida. *Emerging Infectious Diseases* **12**:1873–1879.

Ooper A, Hedlefs R, Ketheesan N *et al.* (2011) Serological evidence of *Coxiella burnetii* infection in dogs in a regional centre. *Australian Veterinary Journal* **89**:385–387.

Deardorff E., Estrada-Franco JE, Brault AC *et al.* (2006) Introductions of West Nile virus strains in Mexico. *Emerging Infectious Disease* **12**, 314–318.

Diniz PP, Schulz BS, Hartmann K *et al.* (2011) 'Candidatus Neoehrlichia mikurensis' infection in a dog from Germany. *Journal of Clinical Microbiology* **49**:2059–2062.

Egberink H, Addie D, Belak S *et al.* (2013) Coxiellosis/Q fever in cats: ABCD guidelines on prevention and management. *Journal of Feline Medicine and Surgery* **15**:573–575.

Eidson M, Thilsted JP, Rollag OJ (1991) Clinical, clinicopathologic and pathologic features of plague in cats: 119 cases (1977–1988). *Journal of the American Veterinary Medical Association* **199**:1191–1197.

Farrar MD, Miller DL, Baldwin CA *et al.* (2005) Eastern equine encephalitis in dogs. *Journal of Veterinary Diagnostic Investigation* **17**:614–617.

Foley JE, Nieto NC (2010) Tularaemia. *Veterinary Microbiology* **140**:332–338.

Furumoto HH (1969) Susceptibility of dogs for St. Louis encephalitis and some other selected arthropod-borne viruses. *American Journal of Veterinary Research* **30**:1371–1380.

Gage KL, Dennis DT, Orloski KA *et al.* (2000) Cases of cat-associated human plague in the Western US; 1977–1998. *Clinics in Infectious Disease* **30**:893–900.

Gasper PW, Barnes AM, Quan TJ *et al.* (1993) Plague (*Yersinia pestis*) in cats: description of experimentally induced disease. *Journal of Medical Entomology* **30**:20–26.

Godsey MS, Amoo F, Yuill TM *et al.* (1988) California serogroup virus infections in Wisconsin domestic animals. *American Journal of Tropical Medicine and Hygiene* **39**:409–416.

Gould LH, Pape J, Ettestad P, Griffith KS *et al.* (2008) Dog-associated risk factors for human plague. *Zoonoses and Public Health* **55**:448–454.

Grankvist A, Andersson PO, Mattsson M *et al.* (2014) Infections with the tick-borne bacterium 'Candidatus Neoehrlichia mikurensis' mimic noninfectious conditions in patients with B-cell malignancies or autoimmune diseases. *Clinics in Infectious Disease* **58**:1716–1722.

Greene CE (2012) *Francisella* and *Coxiella* infections. In: *Infectious Diseases in the Dog and Cat*, 4th Edn. (ed. CE Greene) Elsevier, St. Louis, pp. 476–482.

Hauri AM, Hofstetter I, Seibold E *et al.* (2010) Investigating an airborne tularemia outbreak, Germany. *Emerging Infectious Diseases* **16**:238–243.

Hubalek Z, Halouzka J (1999) West Nile Fever – a reemerging mosquito-borne viral disease in Europe. *Emerging Infectious Diseases* **5**:643–650.

Jahfari S, Fonville M, Hengeveld P *et al.* (2012) Prevalence of *Neoehrlichia mikurensis* in ticks and rodents from North-west Europe. *Parasites and Vectors* **5**:74.

Kawahara M, Rikihisa Y, Isogai E *et al.* (2004) Ultrastructure and phylogenetic analysis of 'Candidatus Neoehrlichia mikurensis' in the family Anaplasmataceae, isolated from wild rats and found in *Ixodes ovatus* ticks. *International Journal of Systematic and Evolutionary Microbiology* **54**:1837–1843.

Keefer GV, Zebarth GL, Allen WP (1972) Susceptibility of dogs and cats to Rift Valley fever by inhalation or ingestion of virus. *Journal of Infectious Disease* **125**:307–309.

Kile JC, Panella NA, Komar N *at al.* (2005) Serological survey of cats and dogs during an epidemic of West Nile virus infection in humans. *Journal of the American Veterinary Medical Association* **226**:1349–1353.

Kokernot RH, Radivojevic B, Anderson RJ (1969) Susceptibility of wild and domestic mammals to four arboviruses. *American Journal of Veterinary Research* **30**:2197–2203.

Lanciotti RS, Roehrig JT, Deubel V *et al.* (1999) Origin of West Nile virus responsible for an outbreak of encephalitis in northeastern United States. *Science* **286**:2333–2337.

Larson MA, Fey PD, Hinrichs SH *et al.* (2014) *Francisella tularensis* bacteria associated with feline tularemia in the United States. *Emerging Infectious Diseases* **20**:2068–2071.

Lichtensteiger CA, Heinz-Taheny K, Osborne TS *et al.* (2003) West Nile encephalitis and myocarditis in wolf and dog. *Emerging Infectious Diseases* **9**:1303–1306.

M'Fadyean J (1894) Louping-ill in sheep. *Journal of Comparative Pathology and Therapeutics* **7**:207–209.

MacKenzie CP, Lewis ND, Smith ST *et al.* (1973) Louping-ill in a working collie. *Veterinary Record* **92**, 354–356.

Magnarelli L, Levy S, Koski R (2007) Detection of antibodies to *Francisella tularensis* in cats. *Research in Veterinary Science* **82**:22–26.

Mares-Guia MA, Rozental T, Guterres A *et al.* (2014) Molecular identification of the agent of Q fever – *Coxiella burnetii* – in domestic animals in State of Rio de Janeiro, Brazil. *Reviews of the Society of Brazilian Tropical Medicine* **47**:231–234.

Marshall ID (1990) Murray Valley encephalitis. In: *The Arboviruses: Epidemiology and Ecology*, Vol. III. (ed. T Monath) CRC Press Inc., Boca Raton, pp. 151–190.

Mellor PS, Hambling C (2004) African horse sickness. *Veterinary Research* **35**:445–456.

Mitten JQ, Remmele NS, Walker JS *et al.* (1970) The clinical aspects of Rift Valley fever virus in household pets. III. Pathological changes in the dog and cat. *Journal of Infectious Disease* **121**:25–31.

Nordstoga A, Handeland K, Johansen TB *et al.* (2014) Tularaemia in Norwegian dogs. *Veterinary Microbiology* **173**:318–322.

Nichols JB, Lassing EB, Bigler WJ *et al.* (1975) An evaluation of military sentry dogs as a sentinel system to Everglades virus (Venezuelan equine encephalitis FE3-7C strain). *Military Medicine* **140**:710–712.

Nichols MC, Ettestad PJ, Vinhatton ES *et al.* (2014) *Yersinia pestis* infection in dogs: 62 cases (2003–2011). *Journal of the American Veterinary Medical Association* **244**:1176–1180.

Obiegala A, Pfeffer M, Woll D *et al.* (2014) Investigations on the transmission paths of *Anaplasma phagocytophilum* and 'Candidatus Neoehrlichia mikurensis' in small mammals and hard ticks. *Parasites and Vectors* **7**: 563.

Pennisi MG, Capri A, Solano-Gallego L *et al.* (2012) Prevalence of antibodies against *Rickettsia conorii*, *Babesia canis*, *Ehrlichia canis*, and *Anaplasma phagocytophilum* antigens in dogs from the Stretto di Messina area (Italy). *Ticks and Tick-Borne Diseases* **3**:315–318.

Pennisi MG, Egberink H, Hartmann K *et al.* (2013) *Yersinia pestis* infections in cats: ABCD guidelines on prevention and management. *Journal of Feline Medicine and Surgery* **15**:582–584.

Pfeffer M, Dobler G (2011) Tick-borne encephalitis virus in dogs – is this an issue? *Parasites and Vectors* **13**:59.

Read RW, Rodriguez DB, Summers BA (2005) West Nile encephalitis in a dog. *Veterinary Pathology* **42**:219–222.

Reisen W, Lothrop H, Chiles R *et al.* (2004) West Nile virus in California. *Emerging Infectious Diseases* **10**:1369–1378.

Rizzoli A, Silaghi C, Obiegala A *et al.* (2014) *Ixodes ricinus* and its transmitted pathogens in urban and peri-urban areas in Europe: new hazards and relevance for public health. *Frontiers in Public Health* **2**:251.

Roest HI, van Solt CB, Tilburg JJ *et al.* (2013) Search for possible additional reservoirs for human Q fever, The Netherlands. *Emerging Infectious Diseases* **19**:834–835.

Taber LE, Hogge AL, McKinney RW (1965) Experimental infection of dogs with two strains of Venezuelan equine encephalomyelitis virus. *American Journal of Tropical Medicine and Hygiene* **14**:647–651.

Tatum LM, Pacy JM, Frazier KS *et al.* (1999) Canine La Crosse viral meningoencephalomyelitis with possible public health implications. *Journal of Veterinary Diagnostic Investigation* **11**:184–188.

Walker JS, Remmele NS, Carter RC *et al.* (1970) The clinical aspects of Rift Valley fever virus in household pets. I. Susceptibility of the dog. *Journal of Infectious Disease* **121**:9–18.

Walker JS, Stephen EL, Remmele NS *et al.* (1970) The clinical aspects of Rift Valley fever virus in household pets. II. Susceptibility of the cat. *Journal of Infectious Disease* **121**:19–24.

Wang X, Liang J, Xi J *et al.* (2014) *Canis lupus familiaris* involved in the transmission of pathogenic *Yersinia* spp. in China. *Veterinary Microbiology* **172**:339–344.

Wheeler SS, Langevin S, Woods L *et al.* (2011) Efficacy of three vaccines in protecting western scrub-jays (*Aphelocoma californica*) from experimental infection with West Nile virus: implications for vaccination of island scrub-jays (*Aphelocoma insularis*). *Vector Borne Zoonotic Diseases* **11**:1069–1080.

Woods JP, Crystal MA, Morton RJ *et al.* (1998) Tularemia in two cats. *Journal of the American Veterinary Medical Association* **212**:81–83.

Yuen JC, Malotky MV (2011) *Francisella tularensis* osteomyelitis of the hand following a cat bite: a case of clinical suspicion. *Plastic and Reconstructive Surgery* **128**:37e–93e.

Printed and bound by CPI Group (UK) Ltd, Croydon, CR0 4YY

24/10/2024

01778285-0012